June 1992

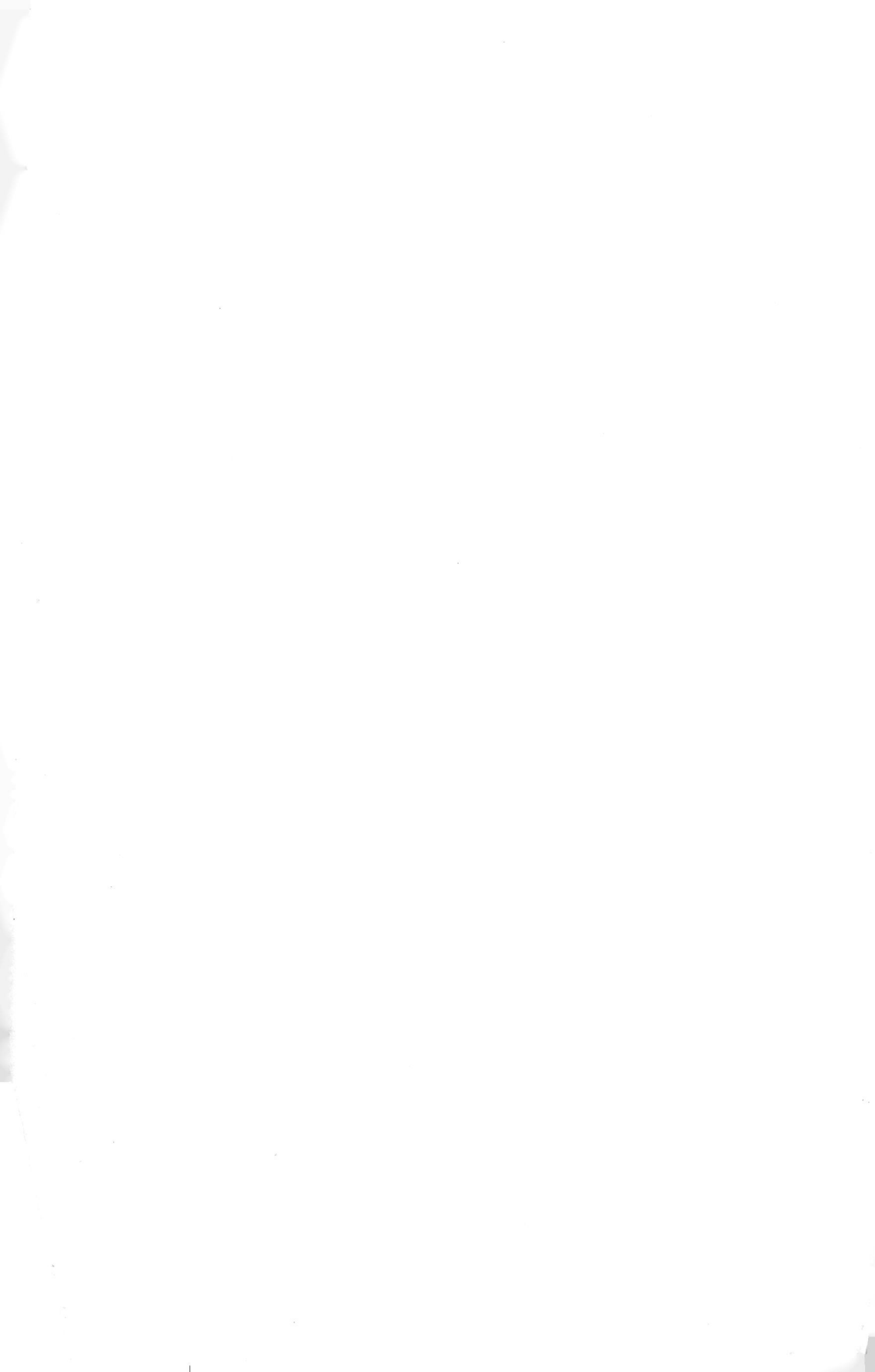

Practical
Blood
Transfusion

Practical Blood Transfusion

Fourth Edition

Douglas W. Huestis, M.D.
Professor of Pathology,
University of Arizona College of Medicine, Tucson;
Chief, Transfusion Medicine,
University Medical Center, Tucson

Joseph R. Bove, M.D.
Professor of Laboratory Medicine,
Yale University School of Medicine;
Director, Blood Transfusion Service,
Yale-New Haven Hospital
New Haven, Connecticut

John Case, F.I.M.L.S.
Vice President, Regulatory Affairs,
Gamma Biologicals, Inc.
Houston, Texas

Little, Brown and Company
Boston/Toronto

Copyright © 1988 by Douglas W. Huestis, Joseph R. Bove, and John Case

Fourth Edition

Previous editions copyright © 1969, 1976, and 1981 by Joseph R. Bove, Douglas W. Huestis, and Shirley Busch

All rights reserved. No part of this book may be reproduced in any form or by any electronic or mechanical means, including information storage and retrieval systems, without permission in writing from the publisher, except by a reviewer who may quote brief passages in a review.

Library of Congress Catalog Card No. 87-83645

ISBN 0-316-37953-0

Printed in the United States of America

MV

Countless lives have been saved through the devoted efforts of those who labor day and night in our blood banks. To them we humbly dedicate this book.

Contents

Preface ix
1. Blood Donation 1
2. Basic Blood Group Immunology 55
3. The Blood Groups 80
4. Testing of Donor Blood 135
5. Pretransfusion Testing 169
6. Red Blood Cell Transfusion 211
7. Complications of Transfusion 249
8. Blood Components, Fractions, and Derivatives 291
9. Hemolytic Disease of the Newborn 348
10. Therapeutic Hemapheresis 367

Addenda 391

Index 395

Preface

Practical Blood Transfusion, Fourth Edition, is intended as a practical book, primarily for physicians and technical personnel regularly concerned with the operation of blood donor or transfusion services and for interns, resident physicians, and medical technology students learning about transfusion medicine. We hope that other physicians, medical students, nurses, and hospital administrators will also find it a valuable general reference to current practices and trends. It is not intended for the specialist in immunology or immunohematology, except to the extent that he or she may be responsible for the day-to-day operation of a blood bank.

We discuss techniques from a general point of view and present enough immunohematology to provide a basis for practical blood banking. This is neither a textbook of immunohematology nor a laboratory manual; other books provide excellent coverage of those fields. Whenever in doubt as to what to include or omit, we have been guided by the word *practical.* This has resulted in a well-balanced presentation, with the emphasis on common sense and clinical reality based on available data. We have avoided fence-sitting and have tried to express our combined opinion on controversial matters, except when definitive data are too few to permit that.

We continue to stress the concept that blood transfusion procedures should be optimal rather than minimal, not only for the safety of patients, but also to ensure the best possible clinical results from transfused blood and components consistent with laboratory and administrative practicability.

We stated much of the above in the preface to our First Edition nearly 20 years ago, and we see no reason now to alter it in any essential respect. Rapid change continues to characterize the field of transfusion medicine, driving us to prepare this Fourth Edition.

We have completely rewritten the book, after extensive consultations and reconsideration of both content and presentation. We again made every effort to keep the book approximately the same size by balancing additions and deletions. The section on blood groups has been rewritten from a new perspective. We have included the latest mandates and trends in screening donor blood and in pretransfusion testing, and hope they will not soon be obsolete. Hemapheresis techniques are now widely used and familiar. Consequently, we deleted the chapter devoted to that topic and substituted appropriate sections in Chapters 1 and 8. However, we decided that the therapeutic applications of hemapheresis were sufficiently new and important to justify a separate chapter. The chapter on blood grouping reagents was eliminated by blending its contents into other parts of the book. Finally, and with little reluctance, we decided that our combined talents were no longer up to the task of summarizing the intricacies of medicolegal considerations. Accordingly, that chapter has been eliminated.

Ave atque vale! We welcome John Case as our new coauthor. John has a wealth of knowledge and experience, backed by a fund of good common sense. He has been instrumental in redirecting many of our attitudes and approaches in this edition. Our long-time friend and former coauthor, Shirley Busch, has "retired" to devote her time to studying primates at the San Diego Zoo. We thank Shirley for all her hard work on the first three editions of this book and for the pleasure of her collaboration; we wish her the best.

We owe a particular debt of thanks to Richard E. Rosenfield, M.D., Harold A. Oberman, M.D., and Delores M. Mallory, MT(ASCP)SBB, each of whom critically read the entire Third Edition and made many useful recommendations for the preparation of this edition. Anne Hoppe, MT(ASCP)SBB, and Christina V. Santos provided invaluable help with the section on automated blood grouping methods. We are also grateful to others who reviewed and criticized parts of the manuscript: Edward L. Snyder, M.D., James J. Corrigan, Jr., M.D., Louis Weinstein, M.D., Marie C. Crookston, B.Sc., Fay Weirich, MT(ASCP)SBB, and H. Neal Smith, Jr., BB(ASCP), and to those among our readers, friends, and colleagues who contributed suggestions for improvement. For the substantial portions of the text that were not prepared on the authors' home computers, we are most thankful for the expert secretarial skills of Terri M. Fiodella and Cynthia Ramírez. Special thanks are due to Drs. Hugh Chaplin, Jr., and John L. Schultz of Washington University, St. Louis, who kindly allowed us to use the Shaffer Conference Room for a face-to-face review of the entire manuscript.

As always, we appreciate the patience and forebearance of our wives, families, and colleagues, who have had to put up with our absentmindedness and preoccupation with the task of writing.

D. W. H.
J. R. B.
J. C.

Practical
Blood
Transfusion

1. Blood Donation

Blood differs from most other tissues used as transplants in that it is fluid and can be put in containers, preserved, and stored. These properties make possible transfusion as we know it today. An intricate system of blood suppliers and users has grown up to serve medical needs; it is sometimes called the *blood service industry*.

Since the transfer of blood directly from donor to recipient is neither convenient nor desirable, a facility for blood storage is necessary. This is called a *blood bank* or *blood center*. Its functions include donor recruitment, blood collection, blood processing, storage, and distribution. Some blood banks, particularly those in hospitals, also do pretransfusion testing of recipients, compatibility testing, and sometimes other diagnostic immunohematologic procedures such as human leukocyte antigen (HLA) typing for tissue transplantation. Many hospitals fulfill all these functions.

Types of Blood Banks

A *community blood bank* is an institution for the collection, processing, and distribution of blood, organized to meet the needs of a community or region. It is usually a nonprofit corporation, often sponsored by a civic or fraternal organization or hospital group. Its size, range of services, and activities are related to the community and its requirements. In many localities, blood services are provided by a regional blood center of the American Red Cross. In others, most of the blood is collected in hospitals, often with supplementation from community blood banks. Large metropolitan areas are likely to have all varieties of blood service.

Some hospital blood banks confine their activities to storage, crossmatching, and transfusion; others carry out every step from donor recruitment to actual transfusion, and may even supply blood to other hospitals in the vicinity.

Since organizations that sponsor blood donor groups and operate blood services have different backgrounds, aims, and philosophies, overall community coordination of blood supplies and needs varies widely in different localities and is sometimes almost nonexistent. Each community's blood service has evolved in response to its needs as envisioned by local medical, hospital, and civic groups, much as other health services have. There is no uniform national program, although limited coordination does take place through three national organizations, the American Association of Blood Banks (AABB), the blood program of the American National Red Cross (ANRC), and the Council of Community Blood Centers (CCBC). These organizations are interested in blood donation and transfusion, and share many attitudes, aims, and purposes.

Blood Donors

Previous editions of this book divided blood donors into two major categories based on whether or not a cash fee was given in payment for the donation. Now, the vast majority of blood donations are from volunteers, i.e., unpaid or altruistic donors. Readers interested in the problems associated with cash-paid blood donation should consult our earlier editions. In the United States, a label on the blood container must indicate whether the blood donor was paid or voluntary.

MOTIVATION

Despite emphatic opinions often expressed on the subject, there has been relatively little scientific investigation of the psychology of blood donor motivation. There have been studies analyzing the motives of those who actually donate and the factors tending to inhibit them [1], but fewer studies directed to the important question of why such a large proportion of the population remains apparently unmoved by repeated exhortations to donate blood. One investigation of donors and nondonors found that donors were more often male, married with children, low risk-takers, very concerned with health, lower in self-esteem, better educated, and (interestingly) of rarer blood types [2] Nondonors had the opposite characteristics. The author concluded that different programs would be needed to attract nondonors as opposed to retaining existing donors, and that attempts to bring in nondonors might be impractical.

An article by Oswalt summarizes much of the literature on these difficult problems and is recommended reading [3]. Among the many points made in this article were that public information could be better directed, that the motivating factors were already well known and had not changed significantly in the previous 20 years, and that advertising campaigns (unless crisis-oriented) are not very effective. He points out that countermotivations are mostly rationalizations of unconscious fear, and that much of that fear could probably be overcome by greater convenience and better organization of blood donation. Fear in potential blood donors may be concealed or unconscious, manifesting itself in such guises as hostility and procrastination. Once someone has successfully donated blood for the first time, it is easier to recruit that person for another donation [4], which reinforces the concept that fear of the unknown is a strong deterrent to the initial donation.

London and Hemphill, in the earlier study, found that motivations vary according to age, sex, income level, and educational status of the donor [1]. Humanitarian motives were more prominent in women, in those of higher educational achievement, and in the older age groups. Men were affected more by practical and economic motives. Young men responded best to dramatic appeals, such as aiding disaster victims. Young people of college age were most responsive to group pressures. In general, humanitarian and altruistic motives seem to play a larger role than practical, security-oriented, or mercenary ones.

Autologous Blood Donation

Donation of blood intended to be given back to the same donor is called *autologous donation* [5]. Usually this person expects to undergo a surgical procedure entailing a likelihood of transfusion. The patient's own blood is preferred because the hazards of foreign antigenic immunization and disease transmission are nonexistent. Autologous transfusion may be necessary when a person has been immunized to some high-incidence blood antigen or to multiple antigens. For a number of reasons, the procedure has been used only to a limited extent. On the whole, it seems to be difficult for surgeons to accept the idea of removing blood from a patient in whom a need for transfusion is anticipated, although many orthopedists and plastic surgeons have done so. Fear of acquired immune deficiency syndrome (AIDS) (see Chap. 7) has stimulated autologous blood usage, although not enough yet to have a significant impact on the transfusion of homologous blood. Autologous transfusion has become easier and more practical with prolonged dating of blood (up to 42 days with additive solutions) and should be strongly encouraged (see Chap. 6).

Recipient-Specific Donations

Donor-Specific Transfusion for Renal Transplants

Blood transfusions before renal transplantation have been shown to cause significant improvement in graft survival, for reasons that remain obscure (see Chap. 6). Some of these transfusions are from unselected donors, as in the case with candidates for cadaveric kidney transplants. For transplants from family members, prior transfusions from the kidney donor may improve graft survival (see Chap. 6).

Directed Donations

Blood donations intended for elective transfusion to a particular patient, e.g., from parents wanting to donate specifically for their own child's surgical procedure, have generally been regarded as an administrative nuisance by blood banks. In past years, such requests have been little more than occasional, and many blood banks refused to accommodate them on the grounds that it was contrary to their policy to reserve special units. Recently, however, as part of the AIDS panic, such requests increased markedly. Blood bankers justifiably feel that all their donors are properly selected and screened, that *directed donations* are illogical, and that the process may even reduce safety by putting undue pressure on friends and relatives of a patient. Refusal of some blood banks to cooperate with requests for directed donations has unfortunately resulted in a great deal of resentment and adverse publicity, and occasionally in coercive legislation. Tennessee, Oklahoma, Illinois, and California require blood banks to provide facilities for directed donations; many other states are

Table 1-1. Opinions For and Against Directed Donations (DDs)*

For	Against
Some patients lack confidence in the blood bank's ability to select safe donors.	The professional blood bank staff is better able to accomplish safe donor selection.
DDs are at least as safe as regular donations. Family and friends will be truthful to prevent harm to the patient.	There is no evidence that DDs are safer. They may be less safe because donors are under pressure and may lie to cover themselves.
Logical or not, DDs relieve patients' anxiety about the possibility of contracting AIDS from transfusion.	Allowing DDs may needlessly keep alive public concern about transfusional AIDS.
DDs encourage volunteering to help a patient.	DDs involve undue coercion and are contrary to the principle of voluntarism.
DDs allow a patient's friends and family to help, with the community blood supply as backup.	DDs create a burden on patients to find enough donors.
DDs bring in new donors who can be recruited for future donations.	DDs interfere with community blood programs because people withhold regular donations in case their blood is needed for friends or family.
Donors feel their effort is appreciated by the patient, and proper consent procedures inform them of any legal risks.	DDs incur increased liability for the donor, who may be known to the patient. Anonymity cannot be assured.
DDs reduce recruiting costs because the donor was recruited by the patient. They can be handled like autologous donations.	DDs create more work and higher costs. Increasing handling increases the chance of error.

*Modified from B. McDonough, Designated donations raise controversial issues. Deerfield, IL: Fenwal Laboratories, *Continuous Flow,* Spring 1986. With permission.

considering such legislation. See Table 1-1 for arguments for and against directed donations.

The blood bank that decides not to permit directed donations is standing on perfectly rational ground and is unquestionably avoiding additional work, confusion, and cost. But we remain unconvinced by arguments that directed donations are less safe than others. After all, blood banks have accepted such donations without question for many years in the provision of platelets and white blood cells for patients with cancer or leukemia. Moreover, many of those who present themselves as donors for a particular patient have already been regular donors.

We believe that directed donations should not be encouraged and that they answer an emotional feeling rather than a rational need. Nevertheless, it is unwise to refuse stubbornly to accede to such requests. Logic to the contrary, the option should be available to patients who are truly worried about pending transfusions. A blood bank will not be harmed by making patients feel better about their treatment, and may reap a few extra benefits as well.

Cadaver Blood

Cadaver blood has been used for transfusion predominantly by some centers in the Soviet Union [6]. Such blood is collected within a few hours of death from persons dying suddenly of conditions in which bacteremia is unlikely. As much as 3,000 ml can be obtained from a cadaver.

Although the idea of using cadaver blood has periodically appealed to some physicians in this country [7] and tends to fascinate the public, cadaver blood has never been widely used outside the Soviet Union and does not seem likely to be. Both legal and medical technicalities stand in the way, and at best, it can be said that the procedure is administratively complicated. Even in the Soviet Union, cadaver blood does not play a prominent role in the overall blood supply.

Blood Donor Recruitment Programs

No single blood donor recruitment program is universally applicable, simply because no two communities are the same, and a system that works well in one locality may not in another. For that reason, our discussion will cover only the broad generalities that should be relevant to almost any program.

Finding Donors

The chances of developing a successful blood donor recruitment program are much higher with groups, because the direct personal appeal can then take place primarily among the members themselves, and guidance can be supplied by the blood bank. The better organized and more closely knit the group, the better the chances for a successful donor program. The approach used must depend, of course, on the organizer's evaluation of the aims, purposes, and psychology of the group, and on the amount of group pressure likely to be brought to bear on each member. No specific blueprint can be offered, but the finger on the group pulse must be sensitive. A good program with one well-organized, prestigious group can serve as a model for others.

Education

Of major importance is the education of the public about blood donation, with the aim of developing favorable attitudes toward blood bank programs and feelings of individual responsibility, and eliminating misconceptions and misinformation. Prospective donors should be informed about what blood is, why there are no substitutes for it, the desirability of volunteer blood donors, and the economics of blood supply and replacement. There are, of course, other

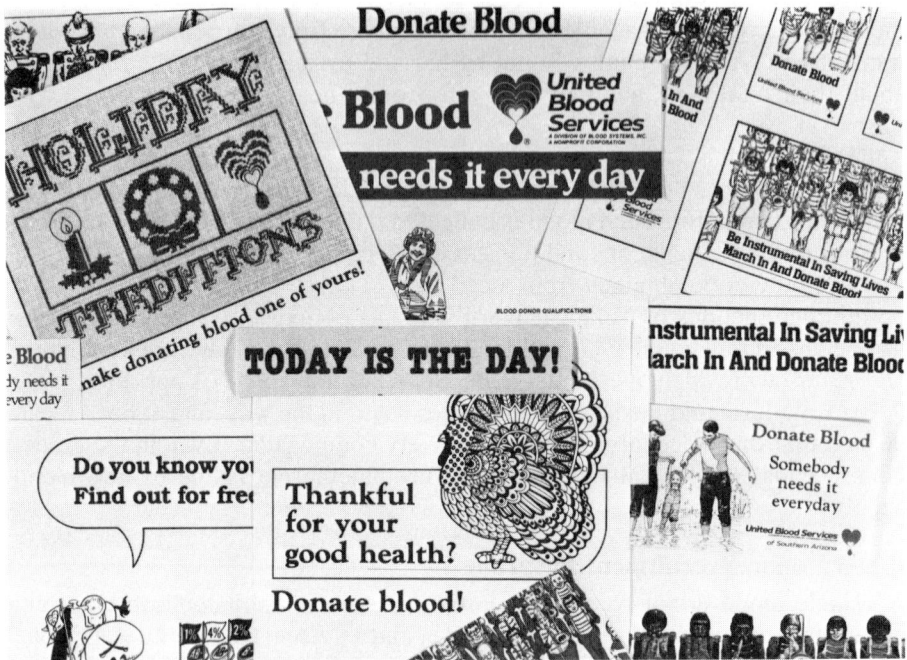

Figure 1-1
A group of posters, brochures, etc., designed to encourage people to donate blood. (Courtesy of Blood Systems, Inc., Scottsdale, AZ.)

aspects that may assume importance in certain communities. The person in charge of such a program must be skilled in public relations, well acquainted with the community, thoroughly familiar with the workings of the public communications media, and well informed about blood banking. Educational programs for schools are highly desirable for the purpose of instilling positive attitudes about blood donation. Figure 1-1 shows a collection of posters designed to encourage people to donate blood.

Donor groups should be kept aware of the ways in which their blood donations are used, of the blood situation in the community at large, and of interesting new techniques, developments, and applications of blood transfusion. They should be encouraged to donate for people with hemophilia, leukemia, heart surgery, or other catastrophic blood needs.

With groups as well as individuals, a call-up system is desirable, so that when the blood bank needs certain types of blood, donors having the needed type may be called on for additional donations. The success of such telephone recruitment depends to a great extent on the skill and personality of the recruiter; not everyone has the right voice or telephone manner to produce re-

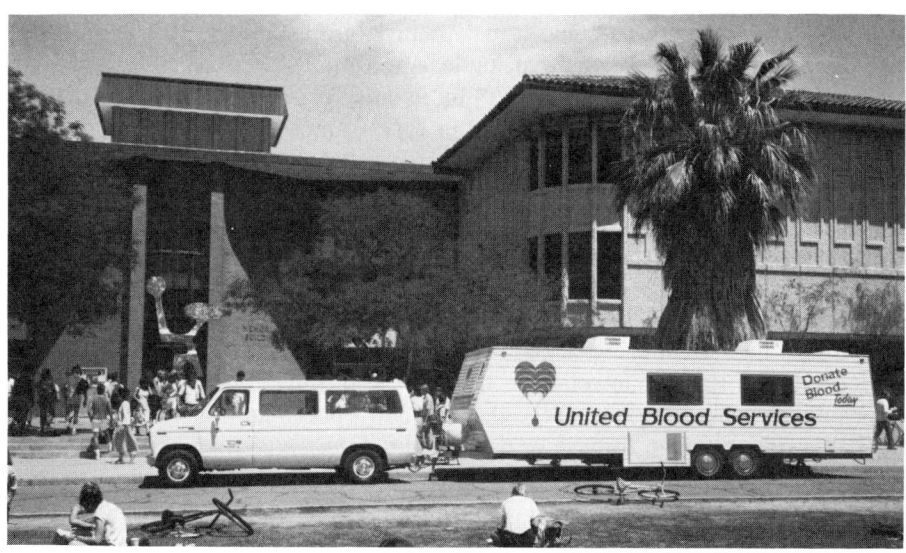

Figure 1-2
A self-contained bloodmobile on the campus of the University of Arizona. (Courtesy of United Blood Services of Southern Arizona, Tucson, AZ.)

sults. Some potentially productive techniques have been developed at the University of Cincinnati [8].

BLOODMOBILES AND SATELLITE STATIONS

Either the blood donor must get to the blood bank, or blood-drawing facilities must be brought to the donor. The circumstances of the two types of blood collection differ considerably. The blood bank maintains fixed facilities that are ready to receive donors at any time, subject only to the availability of personnel. The number of donors that can be taken at a time depends on the blood bank's size and facilities. Donor convenience is vital; at fixed donation sites, donors would like to be able to give blood early in the morning, on evenings, and on weekends [9].

Bloodmobiles offer convenience by bringing the blood bank team to the premises of the sponsoring organization, usually in a large hall, gymnasium, or auditorium, where beds, interviewing tables, and other equipment may be appropriately arranged. This type of mobile unit can carry a great deal of equipment, enabling many donor beds to be set up and thus greatly increasing the blood-drawing potential of even a relatively small blood bank.

Some bloodmobile units actually contain donor beds set up for blood drawing inside the truck (Fig. 1-2). Such vehicles are not as well adapted to large groups, since the number of donor beds is necessarily limited, and even one protracted donor reaction will seriously delay waiting donors. Mobile units do, however, have the advantage that, under appropriate circumstances, they can be used to collect blood from passers-by in cities or from small groups that do not have premises suitable for the larger type of mobile operation.

Although it may seem that bloodmobiles should be used only for groups at some distance from the blood bank, there are times when their use at nearer locations is justified. A blood donor program can be a significant factor in group morale, and this effect is heightened when the group has blood collections on its own premises. Some business or industrial institutions will not give employees time off work to go to the blood bank but are willing to have a bloodmobile operate on their own premises. In this way they achieve not only the morale effect but also the public relations benefits of an obvious gesture of civic responsibility. In short, there are some groups of potential donors who may be available only through the use of the bloodmobile.

A community blood bank may also increase its geographic coverage by the use of *satellite drawing stations*. These are usually small stationary locations, often in a hospital, where blood is collected, but not processed or stored. They should be convenient to large numbers of potential donors, who might otherwise find access to the main blood bank difficult because of distance or inconvenience of transportation.

Community Blood Service Management

In a community blood program involving a central blood provider and a group of hospitals, some central organization must exist. This will involve control of donor intake in proportion to overall blood requirements, distribution of blood within the community on the basis of the estimated needs of each hospital, participation in regional or national inventory-leveling programs, and control of hospital practices with respect to the efficient and appropriate use of blood (see also Chap. 7).

An effective program entails day-by-day reporting to the blood bank of the current status of each unit of blood or blood component assigned to each hospital served by the blood bank. The hospital blood bank must list its component inventory as, for example, unassigned and available, reserved or crossmatched for a particular patient, or already transfused. The community blood service then integrates these data with those from other hospitals it serves, and with its own available and anticipated inventory.

In larger communities, such integration is difficult to accomplish by conventional telephoning and manual listing. It can, however, be done very effectively by computer. A computerized system can keep track of the available blood and component inventory at the community blood center and at outlying hospitals, the anticipated needs of the hospitals, blood units reserved on crossmatch or actually used (and by whom), those units at or nearing expiration, and transfers between hospitals, and can balance all these against the blood bank's planned and anticipated intake, both at the center and at any of its drawing stations or bloodmobiles. The computer can also record individual blood donation data, and in fact, can trace each component from donor to eventual recipient. Such a system increases efficiency and decreases waste, and may even allow smaller inventories.

The application of computers to hospital, community, and regional blood programs has been studied extensively and was stimulated in the early 1970s by government funding of research programs in that area. Computers are being applied more and more to blood programs, because they supply and process information faster and more accurately than any other means. Their associated cost may be largely offset by greater efficiency and decreased waste, but their effectiveness depends on how well the data processing has been programmed and how it is operated. A number of ready-made software programs are now commercially available for both hospital and community blood bank computerization, as well as some elaborate hardware-plus-software combinations. Anyone considering the use of a computer in the blood bank should study the literature carefully, obtain expert disinterested advice, and be sure of exactly what is expected of the computer. Only then should ready-made programs be looked at and compared with respect to how well they will do the job. An important principle, often forgotten, is that the program must fit the blood bank operation, not the other way around.

R. Townsend, whose book *Up the Organization* is filled with commonsense business advice, points out that computers are just "big, expensive, fast, dumb adding-machine typewriters" [10]. Some of his important rules of thumb still apply:

1. At this state of the art, keep decisions on computers at the highest level. Make sure the climate is ruthlessly hard-nosed about the practicality of every system, every program, and every report. "What are you going to do with that report?" "What would you do if you didn't have it?". . . .
2. Make sure your present report system is reasonably clean and effective before you automate. Otherwise your new computer will just speed up the mess.
3. . . . Hire a small, independent software company to come in, plan your computer system, and then get out. Make sure they plan every detail in advance, and let them know you expect them to meet every dollar and time target. . . .
4. Before you hire a computer specialist, make it a condition that he spend some time in the factory and then sell your shoes to the customers. . . .
5. No matter what the experts say, never, never automate a manual function without a long enough period of dual operation. When in doubt discontinue the automation. And don't stop the manual system until the *nonexperts* in the organization think that automation is working. . . .*

---

*Quoted from R. Townsend, *Up the Organization* (copyright Alfred A. Knopf, Inc.). With permission.

Principles of Blood Donor Selection

The safety of any blood transfusion begins with the proper selection of the blood donor. The physician responsible for a blood transfusion service must take care that the removal of blood does not harm the donor. In addition, potential risks to the recipient due to disease conditions in the donor must be kept to a minimum.

The U.S. Public Health Service has long recognized that the safety and purity of blood intended for transfusion are matters affecting public health, and the Food and Drug Administration (FDA) has regulations that are legally binding on all blood banks. These regulations, however, represent only minimum standards, and every blood bank needs additional detailed procedures of its own to guide those engaged in selecting blood donors. In many institutions, rules have been handed down over so many years that the reasons behind them have been forgotten. As a result, interpretation of rules may be difficult, and restrictions may persist for years after medical progress has made them obsolete. We intend to review here the generally accepted regulations applicable to blood donors and to discuss the reasons for them. The reader may then be better able to make an intelligent decision concerning the problems that inevitably arise in donor selection.

The first and most important commandment in blood donor selection is that *the donor shall be in a state of good health*. Like admonitions of love and charity, this concept is so fundamental that it is often forgotten. Most of the questions that arise in donor selection can be solved by reference to this principle. The rule of the healthy donor should not be broken or stretched for reasons of expediency or to avoid hurting a would-be donor's feelings. The number of healthy persons who can donate blood is more than adequate to supply the country's needs, and rather than weaken the standards of donor selection, it is better for hospitals and blood banks to educate the public concerning the ever-present need for blood donors.

There are certain risks that primarily concern the donor's response to bloodletting, others that concern the recipient. The removal of up to 500 ml of blood is easily tolerated by most healthy adults, and no harm should be anticipated. Nevertheless, the procedures associated with blood donation do cause some people to faint (this is more fully discussed later in this chapter). Since the vasovagal phenomenon responsible for fainting cannot be eliminated, all blood donors should be in good enough health to be able to tolerate a short period of hypotension and bradycardia. The donor should also be free of known recurrent diseases, so that a coincidental exacerbation of disease cannot be attributed to blood donation.

There remains the risk that certain disease conditions affecting the donor may be transmitted to a susceptible or weakened patient. Donors who appear fit but may be carriers of some disease transmissible by blood transfusion must therefore be identified (if possible) and excluded from blood donation as a public health measure. As with any medical or surgical procedure, the donor is assessed by his medical history, pertinent physical examination, and certain laboratory tests. The medical history and examination should always be accompanied by a signed statement showing that the risks of blood donation to both donor and recipient were in fact evaluated at the time of donation. A sample donor health review form is given in Fig. 1-3. Since a person's state of health may change from time to time, the entire interview, history, and examination must be repeated and separately recorded each time a donor presents.

Consent

For legal reasons, it is increasingly important that the donor's consent to blood donation be *informed,* that is, that the procedure be explained in such a way that the donor thoroughly understands the process, so that an educated consent is given. The explanation to the donor should be reinforced with printed instructions or a brochure. The same applies to any instructions after donation. In today's litigious climate, this practice is virtually essential.

Age

Blood donation is customarily restricted to adults who have not yet reached their sixty-sixth birthday. Since the donor must be of legal age to consent to the procedure of blood withdrawal, the lower limits of acceptable age depend on the attainment of legal majority. This varies from state to state. In most states, the age of majority is 18 years. However, in 1973, the Red Cross and the American Association of Blood Banks issued a joint statement that they would accept blood donors of age 17 who presented written parental consent. In all matters pertaining to age of majority and competence of blood donors to execute a valid consent, legal advice should be obtained.

From time to time, the question comes up whether to accept a prospective donor who is overage. Although arteriosclerotic conditions are more common in the older age groups, there is no good reason why a healthy older person cannot donate blood. Recent observations indicate that this is indeed so, and that blood banks may be unnecessarily excluding an increasingly large group of willing donors [11]. The decision in any individual case should be made by the blood bank physician.

Temperature

A donor should not have an elevated temperature (above 37.5°C or 99.5°F), because this may indicate disease. The temperature must be taken under valid conditions, that is, the donor must not have been recently smoking or drinking hot or cold beverages. A lower limit of body temperature is not considered necessary.

DONOR # ____________

UNIVERSITY MEDICAL CENTER, BLOOD DONOR AND TRANSFUSION SERVICE, TUCSON, ARIZONA

NAME (LAST, FIRST MIDDLE)						
HOME ADDRESS					HOME TELEPHONE	
CITY, STATE ZIP					BUSINESS TELEPHONE	
DATE OF DONATION	DATE SCR.	DATE OF BIRTH	AGE NOW	SEX ☐ M ☐ F	DATE LAST DON.	
DONATING FOR		PATIENT AT	HT WT	B. TYPE	TEMP	

REMARKS:

Y = YES (EXPLAIN UNDER "REMARKS" = QUESTIONS 3 THRU 32) N = NO

*01 ARE YOU IN GOOD HEALTH		17 EXPOSURE TO INFECTIOUS DISEASE	
02 FEEL WELL TODAY		18 HAZARDOUS OCCUPATION OR HOBBY	
03 COLD, FLU, NOW		19 RHEUMATIC FEVER, VALLEY FEVER, UNEXPLAINED FEVER	
*04 HEART TROUBLE		20 BLEEDING TENDENCY	
05 RECENT SURGERY OR SERIOUS INJURY, LAST 6 MONTHS		21 IMMUNIZATIONS OR VACCINATIONS PAST YEAR	
06 TUBERCULOSIS, COUGH BLOOD		*22 YELLOW JAUNDICE, HEPATITIS	
07 CHEST PAIN, SHORTNESS OF BREATH		*23 EXP. TO JAUNDICE, HEPATITIS, LAST SIX MONTHS	
*08 DIABETES, KIDNEY DISEASE, ULCERS		*24 EXP. TO AIDS PATIENT OR PERSON AT INCREASED RISK OF AIDS	
09 LYMPH GLAND DISEASE, CANCER OR MONO.		*25 POS. HEPATITIS TEST OR AIDS ANTIBODY	
10 PREVIOUS MEDICAL DEFERMENT		26 REC'D. BLOOD, PLASMA, SERUM, TATTOO, LAST 6 MONTHS	
*11 PREGNANCY, MISCARRIAGE OR ABORTION, LAST 6 WEEKS		*27 MALARIA	
12 ALLERGY, ASTHMA, HAY FEVER, NOW		*28 SUPPRESSIVE THERAPY FOR MALARIA	
13 FAINTING, CONVULSIONS, EPILEPSY		29 TRAVEL OUTSIDE OF U.S. WITHIN 6 MONTHS	
*14 TAKING MEDICINE OR DRUGS NOW (INCL. ASPIRIN)		*30 SKIN INFECTION, LUMPS, NODULES	
15 RECENT WEIGHT LOSS, NIGHT SWEATS		31 IMMUNIZED TO HUMAN BLOOD CELL ANTIGENS	
16 MOUTH SORES, PERSISTENT DIARRHEA		*32 PRESENTLY UNDER MEDICAL CARE	

OK obtained from Physician ☐

SIGNATURE OF PHYSICIAN (When required)

X

(SIGNATURE OF DONOR)

INTERVIEWER:

BLOOD DONOR REGISTRATION REV. 8/86 *Complete these items when prescreening donors.

Figure 1–3
A form for the registration and health interview of prospective blood donors.

Weight

Since a person's blood volume is proportional to size, withdrawal of a fixed amount of blood (450 ml in most cases, plus pilot samples) represents a larger proportion of the total blood volume of a small donor than of a large donor (see Chap. 2). Setting a lower limit of acceptable weight is therefore desirable to prevent an excessive number of donor reactions, which to a certain extent relate to the proportion of the donor's blood withdrawn. A full 450 ml of blood should not be taken from a donor weighing less than 50 kg (110 lb). In this country, few adults are below this limit. Although the blood bank may withdraw a smaller amount of blood from such small people, the quantity taken must be at least 90 percent of the amount of blood specified for the volume of anticoagulant in the container. For example, not less than 405 ml of blood should be drawn into the standard container intended for the collection of 450 ml of blood. If a smaller collection than that is indicated, a container with proportionately less anticoagulant must be used. Containers with reduced amounts of anticoagulant are available from some manufacturers. In countries where people are smaller, e.g., Japan, the standard blood collection has been smaller—for example, 200 ml.

Hemoglobin Level

One would not, of course, want to take blood from a person who is anemic. To protect against this possibility, a hemoglobin test, usually done by the copper sulfate specific gravity method, is required for every blood donor at each donation. The blood sample for this test is usually of capillary origin, obtained by pricking the finger or earlobe. The earlobe is popular among donors because of its insensitivity to pain. Unfortunately, the hemoglobin level obtained on blood from the earlobe is significantly higher than that from a finger stick or venous blood, and may therefore show a satisfactory hemoglobin level even though the donor is slightly anemic [12, 13]. We do not recommend the use of an ear stick for this test.

The minimum hemoglobin level acceptable to the FDA is 12.5 gm/dl. The AABB and the Red Cross, on the other hand, have a stricter standard for men (13.5 gm/dl) and retain the federal standard for women (12.5 gm/dl). With some possible reservations, these minimums may also be expressed in terms of the hematocrit reading: we suggest a lower limit of 41 percent packed cell volume for men and 37 percent for women. General experience with these standards has been satisfactory, although from time to time some concern has been expressed about the copper sulfate method, which apparently errs on the side of donor disqualification rather than acceptance [14]. This may at times be an embarrassment or nuisance to the blood bank, but it is in fact an extra protection to the donor. If a person does not pass the copper sulfate test but is found acceptable by a more accurate procedure, he or she need not be disqualified.

An additional means of protecting the donor against the possible development of anemia is the regulation requiring a minimum of 8 weeks between blood donations. Some feel that the 8-week interval is not adequate protection, and some countries require a longer interval. Some donors, particularly women, can be iron-deficient but not anemic [15, 16]. Although the 8-week rule appears to have generally been trouble free, concern over possible iron deficiency persists. The FDA is discussing a limit of four donations per year for women, five for men.

Donor Conditions of Primary Concern to the Recipient

HEPATITIS

Among the infectious diseases that can be transmitted by transfusion, malaria, syphilis, hepatitis, and AIDS are of greatest concern. Of these, hepatitis is the most common, and historically the one that has presented the greatest hazard to blood recipients. More recently, AIDS has preoccupied the minds of both the public and the medical profession, and has virtually eclipsed hepatitis. AIDS, however, is an infrequent transfusion complication. It is still important to focus attention on hepatitis.

We now have a required laboratory test for hepatitis B surface antigen (HBsAg), and other procedures such as tests for hepatitis B core antibody (anti-HBc) and alanine aminotransferase have come into use (see Chaps. 6 and 7). However, they cannot be fully effective, and proper selection of donors is still an important way of diminishing the risk of transmitting the disease. Since hepatitis is serious, and may even be fatal, everyone connected with transfusion must recognize this risk and exert every reasonable precaution in the selection of donors.

Federal regulations prohibit blood donors with a history of viral hepatitis or of a positive test for HBsAg from donating blood for transfusion because some persons carry hepatitis virus in their blood for years after an attack. This makes sense for hepatitis B, but not for hepatitis A. The latter is only rarely transmitted by transfusion (see Chap. 7). Exactly how long a person may remain a carrier of hepatitis B virus is not known, but it appears to be a matter of years. This being the case, it is prudent to assume that the carrier state may be permanent, and that anyone who has ever had diagnosed hepatitis B or non-A, non-B must be regarded as a carrier (with respect to blood donation).

Those who have had close contact with people suffering from hepatitis should be deferred as blood donors for at least 6 months. This time is chosen because the incubation period for viral hepatitis does not ordinarily exceed 6 months. An exception to the 6-month limit is a person exposed to hepatitis who has been given prophylactic hepatitis B immune globulin. Since this may prolong the incubation period when it does not prevent hepatitis, the deferral period should be at least 1 year for people who have been treated with the currently available preparation. Administration of regular (i.e., not hepatitis B–specific) immune serum globulin does not prolong the deferral period.

It is important to be realistic in defining *close contact*. Situations involving significant contact are particularly those within the household, that is, sharing the same kitchen and toilet facilities. Risk also attaches to some institutional contacts, such as may occur in dormitories or military barracks in which there have been multiple cases of hepatitis. Household contact with, or regular medical attendance on, a patient or patients on hemodialysis is also cause for deferral, because of the high incidence of hepatitis in such patients. On the other hand, people experiencing casual contacts, for instance, co-workers or hospital visitors, or medical personnel caring for an occasional hepatitis patient and taking appropriate precautions, are not usually disqualified.

A history of jaundice should be assumed to be due to hepatitis unless proved otherwise. Exceptions do occur, such as jaundice caused by gallstones and that caused by erythroblastosis at birth. In either case, some sort of documentation would be desirable.

Donors Implicated in Transfusional Hepatitis
When a case of hepatitis apparently caused by transfusion is reported to the blood bank, it is difficult to decide what to do about the donors whose blood was received by that particular patient, especially when the patient received multiple transfusions. Certainly, if the patient received the blood of only one donor, that donor should be permanently disqualified and should be notified in writing that he or she must not donate blood again. Some organizations extend this precaution to three donors. When larger numbers of donors are involved, we consider it impractical to implicate all of them, although that may be possible with computerized systems. In implicating multiple donors (admitting that there is not a firm definition of *multiple*), most people would not disqualify all of them, but rather put their names into a retrieval system that would permit disqualification in the event of a second implication. For a discussion and a mathematical approach to this problem, see Ladd and Hillis [17].

Intravenous Drug Abuse
Narcotics users frequently expose themselves to hepatitis, as well as AIDS (see below), by using contaminated needles and syringes, and they cannot be counted on to give a reliable medical history. They include a much higher proportion of hepatitis carriers than the population at large and should be assiduously avoided as blood donors. The informational screening procedure for AIDS may help in excluding such persons (see following section). Since the medical history will rarely disclose addiction, the phlebotomist should search for needle-scarred veins by examining both arms while choosing a vein for blood collection.

Prison Inmates

The nature of the prison population is such that prisoners must be considered unacceptable as blood donors, especially when incentives such as time taken off the sentence are offered by well-meaning prison officials. Prison inmates are at high risk for both hepatitis and AIDS.

Tattooing

This ancient custom persists, although it has been virtually outlawed in some communities. Outbreaks of hepatitis have confirmed that tattooing needles are often unsanitary and that the tattoo parlor client may become a victim or carrier of hepatitis [18]. For these reasons, persons who have exposed themselves to hepatitis in this way must wait at least 6 months before being accepted as blood donors.

Acupuncture

Acupuncture, which has acquired a following in this country, may expose a person to hepatitis. An English report of 36 cases from a home-based practitioner in Birmingham provides justification for concern about this practice, especially if it is carried out without medical supervision [19]. If acupuncture is done with properly sterilized equipment and precautions and under medical supervision, it need not be considered an exposure to hepatitis.

Ear Piercing

An increased incidence of hepatitis has been reported in women who have had their ears pierced by inadequately sterilized needles [20]. It does not appear that this is a significant hazard in male or female blood donors, as long as the piercing was done with sterile disposable equipment.

Blood or Plasma Recipients

Those who have themselves received blood or certain blood products must be considered to have been exposed to hepatitis. Consequently, anyone who has had a transfusion of blood or blood components must be deferred for at least 6 months from the time of the transfusion. Serum albumin, plasma protein fraction, and gamma globulin preparations are blood fractions that carry little or no risk of hepatitis. Naturally, a history of recent treatment with blood or blood fractions, even those that do not carry the hepatitis virus, should lead to a detailed inquiry into the prospective donor's present state of health.

ACQUIRED IMMUNE DEFICIENCY SYNDROME

The sudden appearance and dissemination of this dreaded disease and the evidence that some cases have been spread by blood transfusion have had far-reaching effects on blood transfusion services (see Chap. 7). At times, public anxiety (to the point of hysteria) has been such that procedural changes have been demanded before firm scientific evidence was available to back them up.

The AIDS scare has taken some unexpected turns. A misconception stubbornly persists that people can acquire AIDS by blood *donation,* despite repeated and emphatic public statements to the contrary. A 1985 survey of Maryland residents by the Baltimore *Sun* disclosed that nearly 20 percent of respondents believed this [21]. An AABB survey showed that 34 percent believed so [22]. Also, about 70 percent of those responding in the Baltimore survey expressed little faith in blood-screening techniques. Such attitudes have had their effects on blood donation as well as transfusion in some parts of the country.

Apart from the testing of donor blood (see Chap. 4), screening involves an effort to exclude would-be donors belonging to groups at high risk for AIDS, as well as those who may have been exposed to members of such groups.

High-Risk Donors

AIDS is spread primarily by sexual contact, and about 70 percent of cases have been in homosexual or bisexual men, particularly in large metropolitan areas. This being the case, even though the occurrence of AIDS markers varies among different groups of homosexuals, it is essential to exclude homosexual or bisexual men as blood donors. Obviously, the approach to the donor must be delicate, since people resent interrogation about their sexual preference, and direct or indirect questions of such a nature are generally considered inappropriate. Apart from the hysterical fringe, who would quarantine all homosexuals, there have been serious suggestions that, given the gravity of AIDS, asking highly personal questions of the donor may be justifiable [23]. So far, this has not generally been done.

Other risk groups include intravenous drug abusers, hemophiliacs (who, of course, are not likely to present themselves as blood donors), Haitian or central African entrants to the U.S. (since 1977), persons with AIDS or any signs or symptoms of AIDS, and the sexual partners of any of the above.

Federal authorities, as well as the AABB, Red Cross, and CCBC, advise that literature identifying the risk groups be provided to would-be donors so that they have an opportunity to withdraw from donation or, if they feel compelled to donate, to notify the blood bank in confidence that their blood should not be used for transfusion (Fig. 1–4). The recommendations now avoid using the term *homosexual,* because some men who have sexual contacts with other men do not consider themselves homosexual. The risk group is now defined as those men who have had sex with even one man since 1977. Male and female prostitutes are now also included in the risk groups, with a 6-month deferment for those who have had contact with a female prostitute. The form of donor consent should then include a signed statement that the donor has read and understood the information and considers himself qualified to donate blood for trans-

University Medical Center, Tucson, Arizona

IMPORTANT NOTICE

The incidence of a serious disease called Acquired Immune Deficiency Syndrome (AIDS) continues to increase.

The virus that causes AIDS is now known. Rarely, this disease may be passed on through blood or blood products. **THERE IS NO DANGER TO YOU AS A DONOR,** but there is a potential danger to patients who receive blood and blood products. Federal and state health authorities have recommended that all persons at increased risk of AIDS should refrain from blood donation. We ask your cooperation in carefully reading the following:

Groups at increased risk of transmitting AIDS are:

- Persons with AIDS or with symptoms and signs suggestive of AIDS. These include otherwise unexplained severe night sweating, fevers, weight loss, enlarged lymph nodes (swollen glands), blue or purple spots on or under the skin, white spots or blemishes in the mouth, persistent cough or shortness of breath, or persistent diarrhea.
- Persons with clinical or laboratory evidence of infection with the AIDS virus.
- Any man who has had sex with another man since 1977.
- Present or past abusers of intravenous drugs.
- Sexual partners of the above individuals.
- Hemophiliacs, and their wives or sexual partners.
- Immigrants since 1977 from Haiti or Central Africa.
- Men and women who have engaged in prostitution since 1977 and persons who have been their heterosexual partners within six months.

If you are associated with any of these groups or have engaged in any of these activities, we ask that you PLEASE DISQUALIFY YOURSELF FROM DONATING BLOOD.

You may also disqualify yourself by answering "NO" when the interviewer asks you the question: "Are you in good health today?" You do not need to state a reason. Your voluntary deferral will be kept in the strictest confidence. If you feel compelled to donate blood, please confidentially inform the nurse during the procedure or before you leave, that your blood may be used for research but should not be used for transfusion. You may also phone within an hour after leaving.

If you have questions regarding AIDS, please contact your personal physician or the Blood Donor and Transfusion Service here.

Thank you for helping us maintain a safe blood supply.

Phone number: 626-6294

I have read and understood the contents of this notice.

_____   _____
Signature   Date

Figure 1–4
An information sheet for prospective blood donors, identifying those at increased risk for transmitting AIDS, and requesting self-disqualification of such.

fusion. There is a widespread feeling, backed by some evidence, that this voluntary exclusion process has been reasonably, but not completely, effective [24, 25]. However, human nature being what it is, we should not expect too much of such a procedure, and there is evidence of its fallibility.

The donor interview should include questions designed to detect donors who may already be infected with the human immunodeficiency virus (HIV): night sweats, unexplained fever, persistent cough or sore throat, persistently swollen lymph nodes, blue or purple spots or lumps in the skin or mucous membranes, white patches or other unusual lesions in the mouth, persistent diarrhea, and unexplained weight loss.

In addition, interviewing and phlebotomy personnel should observe donors carefully to detect any evident stigmata, such as skin lesions, fever, weight loss, or evidence of vein abuse. In particular, an environment of confidentiality is essential; otherwise, fear of embarrassment or exposure may lead high-risk donors to conceal a relevant history.

MALARIA

Malaria is readily transmitted by blood transfusion, since the malarial parasites reside within the red cells. In temperate parts of the world, malaria is rare, but it must still be considered by the blood bank because a donor can appear well and yet harbor plasmodia. Transmission of malaria as long as 19 years after the donor's last clinical attack has been recorded [26], but this is rare.

Until recently, people who had ever had malaria were permanently disqualified as blood donors, except as donors for fractions that would not contain red cells. In 1973, however, the Red Cross and the AABB jointly relaxed this restriction. The new standard is that people who have had malaria are deferred for 3 years after becoming asymptomatic or after cessation of therapy. The same 3-year period applies to those who have taken prophylactic antimalarial therapy in an endemic area, have left that area, and have been asymptomatic in the interim, as well as to visitors and immigrants coming from endemic areas. There are two exceptions to this policy: people who are proven carriers of malaria and those who are known to have had quartan malaria (*Plasmodium malariae*) are still permanently excluded, the latter because of the known long latency of the disease. Those who have traveled to endemic areas but who have had no symptoms and have taken no antimalarial medication are deferred for 6 months after their return.

Information about malarious areas can be obtained in a publication from the U.S. Public Health Service, Centers for Disease Control [27]. In fact, transfusional malaria remains a rare occurrence in this country and was so even at the peak of return of service personnel from Vietnam (see Chap. 7). There has been a tendency in the United States to view the malaria hazard with more alarm than it merits.

SYPHILIS

The spirochete of syphilis can be found in the blood of recently infected people. It may also be present in those with active secondary syphilis, although such a person is unlikely to feel well enough to want to donate blood. In any case, blood stored in a refrigerator does not remain infective for more than 97 hours; therefore, transfusional syphilis is for the most part prevented by refrigerated blood storage [28] (see Chap. 7). Donors may be accepted if they neither have active disease nor are under treatment for it.

OTHER INFECTIOUS DISEASES

Although transmission of hepatitis, AIDS, malaria, and syphilis has been the major concern of transfusionists, other infectious diseases must sometimes be considered. Theoretically, any infectious disease characterized by viremia or bacteremia may be transmitted by blood transfusion if the blood is taken at just the proper time. But in fact, at the time when viremia or bacteremia is present, most people do not feel well enough to donate blood.

Virus Diseases

In the case of donors exposed to *measles, German measles, chickenpox,* or *mumps* by family contact, it is prudent to wait one incubation period (about 3 weeks) before accepting the donor. The same recommendation applies to a dormitory population in an epidemic setting, since it should be obvious by the end of this time whether new cases are still occurring. If so, it would be wise to wait until new cases are no longer occurring before accepting members of the group. *Cytomegalovirus* can be spread by transfusion, and there is an applicable test for this condition (see Chaps. 4 and 7), but no way of eliciting a history of it.

Although there is no evidence that *infectious mononucleosis* can be transmitted by blood transfusion, differential diagnosis between this disease and infectious hepatitis is difficult in some cases. Not infrequently, persons with infectious mononucleosis have abnormal liver function tests, and, conversely, patients with viral hepatitis often have atypical lymphocytes in their blood. Since, in addition, people who have had mononucleosis may suffer episodes of lethargy for several months, it is probably best to defer them for at least 6 months after the symptoms have subsided. If there is still doubt whether the person did or did not have infectious hepatitis, permanent disqualification may be advisable.

Babesiosis

Babesia is an intraerythrocytic protozoan parasite, generally spread by tick bites and commonly afflicting cattle or large rodents. Human infections are usually caused by *B. microti,* producing an acute febrile illness that may be fatal (see Chap. 7). In endemic areas, e.g., parts of Long Island in New York and southeastern Massachusetts, it is advisable to defer donors with unexplained fever or history of recent tick bites, babesiosis, or summer residence in affected areas.

Tuberculosis

Persons who have had clinical tuberculosis have customarily been excluded from blood donation. Since only under the rarest circumstances could tuberculosis be transmissible by blood transfusion, the basis for this prohibition is not clear. One consideration may be the fear that a donor suffering a recurrence of the disease might blame the blood donation for it. As long as the donor has no symptoms and is not under therapy, he or she may be accepted.

MISCELLANEOUS DONOR CONDITIONS

Hereditary Red Cell Defects

People with hereditary anemias are not ordinarily accepted as blood donors, since they do not pass the hemoglobin test. Nevertheless, individuals with certain inherited (usually mild) red cell defects, such as glucose 6-phosphate dehydrogenase deficiency, thalassemia minor, and sickle trait, may be unwittingly accepted as blood donors. Although it is possible that their blood may create difficulties with freezing and thawing procedures or with exchange transfusions in infants, or, rarely, be subject to hemolysis after transfusion, there is little evidence that the presence of hereditary red cell defects poses a significant hazard under ordinary circumstances.

Allergies

Allergies may be transferred from donor to recipient by means of plasma, and a recipient could thereupon experience allergic symptoms on exposure to the corresponding allergen. Some blood banks ask donors if they have allergies and may require that they be free of symptoms on the day of donation. We no longer see any compelling reason even to ask this question. Seasonal allergy (hay fever), characterized by rhinitis, is common and relatively benign, and may be disregarded. Donors taking antihistamines may be accepted, since transmission of a significant amount of the drug is unlikely and would in any case be harmless.

Allergies in the donor to drugs and foods are potentially more serious problems than hay fever, since it has been shown that relatively small amounts of donor blood can render the recipient allergic. Despite this, there is little evidence that such donor allergies have caused significant reactions in recipients.

Dental Surgery

Since tooth extractions and oral surgery are sometimes followed by a transitory bacteremia, it is customary to defer prospective donors who have undergone such procedures. A deferral of 3 days is usually advised. This is probably excessive, but gives the donor time to recover from the procedure [29].

Skin Disease

The venipuncture site should be free of any skin disease, and the donor free of skin disease of sufficient extent to pose a risk of blood contamination. Donors with minor lesions of acne, psoriasis, and seborrheic dermatitis do not usually present any risk to the recipient or to themselves as long as the phlebotomy site is clear. The possibility of syphilitic skin lesions, especially secondary ones, should be borne in mind, and doubtful cases should be referred to a physician.

We must add a special note about donors who may be taking *isotretinoin* (13-cis-retinoic acid, or Accutane™) for cystic acne. This drug is a potent teratogenic agent and presents a risk to the fetus if the donor's blood were to be transfused to a pregnant woman. In addition, a blood recipient could suffer significant side effects. Making allowance for the persistence of blood levels of isotretinoin, the FDA advises that donors taking the drug be deferred for at least 1 month after receiving the last dose (E. C. Esber, Letter to all establishments collecting blood, blood components, and source plasma, Office of Biologics Research and Review, FDA, 28 February 1984).

Conditions Affecting the Donor's Response to Phlebotomy

HEART DISEASE

Prospective donors with a history of *coronary heart disease* must be disqualified, since this condition has been responsible for deaths after blood donation [30]. Coronary occlusion may, of course, happen to anyone at any time, but a death coincidental with blood donation would be not only tragic but also fraught with medicolegal and public-relations hazards to the blood program, even if unrelated to blood donation. Hypotension and bradycardia, such as occur after about 1 percent of blood donations, may be dangerous to anyone with narrowed coronary vessels and may lead to myocardial infarction because of poor perfusion of the coronary arteries. Blood banks should therefore question all prospective donors about coronary heart disease, heart attacks, angina pectoris, shortness of breath, etc., to exclude anyone who may have coronary heart disease. This applies also to a history of cardiovascular surgery for such conditions. Persons who have suffered other vascular occlusions, such as a cerebrovascular accident, fall into the same category.

Rheumatic Fever and Rheumatic Heart Disease

Rheumatic fever in childhood is less common nowadays than in earlier times, but a history of rheumatic fever does call for careful evaluation of the donor. In general, the principle to be followed is that the donor must be free of all evidence of rheumatic heart disease. This status can often be ascertained by a careful questioning for symptoms of heart disease. Listening for heart murmurs is not usually feasible in a blood bank. A donor who is under treatment for rheumatic heart disease should not be accepted, for this is good evidence that he is considered likely to have recurrences and is not in a state of good health. If in doubt, the decision should be made by the blood bank physician.

Abnormalities of Pulse and Blood Pressure
Usual practice requires that the donor's pulse be regular and between 50 and 100 beats per minute, and that the systolic blood pressure be between 90 and 180 mm Hg and the diastolic not exceed 100. These are reasonable limits that will include most healthy persons. Many physicians might prefer not to accept donors with a pulse above 90 per minute, or a blood pressure above 160/90, but experience with the wider limits quoted has been satisfactory over the years. Many donors have a rapid pulse and systolic blood pressure above their usual level when they first present themselves. These abnormalities are presumably due to nervousness and should disappear if the donor is allowed to rest quietly for 5 to 10 minutes. If they do not, the donor should be temporarily deferred and advised to see a physician for investigation. Even if the person is only manifesting a deathly fear of blood donation, that in itself is enough reason for deferment. For those taking antihypertensive drugs, see below, under Medications Taken by Blood Donors.

People with high blood pressure (i.e., above the range permissible for donation) are prone to suffer cerebrovascular accidents and attacks of coronary heart disease. Since they might experience such a catastrophe on blood donation, they should be disqualified as donors.

A special note about donors with unduly slow pulse and low blood pressure: Before disqualifying them, it is worth asking whether they indulge in strenuous athletics, which often cause "abnormalities" of this kind. Otherwise, the blood bank might find itself rejecting long-distance runners or other well-conditioned athletes who would probably be excellent donors.

SURGERY
Recent major surgery contraindicates blood donation because the patient may be assumed to be still in a precarious state of health, and a relapse in his basic condition might be blamed on the blood donation. The difficulty lies in the definitions of *recent* and *major*. Since patients undergoing general anesthesia for abdominal or thoracic procedures may also have been given blood or blood components, they may have been exposed to hepatitis. Hence, on this basis as well as that of allowing time for full recovery of the patient, a waiting period of at least 6 months is desirable. A similar period is applicable following severe fractures, burns, or other major traumatic episodes, particularly when extensive blood loss has been involved.

We realize that the foregoing provides no clear definition of donors unaccept-

Table 1–2. Some Surgical Conditions and Procedures in Relation to the Deferral or Acceptance of Prospective Blood Donors

Major* (defer for at least 6 months)	Minor (accept if reasonable time for healing has elapsed and donor feels fully recovered)
Pneumonectomy, heart, or other chest surgery	Appendectomy
Gastrectomy	Herniorrhaphy (inguinal)
Cholecystectomy	Hemorrhoidectomy
Craniotomy	Varicose vein stripping
Hysterectomy	Dilatation and curettage
Intervertebral disk, spinal fusion	Tonsillectomy
Major trauma or fracture (e.g., femur, pelvis), major joint replacement	Removal of skin lesions (e.g., nevuses)
Any condition entailing transfusion of blood or plasma	Suture of laceration

*See p. 25 for policy regarding people treated for cancer.

able because of surgery, but we do not think it possible to offer a hard-and-fast guideline to serve in all cases. Personnel interviewing and examining prospective donors will from time to time encounter persons who have had surgical or traumatic episodes that cannot be clearly classified as major or minor. It is safest to defer them for 6 months unless they can conveniently be evaluated by a blood bank physician. The problem can be partially resolved, and unnecessary referrals and delays avoided, if the blood bank medical director prepares a list of the more common surgical and traumatic conditions, indicating which should be deferred for 6 months and which may be accepted without deferment. Table 1–2 is an example of such a list.

Diabetes Mellitus

Diabetes cannot be transmitted by blood transfusion, and many diabetics have such mild disease that a policy of rigidly excluding all diabetics would result in disqualification of many otherwise suitable donors. On the other hand, donor reactions or other complications of blood donation might be more dangerous to a severely diabetic person. For this reason it is necessary to identify and exclude the more seriously afflicted diabetics among prospective blood donors. A physician can usually decide whether a person has severe or mild diabetes by a detailed medical history, but paramedical staff need a simpler guideline. A useful rule of thumb is to exclude those diabetics requiring medication such as insulin or tolbutamide, and to accept those controlled by diet alone. Some diabetics taking oral hypoglycemic agents can undoubtedly be accepted with safety, but in such a case, the blood bank physician may have to make the decision.

Gout

Hyperuricemic arthritis, or gout, is a common metabolic disease, and donors with a history of gout sometimes present themselves in the blood bank. The increased uric acid in the blood of even severely afflicted people will not harm the recipient. Furthermore, blood donation is unlikely to pose any danger to the gouty donor. Most blood banks, therefore, do not ask specific questions about gout. On the other hand, once such a history is volunteered, the simplest and most effective rule is to consider acceptable those donors who are not currently taking medication.

Acute Respiratory Disease

The donor should be free from acute significant respiratory disease. Although there is no evidence of transmission of respiratory illness by blood transfusion, this precaution will safeguard the donor's health. An upper respiratory infection may progress to pneumonia or other complications, and the donor may think that blood donation was responsible. Many donations are unnecessarily lost because the donor thinks he has a cold; in reality, this may only be dry nasal and laryngeal mucous membranes due to dry indoor atmosphere, especially in winter. If a donor feels well and has a normal temperature, a diagnosis of respiratory infection is not warranted, and he may be accepted.

There is no mandatory waiting period after a cold, flu, sniffles, or sore throat before a donor again becomes acceptable. It is sufficient that the donor feel well and have resumed normal activities.

Gastrointestinal Diseases

A donor suffering from peptic ulcer presents a hazard only to himself. Most peptic ulcers never bleed overtly, and the risks are limited to those that do. Donors who have no history of hemorrhage from the ulcer and no current symptoms, and who are receiving no therapy other than diet and antacids, may be considered acceptable. It is best for this decision to be made by a physician.

Other gastrointestinal conditions, such as rectal polyps, hemorrhoids, and regional enteritis, are not in themselves cause for disqualification. A physician should evaluate the general condition of the donor, who may be accepted if the disease is not active.

Cancer

There is no evidence of cancer transmission by blood transfusion, and it is difficult to see how blood donation could really harm a fully recovered patient. A reasonable guideline, to protect both the prospective donor and the blood bank, is to ensure that the donor has gone at least 5 years without a recurrence, and to confirm this with the donor's physician. Not all authorities agree. The Red Cross, for example, does not accept any former cancer patients as blood donors.

Small skin cancers are common in the sunnier parts of the country, and donors sometimes volunteer the information that they have had one or two of these removed. This need not lead to disqualification unless the neoplasms recur frequently or show evidence of extension. In case of doubt, the donor's physician should be consulted.

Epilepsy or Fits

The prospective donor who gives a history of recurrent epilepsy should be permanently disqualified. There is no risk to the recipient, but some donor reactions are characterized by convulsions and unconsciousness, and neither a person with epileptic tendencies nor the blood bank staff should be subjected to such a hazard. There is also a possibility that an epileptic attack might be provoked by blood donation, although definite evidence is lacking. Our experience is that epileptics often fail to give their diagnosis until questioned about medication.

A history of "fits" in childhood may need individual evaluation. If the fit was associated with fever, the donor need not be deferred. Also, if the donor is no longer under any treatment, the chances are good that he is not now considered epileptic. The blood bank physician may need to make the decision.

Blood Diseases

Since the purpose of blood transfusion is to replace lost or defective blood with healthy blood, prospective donors with any form of blood disease should be excluded. Persons who do not know or understand the nature of their blood abnormality however, may present themselves as blood donors. Furthermore, they are sometimes advised by their physicians to come to the blood bank: "My doctor says it will be good for me to give blood." Any such statement calls for investigation. All donors should be asked if they have any blood disease. An affirmative answer may indicate a blood dyscrasia such as polycythemia or, more commonly, syphilis, and requires explanation before the donor is accepted.

Polycythemia

Patients suffering from various kinds of polycythemia are often treated by repeated bleeding, and blood banks are frequently asked to perform this service. *Polycythemia rubra vera* is a disease of unknown cause, associated with leukemia-like states. Blood from a patient with this disease cannot be given as normal blood and should be clearly identified so that it is not confused with blood from healthy donors. Although on rare occasions the blood from a polycythemic patient may be useful to selected recipients, it is better to regard the "donation" as a therapeutic bloodletting and, as such, a service to the patient. Such blood is rarely used for transfusion nowadays.

SECONDARY POLYCYTHEMIA. Chronic pulmonary disease sometimes results in an increase in total circulating red cells, and some of the patients with this complication are benefited by a moderate program of bleeding. Blood from such patients may be used for transfusion if necessary, with the approval of the recipient and the recipient's physician, but it does not qualify in the usual sense as coming from a healthy donor.

In view of these problems, many blood banks draw blood from polycythemic patients only as a service to that person and under direct instructions from a physician, not as a blood donation. With this we agree.

Bleeding Tendencies

The severely affected hemophiliac will not present himself as a blood donor, but a person with very mild hemophilia or some other undetected abnormality of hemostasis may not be aware of his disease. Questions about any unusual bleeding tendency should be asked of all prospective blood donors, since venipuncture in a person with a bleeding tendency could cause extensive extravasation of blood and consequent tissue damage.

MEDICATIONS TAKEN BY BLOOD DONORS

Prospective donors should be asked if they are taking any medications, and, if so, why. Aspirin, vitamins, antihistamines, reducing pills, thyroid preparations, and oral contraceptives are taken by many physically fit people. Such medications are of little or no consequence in blood donation. In general, the amount of the drug in a unit of blood is negligible, although there could be enough to cause a reaction in an allergic recipient. Antibiotics such as penicillin are generally considered evidence that the donor is not in a state of good health. Antibiotics given for acne are not a cause for deferment, but isotretinoin (Accutane) used in the treatment of cystic acne requires a 1-month deferment after the donor has stopped taking the drug, as discussed above under Skin Disease. The use of *any* medication by a prospective donor should arouse suspicion that he or she may not really be in good health, and the blood bank should find out for what reason medication is being given.

Aspirin has an adverse effect on platelet function, but this effect is nullified by the presence of enough unaspirinated platelets [31], so there is probably no need to screen out donors who have taken aspirin within a few days, unless they are to be subjected to platelet apheresis. In that case, the FDA recommends an aspirin-free period of 36 hours, whereas the AABB has the stricter requirement of 3 days.

Some hypertensive patients taking antihypertensive medication should probably be deferred even if their blood pressure is normal, since they have some circulatory instability, and their response to a vasovagal reaction is unpredictable. Much may depend on the nature of the medication, and the blood bank physician may have to decide (see Table 1-3).

INOCULATIONS AND INJECTIONS

In the case of cell-free vaccines or those containing only killed organisms, donors are acceptable at any time after immunization, providing they feel well enough without medication. This recommendation includes the Salk poliomyelitis vaccine and such inoculations as those for hepatitis B, typhoid, typhus, Rocky Mountain spotted fever, cholera, plague, diphtheria, pertussis, influenza, rabies (duck embryo or human diploid), and tetanus. In the case of live virus vaccines, most authorities recommend a 2-week waiting period after inoculation, since donor viremia within that period could conceivably cause disease in an immunosuppressed recipient. The 2-week deferment applies to oral poliomyelitis (Sabin) vaccine and vaccines for measles (rubeola), mumps, yellow fever, and smallpox.

Longer deferments are generally advised for two other immunizations. One is the vaccination for German measles (rubella), which requires a waiting period of 1 month because of concern over the possible effects of the virus on the fetuses of pregnant blood recipients. The other is the vaccination for rabies. A deferment of 1 year is advisable when the rabies vaccine is given after the bite of a rabid animal, since rabies in those circumstances may have an incubation period of several months (see Table 1–3).

DONOR'S OCCUPATION

Blood donation is not advisable for those who are expecting to return immediately to a hazardous activity, for fear that a delayed reaction might cause an accident. Therefore, persons entrusted with the safety of others (bus drivers, airline crews, operators of power machinery, etc.) should be deferred temporarily, or accepted only when off work (e.g., on weekends or vacations, or after the day's work). The same applies to firemen, workers on scaffolding, and so on, in whom a delayed reaction could have serious consequences. In practice, these recommendations are difficult to follow, for vigorous and active people are the ones most likely to want to donate blood. The exercise of common sense and good judgment may be necessary. At any rate, the possible adverse consequences of blood donation are much less in experienced donors than in those donating for the first time.

WOMEN DONORS

Female donors must be asked about current or recent pregnancy. Childbearing is a burden on the iron stores, and those who are pregnant should be deferred as blood donors until at least 6 weeks after delivery or termination of the preg-

Table 1–3. Acceptance or Deferral of Prospective Blood Donors in Relation to Certain Medications and Immunizations

---

Accept if donor feels well
   Allergy desensitization injections
   Analgesics
   Antibiotics, topical or for acne
   Antidiabetics, oral (with approval of physician)
   Antihistamines and decongestants
   Diet pills (unless in a phase of rapid weight loss)
   Headache remedies with aspirin (except for platelet apheresis)
   Headache remedies without aspirin
   Immunization with cell-free or killed agents (see text)
   Oral contraceptives and other hormones
   Tranquilizers and antidepressants
   Vitamins
Defer
   Antibiotics other than for acne (until several days after therapy is concluded and infection cleared)
   Antihypertensive (until blood pressure is stable without drug)
   Antimalarials (3 years after conclusion of therapy, with no disease in interim)
   Hepatitis B immune globulin (1 year)
   Immunizations, live agent, other than rubella and rabies (2 weeks, see text)
   Immunization, rubella (1 month)
   Immunization, rabies (Pasteur) (1 year after last injection)
   Isotretinoin for cystic acne (1 month after last dose)
Disqualify permanently
   Antiepileptic agents (may accept at discretion of blood bank physician)
   Cancer chemotherapeutic agents
   Drugs used for cardiac failure (digitalis, nitroglycerin, quinidine)
   Insulin for diabetes

---

nancy. Women who are menstruating need not be deferred as long as they feel well and are not experiencing excessive flow.

Responsibility for Donor Selection

The infinite variety among human beings and the multitude of problems and ailments that beset them make it impossible to provide a complete discussion of, and answer for, every dilemma likely to be encountered on a donor service. Judging from questions asked at meetings, and our own experience with blood donors, we believe the foregoing discussion covers the major areas in which difficult decisions have to be made.

Every blood bank needs guidelines to donor selection that can be applied by nonmedical personnel, but these cannot be expected to cover all situations, and the advice of a physician familiar with the problems of blood donation is at times essential. In matters that might affect the health of a blood recipient, the decision to accept a certain donor is the full responsibility of the blood bank physician. Where possible adverse effects of blood donation on a prospective donor are concerned, the blood bank may share the responsibility with the donor's own physician, preferably requiring approval in writing. Nevertheless, the final responsibility for any injury to a donor lies with the blood bank. Many clinicians are not familiar with the practical aspects of blood donation, and the approval of the donor's physician, although it is of medical and legal value to the blood bank, does not absolve the blood bank physician from making the decision in any case.

Blood Collection

Satisfactory transfusion results depend on meticulous blood collection techniques, which are the responsibility of the blood-collecting agency, and rigidly controlled conditions of storage and handling, a responsibility shared by the collecting blood bank and the hospital transfusion service.

Blood-Drawing Area

The blood-drawing area should be pleasant, clean, quiet, and separated from other parts of the blood bank. Because of the possibility of reactions, donors undergoing phlebotomy should not be in view of other donors waiting or being interviewed. Although some people do not like it, soft background music helps relax some blood donors. Blood can be collected satisfactorily from donors on tables, beds, or specially constructed contour chairs, with the donor placed high enough so that the phlebotomist can work without having to bend over. In all cases, washable surfaces are essential. A table, either stationary or on rollers, is needed for supplies. Every part of the donor area should be scrupulously clean and uncluttered.

Blood Containers

Plastic containers for blood have now replaced glass bottles. The principal advantages of plastic are compactness and lightness in storage and shipment; flexibility, which allows rapid infusion by external pressure with almost no hazard of air embolism; and the possibility of making containers with two, three, or more integrally connected secondary bags. This greatly facilitates component preparation or removal of portions of the original blood without entering the primary container. Integrally connected multiple plastic containers are more expensive than single ones, but the additional cost is justified because it permits maximum salvage of blood components or of fractional blood units,

Table 1-4. Major Plastics and Plasticizers in Current Use

Plastic, Plasticizer	Application	Trade Designs
Polyvinyl chloride with di(2-ethylhexyl) phthalate	Primary collection bag	PL-146 (Fenwal) XT-150 (Terumo)
Polyvinyl chloride with di(2-ethylhexyl) phthalate (reduced thickness)	Satellite bag for platelets	T-612 (Terumo)
Blow-molded polyolefin without plasticizer	Satellite bag for platelets	PL-732 (Fenwal)
Polyvinyl chloride with tri(2-ethylhexyl) trimellitate	Satellite bag for platelets	PL-1240* (Fenwal) CLX (Cutter)

*Not widely used in the United States; more common in Europe.

which are often used, for example, in the transfusion of small children or babies.

Plastic blood bags are for the most part manufactured from polyvinyl chloride (PVC) with stabilizing agents and plasticizers added. To ensure appropriate flexibility and pliability, as much as 40 percent of the bag weight may be plasticizer, usually di(2-ethylhexyl) phthalate (DEHP). This material does leach from the plastic, and levels of DEHP may reach 6 mg/dl in stored blood [32]. The chemical has been isolated from the tissues of transfused patients, but there is no evidence that toxic effects occur. The wide use of PVC transfusion equipment for over 20 years without evidence of toxicity certainly suggests that this plastic is safe. The demonstrable leaching of the plasticizer, however, is disturbing, and for this reason blood containers of different plastics are being evaluated.

Satellite bags made of special plastics that permit better gas exchange now make possible the storage of platelet concentrates for 5 days or even longer (see Chap. 8). Table 1-4 gives a listing of some of the plastics used in blood collection and storage.

Samples for Laboratory Testing and Crossmatching

Laboratory testing of donor blood and subsequent crossmatching must be possible without entering the primary container. Samples for processing are collected at the time of blood donation. The collection system must ensure that the blood in the samples is from the same donor as that in the container. Ideally, this is accomplished by having the processing tube integrally connected with the primary container as an in-line tube. There must be assurance of absolute identity of donor container and pilot sample. For crossmatching, blood from the integral donor tubing should be used. For this reason, the full length of tubing should be left attached to the bag on the completion of phlebotomy.

DONOR IDENTIFICATION

The container of blood must be identified accurately with the donor from whom it was collected. To this end, blood banks attach a number to the container, processing tubes, and donor record before phlebotomy. The phlebotomist must make sure that the numbers on the container and its tubes are identical to the number on the donor record, and that the record is that of the person being prepared for venesection. To be certain, the donor and his record and blood container should be kept together and positively reidentified before the venipuncture.

INFORMATION PROVIDED TO THE DONOR

Before venipuncture, the prospective donor must be told about the procedure and its potential risks and complications. This is done to allow the donor to give *informed* consent before the procedure and to make a rational decision whether to participate. The current legal climate is such that most large blood-collecting organizations have prepared a simple but relatively complete brochure which the donor reads before giving permission. This is a good idea, and we encourage it. Additional predonation information sheets regarding the risks of AIDS transmission and donor self-exclusion are now virtually mandatory (see Fig. 1–4). A brochure with postphlebotomy instructions, as in Table 1–5, is also recommended.

VENIPUNCTURE SITE

A large vein in the antecubital region is used for phlebotomy. Both the donor's arms should be examined, not only to select the best vein, but also to detect possible signs of drug injection, exemplified by scarred veins with many small puncture marks. Pressure is applied to the upper arm by means of a blood pressure cuff, which provides better control than a rubber tourniquet. The cuff is adjusted to a level just about the diastolic pressure, and the donor clenches his fist. The veins will then distend, and the most suitable one can be chosen. Whenever possible, veins in the center of the antecubital fossa are used, since those along the side of the arm are less firmly fixed and more likely to roll when touched by the needle. The selection of a good vein is important, not only because it will provide an uninterrupted flow of blood, but also because frequent manipulation and adjustment of the needle may be necessary in a poor vein, and this may disturb the donor sufficiently to trigger a reaction. Once the vein has been chosen, the pressure may be released.

The area to be used for venipuncture must be cleaned thoroughly to ensure asepsis. This is done by first washing with a soap solution, then removing the soap and applying an appropriate disinfectant. Povidone-iodine is probably the best disinfectant. Sterile techniques and supplies are used throughout, as for a surgical procedure. Hemostats or forceps, stored in an antiseptic solution, are

Table 1–5. Advice to Donors after Blood Donation

Many thanks for donating your time and blood. As a donor, you are vitally important to us and to our patients, so we want you to take good care of yourself after your donation. Most people have no trouble, but we advise the following as commonsense precautions:

1. Do not smoke for at least half an hour.
2. Have a good meal afterward.
3. Leave the bandage in place for a few hours.
4. You may resume most normal activities after donating, but you should preferably avoid strenuous arm work or exercise for the rest of the day, as it could cause your vein puncture to bleed.
5. If any bleeding occurs at the needle site, raise your arm and apply light pressure directly to the bleeding site.
6. If a bruise develops at a needle site some time after the procedure, pressure with an ice pack will help in the early stages. Later, a bruise will be slightly painful for about a week. If it bothers you at this stage, hot packs will speed up its disappearance.
7. If you have any problems or questions, please call us at _____.

---

used to hold the gauze or cotton balls. At no time should the fingers of the phlebotomist touch the sterile applicators or the prepared area of the skin.

PHLEBOTOMY

The technique of venipuncture in blood donation differs from that used to collect small blood samples. A large, 15- to 17-gauge needle is used and must remain in the vein for 4 to 7 minutes, maintaining a free blood flow the entire time.

The blood container must be kept below the level of the needle in the arm to ensure adequate gravity flow. To facilitate the mixing of blood and anticoagulant, the container should be in an inverted position during collection; occasional agitation is important. Mechanical agitators are now commonly used, generally with a weight-balance calibrated to shut off the blood flow when the proper amount of blood has been collected.

When the bleeding is completed, it is necessary to seal the container and prepare the appropriate pilot samples. In all cases, the donor tubing should be clamped before the needle is removed or the tubing cut. The pressure cuff is now deflated and removed from the arm, the needle is withdrawn, and a sterile gauze pad is placed on the venipuncture site. Enough donor tubing is left attached to the bag to allow preparation of a sufficient number of segments, after which blood from the attached tubing is stripped into the bag several times so as to fill the tubing with anticoagulated blood. The tubing is then divided into multiple segments by a dielectric sealing device. The segments remain connected to the bag and to each other and are used for crossmatching.

After the removal of the needle, the donor raises the arm (straight, not bent) and applies gentle pressure with the fingers of the other hand. Three or four minutes of manual pressure usually suffice to close the wound, after which a small tape bandage may be applied. During the phlebotomy and for at least 10 minutes afterward, the donor should be continuously observed by a member of the staff. Abrupt changes of position, from lying to sitting or from sitting to standing, should be avoided because they may cause dizziness.

REFRESHMENTS

Most blood banks provide refreshment for the donor. The area used should be supervised so that immediate aid can be given in case of delayed donor reactions. Smoking immediately after donation should be discouraged, and alcoholic beverages prohibited, because both nicotine and alcohol may cause syncopal reactions.

Adverse Reactions to Blood Donation

When blood collection is confined to adults of average size and good health, untoward reactions occur in less than 1 percent of blood donations. Reactions are more common in persons of small size, in whom the standard donation represents a larger proportion of the total blood volume.

FAINTING (SYNCOPE)

By far the most frequent type of reaction is a simple faint. It is caused by a neurophysiologic response to blood loss but is decidedly aggravated by psychologic factors. In the latter respect, it may resemble the fainting that sometimes follows psychic shock, such as the receipt of bad news. The psychologic component is illustrated by prospective donors who faint at the mere sight of blood, or when their fingers are pricked. Another example is the "contagious" fainting that sometimes occurs in large groups of excitable donors, especially young people. Fainting is also more common in first-time donors, probably partly because of fear. But despite these evident psychologic aspects, there is no doubt that fainting is for the most part triggered by the blood donation itself.

The donor is lying or reclining during and immediately after donation, and the evidence of impending collapse can be easily missed if the phlebotomist is not alert. The first complaints are usually a feeling of dizziness or lightheadedness, often accompanied by tingling of the fingers and a cold, clammy feeling in the palms of the hands. The observer notices an almost greenish pallor of the donor's face, cold sweaty palms, and beads of sweat, appearing first on the upper lip. The donor then usually loses consciousness for a few moments or longer. During the reaction, the blood pressure usually falls, often to a systolic level of 50 to 60 mm Hg, sometimes with imperceptible diastolic pressure, and the pulse slows to as low as 40 to 60 beats per minute. In milder reactions, hypotension and bradycardia may not occur or are transitory, but they sometimes persist for an hour or even longer. In prolonged reactions, the donor may feel well after his pulse and blood pressure return to normal, but dizziness and light-headedness will recur on arising.

REACTION VARIATIONS

Only occasionally are reactions rated as severe by the persons in attendance, mostly on the basis of prolonged recovery time. About one-third of severe reactions entail vomiting, a distressing complication to the donor and alarming and upsetting to other donors. Vomiting is a puzzling phenomenon, apparently unrelated to the severity of the other signs and symptoms of the reaction. Most such donors have recently eaten, but this is not always the case, and some donors retch miserably on an empty stomach. Like other reactions, it may have a psychologic component.

Approximately another third of the severe reactions include some form of increased neuromuscular excitability, usually associated with hyperventilation. Excessively deep breathing is probably related to fear, and its onset during blood donation is insidious. It results in rapid depletion of CO_2 in the alveolar air and in the blood, and a consequent rise in blood pH (alkalosis). The latter directly causes increased neuromuscular excitability, producing spasm of the muscles of the hands and feet (carpopedal spasm) and stiffness of the face and lips. Occasionally this leads to more generalized convulsive movements.

One variant that may have serious consequences is the delayed syncopal reaction, in which fainting may occur as late as 30 minutes to an hour after donation, by which time the donor has usually left the blood bank or hospital. The donor may fall and be injured, and fainting may be dangerous if the donor is engaged in some potentially hazardous occupation (see p. 28). Paradoxically, the "hazardous occupation" concept is not extended to the driving of a personal motor vehicle, surely a risky enough procedure. However, in practice, reactions under such circumstances do not seem to be a significant problem.

TREATMENT OF REACTIONS

Measures to relieve symptoms usually suffice. If the bleeding is still in progress, it should be stopped. If the container is nearly full, it is reasonable to try to obtain a processing sample, since the additional small blood loss will be inconsequential. To improve cerebral circulation, the feet should be raised or the head lowered. Many donor beds have a special arrangement for accomplishing the change in position; otherwise, blocks may be placed under the foot end of the bed. Donors who have already left the bed should be placed supine with the legs somewhat elevated, and if possible, screened from the view of other donors. Constant observation is essential until recovery is complete. The person in charge, preferably a nurse or physician, must record in writing the signs and symptoms, time, and duration of the reaction, and preferably also periodic readings of pulse and blood pressure. This report becomes a part of the permanent donor record. It is essential to have arrangements for medical care in the event of severe or prolonged donor reactions.

Management of convulsive seizures can be difficult, because the onset may be rapid and the victim often manifests unexpected muscular strength, the uncontrolled and unexpected application of which can injure the donor or members of the blood bank staff. Prevention of injury is the primary consideration. A padded object, such as a wooden tongue depressor wrapped in gauze, should always be in the donor room. In the event of a seizure, this object is inserted between the donor's teeth, if possible, to prevent biting of the tongue. Total immobilization of the donor is usually impossible, but partial restraint is appropriate to prevent the donor from falling off the bed or striking potentially dangerous objects. If the phlebotomist has help, someone should attempt to remove the needle, since tissue damage and hemorrhage are otherwise likely. A physician should be called at once to assist in the immediate handling of the donor, to examine for possible injury, and to add notes to the reaction report. Parenteral administration of a sedative (see below) may be required.

Medication

Most donor reactions are over in 10 to 20 minutes and require no medication. A brief inhalation of spirits of ammonia, sufficient to make the donor cough, is often helpful. When the reaction is severe enough not to respond to this, further treatment should be under the direction of a physician. The medical director should decide on the contents of an emergency kit, to be available at all times. This might include oxygen and various injectables, such as an antiemetic, a barbiturate, vasopressor agents, coronary vasodilators, bronchodilators, and antihistamines. It is worth stressing, however, that drugs or more radical therapy will rarely be necessary.

HEMATOMAS

Small hematomas sometimes occur at the phlebotomy site, particularly when there has been difficulty entering the donor's veins. Subcutaneous bleeding can usually be seen without difficulty and may be prevented from extending by means of firm pressure on the site, after removal of the needle. Most such extravasations result only in slight bruising of the antecubital fossa, but a few progress to larger and more unsightly hematomas. Donors experiencing such bleeding usually call the blood bank to complain about it, whereupon the circumstances should be written on the donor's record. If it seems necessary, the donor may then be referred to a physician for further treatment. If bruising is noticed at the time of donation and successfully arrested, it is still wise to warn the donor that the area will probably be slightly tender for a few days or even a week. This prevents undue worry.

Prevention of Donor Reactions

There is a strong undercurrent of fear and nervousness in donors who have had reactions. This being the case, the attitudes of the blood bank staff toward donors are extremely important. A warm and friendly approach with just the right amount of calm self-confidence, particularly on the part of the phlebotomist, will do much to allay fear. Excessive jocularity and mutual teasing among prospective donors should be firmly discouraged; this type of behavior, particularly in young people, is associated with anxiety and tension and leads to an increased incidence of reactions. Experienced personnel are usually able to detect nervous and fearful donors and can often prevent reactions by personal attention and friendly conversation. Since in our experience donor reactions are especially frequent in first-time donors and in women, both these groups may require particular attention.

Donors who have had severe reactions should be discouraged from future attempts at blood donation. Some blood banks notify them to that effect by a tactfully worded letter, offering to provide details about the reaction to the donor's physician. We usually disqualify any donors who have experienced severe delayed or prolonged reactions or who have had convulsions. Those who have had mild reactions should be given a second chance, if they wish.

Record of Donor Reaction

As with all untoward incidents, the important details of a donor reaction should be reported, signed by the person in attendance, and filed with the donor record so as to be available if the donor presents himself at another time. A simple form for this purpose will ensure proper completion of the essential details, including the description of the reaction, time of onset, pulse and blood pressure during the reaction and after recovery, duration of the reaction and subsequent period of rest and observation, physician's notes, and any special circumstances that may seem important. Severe or repeated reactions should be drawn to the attention of the blood bank physician. If the donor is to be disqualified from future blood donations, the record should be so marked. In the case of any reaction in which the donor sustains an injury, or in which it seems possible that litigation will ensue, full details should be provided in writing to the proper authorities of the hospital or blood bank.

Blood Donation by Hemapheresis

These are systems by which, at one sitting, whole blood is taken from a person, part of it is separated and retained, and the remainder is returned to the individual's bloodstream. Such procedures can be used to obtain certain blood components for transfusion, or to remove unwanted or harmful components from patients' blood (see Chap. 10). Those interested in the historical development of these machines and the hardware available up to 1980 may consult the third edition of this book. The same applies to the etymology and spelling of the various *apheresis* words, the correct versions of which are now generally used. One exception is the term *thrombocytapheresis,* which we had preferred for platelet collection by apheresis, but which does not seem likely to survive. *Platelet apheresis* is an easier and equally acceptable alternative, and we prefer it to the widely used *plateletpheresis*. We still consider *pheresis* to be jargon that should not be used by careful writers, despite its government-sponsored application to some blood components and procedures (". . . Platelets, Pheresis"*).

Manual Methods

The term *manual* is used to describe component collection systems not requiring a blood cell separator. The removal of a regular unit of blood from a donor, centrifugation to separate and remove the plasma, then return of the red cells to the donor is called *plasmapheresis*. In this manual procedure, plasma is separated off-line in a regular blood bank centrifuge. By a special array of integrated plastic bags and tubing, plasmapheresis can be accomplished twice at a single half-hour session with one venipuncture. Manual plasmapheresis is still the major method of commercially harvesting plasma for fractionation by the pharmaceutical industry, because the process is economical, quick, and adaptable to collection from large numbers of donors. Millions of liters of Source Plasma (a product intended for further processing) are obtained this way annually.

Obviously, donors must be protected from excessive loss of plasma, such as might lead to hypoproteinemia and consequent health impairment. Most developed countries therefore have regulations governing the amount of plasma that can be removed in a period of time.

In the U.S., the federal government, various state agencies, and the AABB have drawn up standards and regulations, under which it is legal to remove as much as 60 liters of plasma per year from normal donors. Few donors in plasmapheresis programs reach such high levels, but many people are concerned that current allowances are too liberal and that continued losses of 1,000 to 1,200 ml of plasma per week have the potential to deplete plasma proteins seriously [33]. On the other hand, studies have shown that intensive plasmapheresis of healthy subjects is well tolerated, and several donors have given as much as 1,000 ml per week for 32 months without obvious ill effect [34]. Standards in most European countries are more restrictive [35, 36].

There is no definite evidence that present practices in this country are ill founded, but all subjects in long-term plasmapheresis programs must be monitored for evidence of protein depletion or abnormality. In addition, since the

---

*U.S. Food and Drug Administration, Revised Guidelines for the Collection of Platelets, Pheresis. Washington, D.C.: January 1985.

red cell loss in tubing or samples can be enough to cause anemia or iron deficiency, hemoglobin or serum iron values should also be measured and evaluated periodically.

Manual Platelet Apheresis
It is possible to do an adequate platelet apheresis by a manual method analogous to manual plasmapheresis. Usually, 4 units of whole blood are collected in succession from a donor, each time returning the red cells but retaining the platelets and sometimes also the plasma [37]. The platelet yield by this procedure averages about 6×10^{10} per unit of blood; thus about 2.4×10^{11} platelets could be expected from a 4-unit platelet apheresis. This transfusion dose, equivalent to about three or four conventional platelet concentrates, is small, but offers the usual advantages of single-donor platelets (see Chap. 8). The procedure is cumbersome, requiring multiple centrifugations, and it is potentially hazardous if there is more than one donor at a time (there is always the possibility of returning the wrong red cells). Nonetheless, it is an available method of providing single-donor platelets in institutions that do not have access to an automated system.

AUTOMATED HEMAPHERESIS

Centrifugation Systems
Over the past 20 years or so, hemapheresis machines (blood cell separators) have been developed. These are devices with an extracorporeal blood circuit, through which the donor's blood moves with the aid of pumps, the separation of plasma or blood cells taking place by means of centrifugation in the machine, or by some other process, while the blood is in passage. In general, such machines are comparatively expensive and some are difficult to operate, but they can process more blood per unit of time than is possible in manual hemapheresis. Centrifugation systems can be broadly classified as *continuous flow* (CFC), in which donor blood flows through the extracorporeal circuit and cell separation device and returns to the donor without interruption; or *intermittent,* or *discontinuous, flow* (IFC), which processes donor blood in batches.

Just as plasma and red cells can be separated by centrifugation because of their relative differences in specific gravity or density, so the composition of the various cells in the buffy coat can be changed during centrifugation of whole blood, depending on variables of cell density and, in turn, on the strength and duration of centrifugal force. In order of increasing density in centrifuged whole blood, plasma will be on top, then platelets, lymphocytes, monocytes, granulocytes, and finally young and old red cells in that order. These are not to be thought of as sharp layers, but rather as overlapping bands. The composition of the buffy coat formed during centrifugation depends on many variables, including the centrifuge geometry, the presence or absence of macromolecular agents, the centrifugal force, and the rate at which the blood moves through the centrifugal field. In any particular centrifugal system, combinations of blood-flow rate, centrifugal force, and anticoagulant mixture can be developed for the collection of buffy coats of a desired composition.

Donor blood passing through an extracorporeal circuit must be prevented from clotting. When platelets, lymphocytes, and plasma are being collected, a conventional citrated anticoagulant is usually used, such as acid-citrate-dextrose (ACD) (formula A or B, depending on the desired proportion of anticoagulant to blood). When the aim is to collect granulocytes, citrate is added to an appropriate macromolecular agent (to be discussed later).

Centrifugal Devices, Updated

The available hardware for blood centrifugation was discussed and described in considerable detail in our third edition. Since that time, no basically new machines have appeared, so the discussion will not be repeated here. An Italian firm (Dideco) has produced blood cell separators of both intermittent-flow and continuous-flow types, concerning which few data have been published (Dideco, c/o Cryosan, Inc., Dedham, MA 02026). The IBM 2997 is now sold and serviced by Cobe Laboratories (and should henceforth be referred to by the latter name: Cobe Labs., Inc., Lakewood, CO 80215). The Fenwal CS-3000 (Fenwal Labs., Deerfield, IL 60015) is now well established (Fig. 1–5), but the Celltrifuge II is no longer being manufactured.

The IFC Haemonetics system now includes an updated but nonautomatic model 30S, very similar to the model 30 detailed in our third edition, as well as a versatile and fully automated model V50. The V50 features an elutriation system that shunts a rapid surge of plasma into the bowl at the time of collection of the buffy coat [38]. The effect of this "surge" technique is to concentrate the platelet layer in such a way that it is separated with fewer contaminating lymphocytes or red cells, a definite improvement over the concentrates obtained from the model 30 systems. Experience with the V50 seems to indicate that it is effective and reliable.

In addition to its use in the platelet surge system, centrifugation combined with *counterflow elutriation* has had considerable application for the production of purified cell suspensions in research [39]. The technique has potential for the production of suspensions of one isolated cell type, which is desirable for such purposes as adaptive immunotherapy with lymphocyte or monocyte lines, concentration of stem cells from peripheral blood, or removal of T lymphocytes from bone marrow collected for transplantation. The same principle has been applied to the purification of granulocyte concentrates for transfusion.

Membrane Systems

Technology that permits the passage of small molecules through a membrane while barring proteins and blood cells has been used primarily in hemodialysis

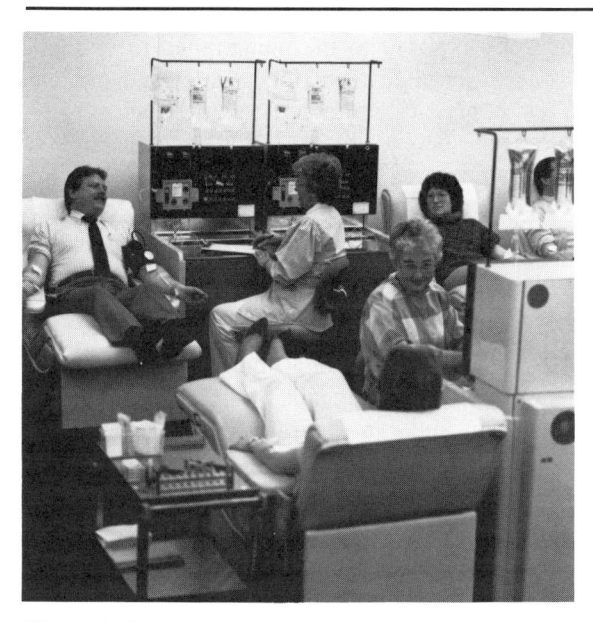

Figure 1-5
A group of Fenwal CS-3000 blood cell separators in use for platelet apheresis at a busy blood donor center. (Courtesy of Fenwal Laboratories, Deerfield, IL.)

for the removal of non-protein-bound solutes from blood. Recently, with membranes of coarser porosity, the principle has also been used in therapeutic plasmapheresis to remove protein-bound pathogenic substances (see Chap. 10). Such a system could not be used to collect cellular blood components, but could be applied to plasma collection.

The membranes used are plastic structures of various thickness and porosity, sometimes with a thicker supporting membrane [40]. The configuration of devices using such membranes is that of blood flowing either between flat sheets of membrane (the *sandwich* type) or through multiple capillary-like membranous tubules (*hollow-fiber* type). With either type, the blood flow is parallel to the membrane surfaces, with the flow of filtered plasma therefore at right angles, or perpendicularly, through the membrane. This results in a convective force toward the surface, which is countered by a tendency for blood cells to pile up against the membrane, forming in effect a secondary membrane, the properties of which vary according to existing geometry and operating conditions [41]. Mathematical formulas relating such variables have been derived. Another possible complicating factor is that of polarization concentration of protein molecules at the membrane surface. Factors affecting the efficiency of membrane separators are given in Chapter 10, Table 10-1.

The membranes must, of course, be biocompatible. There should be minimal or no adverse effects on blood cells exposed to the membrane, no systemic toxic effects, no harmful substances leached from the plastic, and minimal complement activation [42]. Various plastics and polymers are used.

A few of these devices have been specifically made for the collection of plasma for fractionation. For commercial use, they must be economically competitive with manual plasmapheresis, and it remains to be seen how successful they will be. Hemascience Laboratories, Santa Ana, CA, has produced an ingenious modification of a flat plate device in which the very small membrane is of cylindrical configuration, inside a somewhat larger cylinder, and supported by an internal fluted cylinder to conduct away the filtered plasma [43]. Blood flows into the external chamber while plasma filters through into the center. The membrane is constantly rotated by means of a magnet. This machine is operated by a microprocessor and can separate 500 ml of plasma in about 30 minutes (see Fig. 1–6). In addition to the latter, a hollow-fiber device for plasma collection has been manufactured by Organon-Teknika, a Dutch firm (Organon Teknika Corp., Durham, NC 27701).

CYTAPHERESIS PROCEDURES

We will not give methodologic details in this edition because there is an abundance of pertinent literature, scientific as well as practical. Furthermore, the equipment manufacturers all have detailed and well-prepared operational manuals.

The use of granulocyte transfusions has sharply declined in the past few years, whereas the clinical use of platelets has increased greatly. Consequently, platelet apheresis is the most frequent cytapheresis procedure today, and more and more platelet transfusions are being supplied by this procedure (see Chap. 8). It is therefore of some importance to review the donor qualifications and the effects of platelet (and leukocyte) apheresis on the donor.

Donor Selection

Cytapheresis procedures take more time than regular blood donation, often require two venipunctures, involve the establishment of an extracorporeal circuit with inflow and outflow of saline and anticoagulant, and sometimes make even healthy young donors felt tired and worn out. In some cases, particularly with intermittent flow procedures, the extracorporeal blood volume may exceed 500 ml, especially toward the end of a procedure. Consequently, although basically the same criteria are applied as for regular blood donation, the many other variables involved require donor selection procedures to be established by a nurse and physician experienced in hemapheresis.

The interval between cytapheresis donations is not firmly established. Some blood banks use the same interval as regular whole blood donation, thus avoiding undue pressure on the available donors. But a greater frequency is

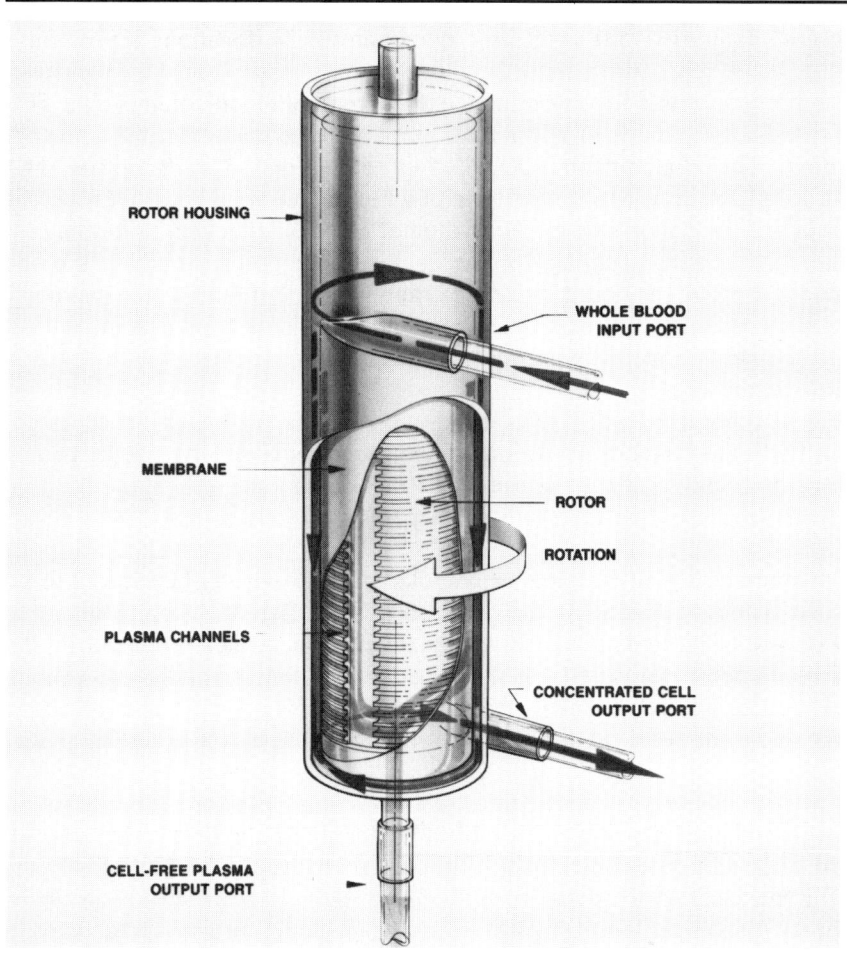

Figure 1–6
The Fenwal (Hemascience) Plasmacell-C® membrane plasma-collecting device. See text for description. (Courtesy of Fenwal Laboratories, Deerfield, IL.)

used by others. The FDA's *Revised Guidelines for the Collection of Platelets, Pheresis* (5 January 1985) suggests a maximum of 24 donations a year for a donor.

If the procedure will involve a large extracorporeal blood volume, as in IFC cytapheresis, the donor's size and total blood volume must be taken into consideration. The Haemonetics Corporation (400 Wood Rd., Braintree, MA 02184), for example, advises avoidance of an extracorporeal volume exceeding 15 percent of the donor's own blood volume; a useful guideline. A formula for calculating the extracorporeal volume as a percentage of the donor's blood volume is based on the donor's size, sex, and hematocrit, and on the geometry of the Haemonetics centrifuge bowl (formula available from Haemonetics). Extracorporeal volume problems are considerably less common with continuous flow separators.

The best screening test for successful cytapheresis is a history of repeated, uneventful blood donation. With that background, even elderly people can be accepted, particularly if they are in robust health and are well motivated.

ABO Group

ABO incompatibility of platelets or granulocytes can usually be ignored to no great disadvantage as long as the concentrates are free of visible contamination with red cells, as is the case with platelet concentrates produced by the newer blood cell separators (see Chap. 8). Platelet collections that do contain obvious red cells can be centrifuged slowly (e.g., 150 g for 7 minutes at 20 to 24°C) to allow the removal of red cells, although there is some platelet loss as well.

Virtually all *leukocyte* concentrates contain a large number of red cells, but because of the presence of a macromolecular agent (e.g., hydroxyethyl starch), the red cells will sediment rapidly without centrifugation and are easily removed if necessary.

"Minor" incompatibility (anti-A or anti-B in donor plasma) is actually a greater problem, and transfusion of, for example, group O platelets to a patient of Group A can and often does cause sensitization of the patient's red cells and a positive direct antiglobulin test after transfusion (see Chap. 7). To prevent these problems, unless the concentrate is compatible with the patient's red cells, excess plasma should be removed after moderate centrifugation (e.g., 3,000 g for 5 minutes at 22°C).

Obviously, the foregoing problems will not occur if donors are of the same ABO type as the recipient. When this is practical, it is undoubtedly best.

Rh Type

Rh antigens occur only on red cells. Consequently, the Rh type of either granulocyte or platelet concentrates is generally not taken into account for recipients who are not Rh-immunized, when such transfusions are given for leukemia and cancer. An exception is made for young women in whom a long remission of disease is likely. When Rh-positive platelet or white cell donors are used for Rh-negative recipients, Rh immunization does sometimes occur, but not often [44, 45]. The administration of prophylactic Rh immune globulin should be considered (see Chap. 8). In the case of patients who already have antibody to Rh or some other red cell antigen or antigens, the donor may be selected by red cell phenotype, or (more easily) the red cells may be removed from the concentrates, or techniques may be used that give red cell–free apheresis concentrates.

HLA Type

HLA matching for platelet transfusions is covered elsewhere (see Chap. 8). In the case of granulocyte transfusions, HLA matching is not necessary unless the patient is already demonstrably immunized.

DONOR BLOOD MODIFICATION IN LEUKAPHERESIS

Macromolecular Agents

Neutrophils are very close to erythrocytes in density. Consequently, when normal donor blood is anticoagulated with citrate (e.g., ACD) and centrifuged, the resultant buffy coat includes platelets and lymphocytes as well as neutrophils; in fact, lymphocytes usually predominate. The addition to the blood of a macromolecular agent greatly increases the number of granulocytes in the buffy coat, apparently by altering the sedimentation characteristics of the red blood cells. The agents used include the dextrans [46], hydroxyethyl starch (HES) [47], and various modified fluid gelatins (MFG) [48]. These are added to the donor blood with the anticoagulant (usually a concentrated citrate mixture) as it enters the tubing leading to the centrifuge. Aside from an occasional idiosyncratic reaction and continued concern over the possible harmful effects of long-term persistence of traces of HES, these agents are generally considered harmless to the donor (see p. 48). The persistence of HES has been a concern to many, even though harmful effects have not been shown. A new type of lower molecular weight HES has been developed; this seems to be completely eliminated in a relatively short time [49].

Dextrans of lower molecular weight (40,000 to 150,000), HES, and the various MFGs can be used more or less interchangeably, the choice being based largely on the availability of the agent. For example, HES is used in the United States, MFG and HES in continental Europe, dextran and HES in Great Britain, and dextran in Australia. The anticoagulant is most often trisodium citrate, with a small amount of citric acid in the same proportion as in ACD. To prevent clots or aggregates from forming, the anticoagulant must be in the correct proportion to donor blood, either by adjusting the concentration of the anticoagulant itself, or by varying the anticoagulant-to-blood ratio, depending on the machine being used. Heparin offers no particular advantage.

The effectiveness of granulocyte transfusions in appropriate clinical situations is somewhat debatable and will be discussed in Chapter 8. However, it is reasonably clear that inadequate doses will give rise to all the complications but few or no benefits [50]. To carry out leukapheresis without using a macromolecular agent guarantees inadequate granulocyte yields; consequently, the use of one of these agents is a sine qua non of granulocyte transfusion.

Steroid Stimulation of Donors

The number of granulocytes obtained by leukapheresis is roughly proportional to the donor's original peripheral granulocyte count. Therefore, if the donor's granulocyte count can be artificially or physiologically elevated before and during leukapheresis, an increased yield usually results [51, 52]. This has been shown with physical exercise [53] and with the administration of various corticosteroids, e.g., hydrocortisone, dexamethasone, prednisone, methylprednisolone, and etiocholanolone [54]. Even epinephrine has been used (e.g., in the Soviet Union). Epinephrine and physical exercise (the latter, of course, exerts its effect by the release of endogenous epinephrine) appear to work primarily by demarginating leukocytes from the endothelial surfaces, and this effect is rapid and transitory. The corticosteroid mechanism is not fully understood, but is probably a combination of demargination, release of additional granulocytes from the bone marrow reserve, and inhibition of granulocyte egress from the circulating pool. Different steroids may act by various mechanisms.

If corticosteroids are to be effective in stimulating leukocyte donors, they must be given in appropriate doses, and on a time schedule that ensures continuation of leukocytosis during the anticipated period of the leukapheresis. This may be effected by a single dose given at least 2 hours before the start of the procedure. But the most effective stimulation seems to be achieved by two or more oral doses of dexamethasone or prednisone given over the 2 to 17 hours preceding leukapheresis [51, 52].

Finally, a number of studies have shown that neither the use of macromolecular agents in cell collection nor the steroid premedication of donors adversely affects the function of either platelets or neutrophils collected by centrifugal methods [55, 56]. Neither of these agents is necessary in the collection of platelets, for which simple citrate anticoagulant solutions are adequate (e.g., ACD).

FILTRATION LEUKAPHERESIS (FL)

The adherence of granulocytes to nylon fibers has long been used as a means of reducing the number of leukocytes in blood intended for transfusion to patients with leukocyte antibodies. The use of this technique as a means of collecting and subsequently eluting neutrophils for transfusion was developed by Djerassi, who constructed a mechanical, pumpless device for that purpose [57]. Filtration leukapheresis is easy technically, the machine is simple and cheap, and large numbers of granulocytes can be obtained. These attractive features, sufficient in themselves to encourage many to make use of filtration, are counterbalanced by a number of disadvantages: increased reactions in donors as well as recipients, the need to heparinize donors and neutralize the heparin, inability to supply platelets from the same donation, and damage to the granulocytes collected.

The disadvantages of filtration leukapheresis outweigh the advantages, and unless new data or procedural modifications bring about effective improvement, the procedure is likely to remain in disuse in this country. In any case, newer centrifugal methods seem to be able to produce as many granulocytes without the above disadvantages.

Effects of Hemapheresis on Donors

REACTIONS

Most of the reactions to hemapheresis encountered in the donor are much the same as those seen in regular blood donation, that is, vasovagal responses relating partly to extracorporeal blood volume and partly to ill-defined psychologic causes (predominantly fear) [58, 59]. These reactions are more common when a larger extracorporeal volume is involved, as in the IFC procedure. The same general measures are applied as in regular blood donation, but the operator has the advantage of being able to counter hypovolemia by increasing the return flow of blood or simply running more saline, and can usually halt the reaction without interfering with the procedure. In this sense, cytapheresis is more controllable than regular blood donation. In general, platelet apheresis is simpler than leukapheresis, in that neither a macromolecular agent nor steroid stimulation is used. In manual procedures, only citrated red blood cells are usually returned to the donor, as in simple plasmapheresis, whereas in cytapheresis, most of the plasma is returned as well, thus increasing the dose of citrate received by the donor. Table 1–6 lists the major complications of donation by hemapheresis.

Citrate

Rapid infusion of citrated blood can overwhelm the usually very fast breakdown of citrate, leading to chelation of calcium, diminished ionized calcium in the blood, and even electrocardiographic changes (see Chap. 7). The donor experiences chilliness, circumoral paresthesias, a vibratory feeling in the chest, sometimes nausea, and rarely, overt tetany. The operator can control this by slowing the reinfusion rate or the blood flow rate, or (in the case of continuous

Table 1-6. Actual and Potential Complications of Component Donation by Apheresis

Procedural	Vascular	Component Depletion	Specific to Leukapheresis
Vasovagal reaction	Hematoma	Red blood cells	Hypervolemia, edema
Citrate reaction	Sclerosis	Platelets	Skin manifestations
Hypovolemia	Thrombosis	Lymphocytes*	HES accumulations
Hypervolemia	Fistula	Plasma proteins*	Steroid effects
Hemolysis		Immune globulins*	Filtration apheresis:
Chilling		Clotting factors*	Perineal effects
Allergy, anaphylaxis			Complement activation
			Priapism

*Data are lacking as to real clinical effects of depletion of these items in donor plasmapheresis or cytapheresis.

flow centrifugation [CFC]) by diminishing the proportion of anticoagulant. Of course, enough anticoagulant flow must be present to prevent clotting or platelet aggregation. In most systems, a reduction in blood flow rate also reduces or eliminates the citrate effect. Exogenous calcium in the form of milk or a 1 gm oral tablet of calcium gluconate is considered a useful adjunct by some. Chilliness is alleviated by a blanket or a blood warmer.

Steroid

When used to stimulate granulocytosis, steroids may give rise to mild headache, insomnia, flushing, palpitations, or euphoria. These effects are transitory and appear to be dose-related. Donors who seem to be unusually sensitive to such effects should not be given steroid. The same applies to those with any condition known to be aggravated by steroid, e.g., diabetes, peptic ulcer, tuberculosis, glaucoma, and perhaps hypertension.

Other Types of Reaction

A few allergic-type reactions have been reported, including sneezing and sniffling, and rarely, anaphylactoid signs and symptoms. The nasal manifestations may be ascribed to citrate or to HES. Such reactions are not necessarily repeated on reexposure to HES and a cause-and-effect relationship to HES is unproved. A case of lichen planus in a leukapheresis donor was tentatively blamed on HES [60], but again the connection was not proved, and another case of lichen planus was reported in an apheresis donor who had *not* received HES [61]. There have also been cases of persistent skin itching associated with HES. HES does cause plasma expansion [62, 63], particularly when donors receive it frequently. Headaches and even edema may then occur [64]. Mild hemolysis has occasionally been encountered. One group has encountered hypersensitivity-type reactions apparently caused by exposure to ethylene oxide gas that had been used to sterilize the disposable plastic apheresis kits [65].

Most reactions to cytapheresis are mild and readily controlled by the operator, probably to a greater extent than is possible in regular blood donation.

Reactions Associated with Filtration Leukapheresis

As with dialysis membranes, strange things happen when donor blood passes through nylon fibers. There is an initial drop and then a rise in the donor's neutrophil count [66]. Certain complement components become activated, leading to sequestration of granulocytes in the pulmonary capillaries. Some donors, particularly women, experience crampy abdominal or perineal pain. Two male donors have had priapism that required surgical intervention [67]. Reactions to heparin have been encountered, as well as to the protamine used to neutralize heparin. Steroid premedication may reduce the number, and mitigate the effects of, such reactions. The increased incidence of reactions associated with filtration leukapheresis, particularly the occurrence of priapism and complement activation, has undoubtedly contributed to the near disappearance of this technique in the United States in the past few years.

CELL DEPLETION AND FREQUENCY OF DONATION

A normal person produces granulocytes far faster than we can remove them by cytapheresis, whereas platelets, red cells, plasma, and perhaps even certain types of lymphocytes can be depleted. But how often can a donor undergo hemapheresis, and what amounts of components can be safely collected per

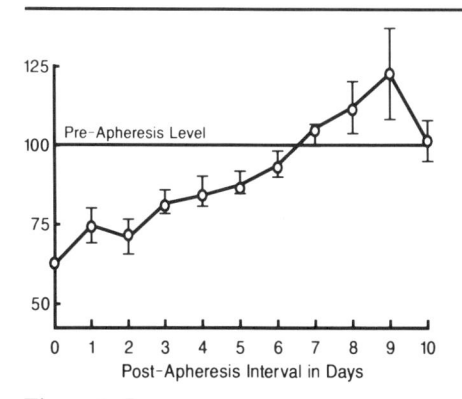

Figure 1-7
Donor preapheresis platelet counts compared with the same donor's preapheresis count at a second procedure 1 to 10 days later (expressed as a percentage of the first count). Total of 206 observations. Vertical lines indicate standard error of mean.

Table 1-7. Monitoring Criteria for the Prevention of Excessive Blood Component Depletion in Donor Cytapheresis

Component	Criterion, or Minimal Acceptable Level
Red blood cells	Hemoglobin above 12.5 gm/dl
	Removal of < 200 ml RBC/month
Plasma	Removal of < 1,000 ml/week
Serum protein	Above 6.0 gm/dl
Platelets	Count above 150,000/µl
Lymphocytes	Absolute counts above 1,200/µl
Granulocytes	No criterion: cannot be depleted

Criteria in part from reference 70, in part extrapolated from U.S. federal regulations and AABB standards, and influenced by what the authors consider reasonable. Note that no special monitoring is necessary if the donations conform to the regulations for whole blood donors, but that extensive monitoring may be needed when donors are subjected to very frequent cytapheresis.

procedure? Plasma loss is regulated in many countries, and, therefore, the plasma included in cytapheresis collections should in general be kept within those limits. Likewise, any red cell loss should be kept within the limits permitted for whole blood donors.

Platelets

After a platelet donation, it takes 6 or 7 days for the platelet count to return to its preapheresis level, as shown in Fig. 1-7 [68]. This places obvious limits on the frequency with which platelets may be collected. When platelets are donated several times within a week or two, the platelet count can quickly be lowered (e.g., to 100,000/mm^3 or even less). Further platelet apheresis will then be unproductive and should be stopped, at least until the platelet count has recovered (e.g., to at least 150,000/mm^3). There is probably not much of a hazard to the donor. The poor harvest of platelets from a donor with a low platelet count undoubtedly protects against potentially serious depletion. Leukapheresis, too, leads to platelet depletion, and platelet counts should be monitored in donors undergoing repeated procedures.

Lymphocytes

Depending on the collection technique, platelet apheresis may remove donor lymphocytes as well. Although recent data seem to show no significant change in the donor's lymphocyte count or general state of health, the theoretical possibility remains that lymphocyte depletion may exert some longer-term deleterious effect [69].

Table 1-7 lists some suggested criteria for monitoring blood component losses in donors who are subjected to cytapheresis procedures at donation intervals more frequent than those of routine blood collection [70].

References

1. London P, Hemphill BM. The motivations of blood donors. *Transfusion* 1965; 5:559–68.
2. Burnett JJ. Examining the profiles of the donor and nondonor through a multiple discriminant approach. *Transfusion* 1982; 22:138–42.
3. Oswalt RM. A review of blood donor motivation and recruitment. *Transfusion* 1977; 17:123–35.
4. Condie S, Maxwell N. Social psychology of blood donors. *Transfusion* 1970; 10: 79–83.
5. Milles G, Langston HT, Dalessandro W. *Autologous Transfusions.* Springfield, IL: Thomas, 1971.
6. Vaughn J. Blood transfusion in the U.S.S.R. *Transfusion* 1967; 7:212–29.
7. Kevorkian J, Marra JJ. Transfusion of human corpse blood without additives. *Transfusion* 1964; 4:112–7.
8. Hayes TJ, Dwyer FR, Greenwalt TJ, Coe NA. A comparison of two behavioral influence techniques for improving donor recruitment. *Transfusion* 1984; 24:399–403.
9. American Association of Blood Banks, Arlington, VA. Value improvement program study finds convenience top priority. *Blood Bank Week* 1986; 3(39):9–10.
10. Townsend R. *Up the Organization.* New York: Knopf, 1970.
11. Pindyck J, Avorn J, Kuriyan M, et al. Blood donation by the elderly. Clinical and policy considerations. *JAMA* 1987; 257:1186–8.
12. Avoy DR, Canuel ML, Otton BM, Mileski EB. Hemoglobin screening in prospective blood donors. A comparison of methods. *Transfusion* 1977; 17:261–4.
13. Coburn TJ, Miller WV, Parrill WD. Unacceptable variability of hemoglobin estimation on samples obtained from ear punctures. *Transfusion* 1977; 17:265–8.
14. Keating LJ, Gorman R, Moore R. Hemoglobin and hematocrit values of blood donors. *Transfusion* 1967; 7:420–4.
15. Milman N, Søndergaard M. Iron stores in male blood donors evaluated by serum ferritin. *Transfusion* 1984; 24:464–8.
16. Skikne B, Lynch S, Borek D, Cook J. Iron and blood donation. *Clin Haematol* 1984; 13:271–87.
17. Ladd DJ, Hillis A. A new method of evaluating the hepatitis risk of the multiply-implicated donor. *Transfusion* 1984; 24:80–2.
18. Mowat NAG, Albert-Recht F, Brunt PW, Walker W. Outbreak of serum hepatitis associated with tattooing. *Lancet* 1973; 1:33–4.
19. Boxall EH, Acupuncture hepatitis in the West Midlands, 1977. *J Med Virol* 1978; 2:377–9.
20. Johnson CJ, Anderson H, Spearman J, Madson J. Ear piercing and hepatitis. Nonsterile instruments for ear piercing and the subsequent onset of hepatitis. *JAMA* 1974; 227:1165.
21. *Baltimore Sun,* 1 December 1985. (Also quoted in *Blood Bank Week,* American Association of Blood Banks, 6 December 1985.)
22. Berkman EM. News release. American Association of Blood Banks, Arlington, VA, 10 January 1986.
23. Miller PJ, O'Connell J, Leipold A, Wenzel RP. Potential liability for transfusion-associated AIDS. *JAMA* 1985; 253:3419–24.
24. Pindyck J, Waldman A, Zang E, et al. Measures to decrease the risk of acquired immune deficiency syndrome by blood transfusions: evidence of volunteer blood donor cooperation. *Transfusion* 1985; 25:3–9.
25. Wykoff RF, Halsey NA. The effectiveness of voluntary self-exclusion on blood

donation practices of individuals at high risk for AIDS. *JAMA* 1986; 256:1292–3 (letter).
26. Black RH. Investigation of blood donors in accidental transfusion malaria. *Med J Aust* 1960; 2:446–9.
27. Centers for Disease Control. *Health Information for International Travel.* Washington, DC: Government Printing Office, Superintendent of Documents, 1985.
28. Walker RH. The disposition of STS-reactive blood in a transfusion service. *Transfusion* 1965; 5:452–6.
29. Ness PM, Perkins HA. Transient bacteremia after dental procedures and other minor manipulations. *Transfusion* 1980; 20:82–5.
30. Zuckerman CM. Fatality in a blood donor: a case report, with a review of the literature. *Ann Intern Med* 1947; 26:603–8.
31. Stuart MJ, Murphy S, Oski FA, et al. Platelet function in recipients of platelets from donors ingesting aspirin. *N Engl J Med* 1972; 287:1105–9.
32. Jaeger RJ, Rubin RJ. Migration of a phthalate ester plasticizer from polyvinylchloride blood bags into stored human blood and its localization in human tissues. *N Engl J Med* 1972; 287:1114–8.
33. Lundsgaard-Hansen P. Volume limitations of plasmapheresis. *Vox Sang* 1977; 32:20–5.
34. Cohen MA, Oberman HA. Safety and long-term effects of plasmapheresis. *Transfusion* 1970; 10:58–66.
35. Society Transactions: Meeting on the utilization and supply of human blood and blood products. *Vox Sang* 1977; 32:367–73.
36. Smit Sibinga CT, Huestis DW, Valbonesi M. The apheresis donor: how much and how often. *Vox Sang* 1984; 46:40–7.
37. Schiffer CA, Buchholz DH, Wiernik PH. Intensive multiunit plateletpheresis of normal donors. *Transfusion* 1974; 14:388–94.
38. Hogge DE, Schiffer CA. Collection of platelets depleted of red and white cells with the "surge pump" adaptation of a blood cell separator. *Transfusion* 1983; 23:177–81.
39. Gao IK, Noga SJ, Wagner JE, et al. Implementation of a semiclosed large scale counterflow elutriation system. *J Clin Apheresis* 1987; 3:154–60.
40. Stromberg RR, Hardwick RA, Friedman LI. Membrane filtration technology in plasma exchange. In: MacPherson JL, Kasprisin DO (eds). *Therapeutic Hemapheresis*, Vol. 1. Boca Raton, FL: CRC Press, 1985; 135–47.
41. Chmiel H. The effects of pressure, flow conditions, and surface composition on the filtration properties of plasma separation modules. *Plasma Ther Transfus Technol* 1983; 4:387–96.
42. Wegmüller E, Kazatchkine MD, Nydegger UE. Complement activation during extracorporeal blood bypass. *Plasma Ther Transfus Technol* 1983; 4:361–71.
43. Roch G, Tittley P, McCombie N. Plasma collection using an automated membrane device. *Transfusion* 1986; 26:269–71.
44. Goldfinger D, McGinniss MH. Rh incompatible platelet transfusion—risks and consequences of sensitizing immunosuppressed patients. *N Engl J Med* 1971; 284:942–4.
45. Lichtiger B, Surgeon J, Rhorer S. Rh-incompatible platelet transfusion therapy in cancer patients. *Vox Sang* 1983; 45:139–43.
46. Lowenthal RM, Park DS. The use of dextran as an adjunct to granulocyte collection with the continuous-flow cell separator. *Transfusion* 1975; 15:23–7.
47. Mishler JM. *Pharmacology of Hydroxyethyl Starch.* Oxford, UK: Oxford U Pr, 1982.

48. Huestis DW, Loftus TJ, Gilcher R, et al. Modified fluid gelatin. An alternative macromolecular agent for centrifugal leukapheresis. *Transfusion* 1985; 25: 343–8.
49. Strauss RG, Hester JP, Vogler WR, et al. A multicenter trial to document the efficacy and safety of a rapidly excreted analog of hydroxyethyl starch for leukapheresis with a note on steroid stimulation of granulocyte donors. *Transfusion* 1986; 26:265–8.
50. Huestis DW. Technical aspects of cell collection—donor considerations. *Clin Oncol* 1983; 2:529–47.
51. Winton EF, Vogler WR. Development of a practical oral dexamethasone premedication schedule leading to improved granulocyte yields with the continuous-flow centrifugal blood cell separator. *Blood* 1978; 52:249–53.
52. Hinckley MH, Huestis DW. Premedication for optimal granulocyte collection. *Plasma Ther Transfus Technol* 1981; 2:149–52.
53. Söderlund I, Engstedt L, Paléus S, Unger P. Induction of leukocytosis by means of hydrocortisone and/or muscular exercise. In: Goldman JM, Lowenthal RM (eds). *Leucocytes: Separation, Collection and Transfusion*. New York: Acad Pr, 1975; 97–103.
54. Mishler JM. The effects of corticosteroids on mobilization and function of neutrophils. *Exper Hematol* 1977; (suppl.) 5:15–32.
55. Glasser L, Huestis DW, Jones JF. Functional capabilities of steroid-recruited neutrophils harvested for clinical transfusion. *N Engl J Med* 1977; 297:1033–6.
56. Slichter SJ. Efficacy of platelets collected semi-continuous flow centrifugation (Haemonetics model 30). *Br J Haematol* 1978; 38:131–40.
57. Djerassi I, Kim JS, Mitrakul C, et al. Filtration leukopheresis for separation and concentration of transfusable amounts of normal granulocytes. *J Med (Basel)* 1970; 1:358–64.
58. Huestis DW. Complications of frequent donor cytapheresis and plasma exchange. *Plasma Ther Transfus Technol* 1985; 6:541–6.
59. Sandler SG, Nusbacher J. Health risks of leukapheresis donors. *Haematologia* 1982; 15:57–69.
60. Bode U, Deisseroth AB. Donor toxicity in granulocyte collections: association of lichen planus with the use of hydroxyethyl starch leukapheresis. *Transfusion* 1981; 21:83–5.
61. Newman RS, Barr RJ, Ocariz JA, Kaplan HS. Does hydroxyethyl starch cause lichen planus? Lichen planus in a long-time routine blood donor never exposed to hydroxyethyl starch. *Transfusion* 1983; 23:531–2.
62. Rock G, Wise P. Plasma expansion during granulocyte procurement: cumulative effects of hydroxyethyl starch. *Blood* 1979; 53:1156–63.
63. Strauss RG, Koepke JA. Chemistry, pharmacology, and donor effects of hydroxyethyl starch as used during leukapheresis. *Plasma Ther Transfus Technol* 1980; 1(3):35–4.
64. McCredie KB, Freireich EJ, Hester JP, Vallejos C. Increased granulocyte collection with the blood cell separator and the addition of etiocholanolone and hydroxyethyl starch. *Transfusion* 1974; 14:357–64.
65. Leitman SF, Boltansky H, Alter HJ, et al. Allergic reactions in healthy plateletpheresis donors caused by sensitization to ethylene oxide gas. *N Engl J Med* 1986; 315:1192–6.
66. Hammerschmidt DE, Craddock PR, McCullough J, et al. Complement activation and pulmonary leukostasis during nylon fiber filtration leukapheresis. *Blood* 1978; 51:721–30.

67. Dahlke MB, Shah SL, Sherwood WC, et al. Priapism during filtration leukapheresis. *Transfusion* 1979; 19:482–6.
68. Huestis DW. Adverse effects of granulocyte donations. In: Vogler WR (ed). *Cytapheresis and Plasma Exchange: Clinical Indications.* New York: A. R. Liss, 1982; 101–4.
69. Blanchette VS, Dunne J, McPhail S, et al. Immune function in blood donors following short-term lymphocytapheresis. *Vox Sang* 1985; 49:101–9.
70. Strauss RG, Huestis DW, Wright DG, Hester JP. Panel V: cellular depletion by apheresis. *J Clin Apheresis* 1983; 1:158–65.

2. Basic Blood Group Immunology

A knowledge of the basic principles of immunology is essential for a true understanding of blood transfusion serology. For one thing, the blood groups are antigens, and their reactions with corresponding antibodies are antigen-antibody reactions typical of those seen in other branches of immunology. In addition, many of the important concepts that laid a foundation for present thinking in immunology were developed through the study of the blood groups and their serologic reactions.

In 1798, Edward Jenner published the results of his experiments using vaccination to induce immunity to smallpox. Before Jenner's time, it had been common knowledge that those who survived an infectious disease almost never had a second episode of that particular disease, although there was no understanding of the mechanism by which this protection was brought about. Jenner, and later Pasteur, showed that the deliberate treatment of persons with disease-causing agents that had been modified, or even with a different but related bacterium, could lead to the same kind of protection without causing the disease. Neither Jenner nor Pasteur understood the mechanism by which such immunization led to protection against disease. A beginning knowledge was obtained in the late 1800s, when a substance that neutralized bacteria or bacterial extracts was found in the blood of "immune" animals. This protective material was named *antitoxin* or *antibody*. Shortly thereafter, it was shown that antibody not only had the power to protect against disease, but also could react with its specific bacterium (the antigen) in certain laboratory tests. This was the beginning of immunology, the study of antigens, antibodies, and antigen-antibody reactions.

The science of immunology has grown in scope and complexity and has become central to many areas of medical thought. Definitions of immunity have been broadened from the original observation that those who recovered from an infectious disease were no longer susceptible to it to the modern-day concept that one central feature of an immune reaction is the ability of an organism to recognize "self" and "not-self" and, in so doing, to identify and react to foreign substances. New, too, is the knowledge that these reactions are mediated by two separate, but related, systems and controlled by the complex interactions of several groups of cells and hormones, all of which, taken together, initiate and control the body's immune response. The two systems, *cell-mediated* and *humoral,* act together to bring about the many reactions, conditions, and diseases that are the province of modern immunology. Clinical immunology has also expanded to include disease entities marked by a failure of the self-recognition mechanism, which, in turn, leads to a self-destructive, or *autoimmune,* process.

Reactions that characterize the immune response are mediated by the interaction of foreign substances called *antigens* with selected cells—either the *macrophages,* which process the antigen in a way that makes it available to the various other cells in the immune system, or the *B lymphocytes,* which ultimately produce antibody. When the final product is circulating antibody—as is the case in those reactions involved in traditional blood bank work—the ultimate antibody-producing cells (B lymphocytes) are derived from the blood, and the process is known as *humoral immunity.* In other cases, viral or fungal infections or tissue rejection, for example, the antigens interact predominantly with *thymus-derived* or *T lymphocytes,* and the process is known as *cellular immunity.* Blood transfusion serology is based on the reactions of blood group antigens with antibodies produced by B lymphocytes. Cell-mediated immune reactions are undoubtedly important as well, but do not, at present, enter into those areas considered basic blood group immunology. Rather, the interaction of blood group antigens and their B cell–derived antibodies is the essential constituent of the reactions, both in vitro and in vivo, that concern blood bankers.

Antigens

Antigens are substances that can, under proper circumstances, elicit a specific immune response when introduced into the tissues of an animal [1–3]. Most are of biologic origin, and all organisms, from the human to the simplest bacterium, have numerous different antigens. Usually, antigens are proteins, but they may also be lipids, polysaccharides, or even nucleic acids. Inherent properties, such as molecular weight, size, and complexity, determine which substances are antigens.

The usual immune response elicited by antigens, and the one of most interest to blood bankers, is the formation of circulating antibody. For an antigen to give rise to antibody formation it must possess certain of the intrinsic properties described above, but it must also be foreign to the host. Except in autoimmune disease, an animal cannot produce antibodies against antigens that are part of its normal body structure. The mechanism by which whole cells are recognized as foreign involves various cell membrane markers coded for by genes of the human histocompatibility (HLA) system. To stimulate an immune response in a normal individual, the antigen must be recognized as foreign; in general, the more foreign, the greater is its potential to stimulate. For example, duck albumin produces no immune response in the duck, a weak one in the chicken, and a strong one in the rabbit. An antigen may be thought of as having at least two components: the reactive site and the remainder of the structure. Each reactive site contains at least one area, known as an *epitope* (formerly, *antigenic determinant*), which is specific for that site alone. The epitope is responsible for the unique individuality of that portion of the antigen and is the locus for specific antibody binding. Each antigen can, and usually does, have multiple epitopes. This is true of natural antigens as well as those prepared in the laboratory. Thus, one expected characteristic of antigens is multispecificity, that is, the ability to react with more than one antibody. The second portion of the antigen, the *carrier,* is responsible for other functions, including antibody-stimulating activity (*immunogenicity*). Molecules containing reactive sites (epitopes) can be coupled to a carrier protein in the laboratory. In such a case, the reactive portion is called a *hapten* and, like a naturally occurring site, it determines specificity.

Antibodies

Antibodies are serum proteins that have been produced in response to antigenic stimulation [1–4]. They are usually found in plasma, although some kinds of antibody do not appear to circulate, but are fixed to body tissues or cells. Nearly all antibodies are in the gamma globulin fraction of the serum proteins, but a few are nongamma proteins. The term *immunoglobulin* applies to all proteins that are antibodies, and to certain proteins related to them by molecular structure.

Immunoglobulins

The basic immunoglobulin structure is a protein molecule built up from two pairs of polypeptide chains held together by disulfide bonds (Fig. 2–1). One pair of peptide chains, called the *light chains,* consists of 214 amino acids. Light chains can be either of two different antigenic types, called *kappa* and *lambda.* These light chains are common to all classes of the immunoglobulin molecules, although the ratio of kappa to lambda types will vary. Every light chain, whether kappa or lambda, has two regions known as *domains.* The region nearest the distal, or amino, terminal has varying amino acid configurations depending on the antibody specificity. It is known as the *variable region* or *domain* and extends to amino acid number 107. The region of the light chain from amino acid 108 to 214 is nearly identical in all light chains and is known as the *constant domain.* These domains are aligned with variable and constant domains of *heavy chains* (see below). The variable regions are associated with antibody specificity and antigen (epitope) binding.

The second pair of chains in the immunoglobulin structure, heavy chains, are built up from 330 or 440 amino acids and are structurally different for each immunoglobulin class and subclass (Tables 2–1 and 2–2). Heavy-chain differences provide the basis for the distinction among the five different classes of immunoglobulins, as well as among the four subclasses of IgG, the two subclasses of IgA, and the two subclasses of IgM.

Although subclass differences were originally demonstrated by dissimilar antigenic structure, there are also important biologic consequences of the various subclasses. For example, complement activation is greatest with antibodies of subclass IgG_3, less so with IgG_1, slight with IgG_2, and nonexistent with IgG_4. Rh antibodies are predominantly IgG_1 and IgG_3, which may seem paradoxical,

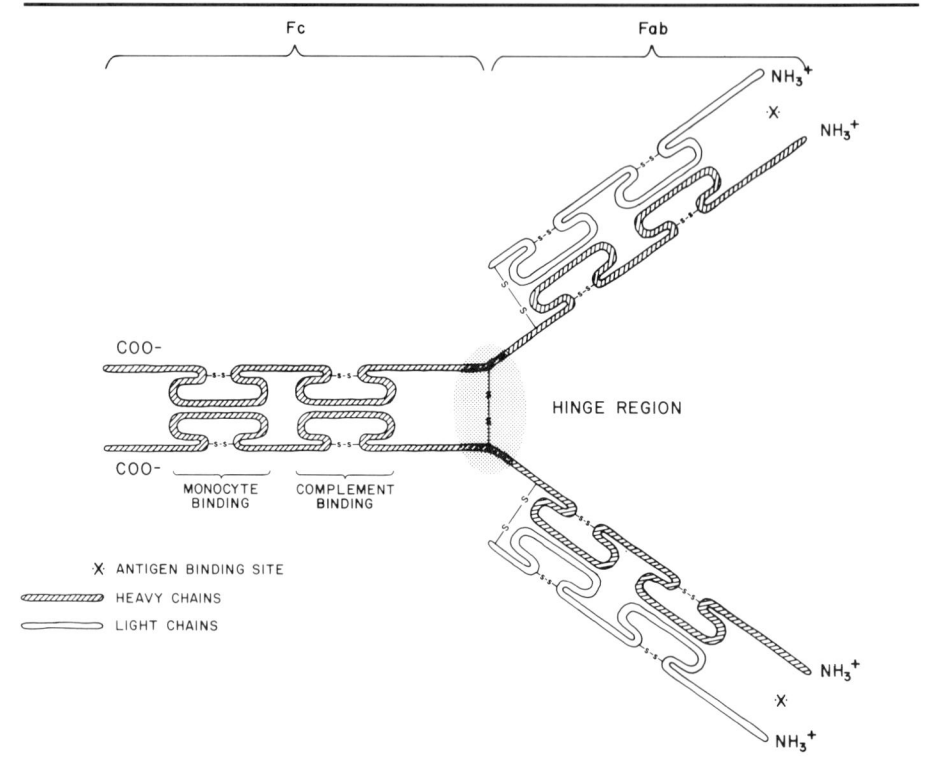

Figure 2–1
Schematic representation of the immunoglobulin G molecule.

since Rh antibodies are known not to activate complement in the traditional sense. This is probably attributable to the fact that there are relatively few Rh binding sites on red cells compared, for example, to the number for A or B.

The immunoglobulin structure, shown schematically in Fig. 2–1, is basic to all classes. The IgM molecule is a pentamer of such structures (each with μ heavy chains), whereas IgA is either a monomer or a polymer of two to five such structures (each with α heavy chains). IgA in secretions is a dimer, whereas serum IgA may be a monomer or a polymer of two to five units. Both IgM and IgA contain an additional polypeptide, the *J chain* or *joining piece*, with a molecular weight of about 15,000 daltons. The biologic role for the J piece appears to be initiation of polymerization of IgA or IgM.

One area of immunoglobulin molecules, the *hinge region,* is flexible and actually allows for some movement of the Fab segments (see below) when antibody combines with antigen.

Various chemical, electrophoretic, and immunologic techniques have been

Table 2-1. Classification of the Immunoglobulins

Recommended Term*	Other Terms	Heavy Chains	Light Chains	Number of Subclasses
IgG	γG, $7S\gamma$, γ_{ss}	γ	κ, λ	4
IgM	$\beta_2 M$, $\gamma_1 M$, $19S\gamma$	μ	κ, λ	2
IgA	$\beta_2 A$, $\gamma_1 A$	α	κ, λ	2
IgD	γD	δ	κ, λ	1
IgE	γE	ϵ	κ, λ	1

*World Health Organization, 1972.

used to study the immunoglobulins. Treatment with the enzyme papain breaks the immunoglobulin molecule into three pieces. Two are identical; they contain the antigen-reactive site and are known as the *Fab* (antigen-binding) *fragments*. The third, called *Fc,* contains portions of heavy chains only and is known as the *constant fragment,* since it is identical within each immunoglobulin subclass, even though the antibody specificity, and hence the Fab fragments, are different.

The immunoglobulin molecule can also be broken into its light and heavy chain components by reduction in the presence of urea. Reduction breaks the disulfide (S-S) bonds, and urea interrupts the hydrogen bonds.

Mild reduction increases flexibility of the IgG molecule, making it more suitable for hemagglutination and hence, in some circumstances, a more useful reagent for blood typing [5].

Table 2-2. Chemical and Physical Properties of the Immunoglobulins

Characteristic	IgG	IgM	IgA	IgD	IgE
Molecular weight (daltons)	150,000	900,000	150,000*	170,000–200,000	190,000
Sedimentation constant (Svedberg units)	7	19	7*	7	8
Carbohydrate content (%)	3	12	7	12	12
Electrophoretic mobility	Gamma	Between gamma and beta	Slow beta	Between gamma and beta	Slow beta
Normal concentration (mg/dl)	700–1,700	70–210	70–350	3	0.03
Percent total globulin	70–80	5–10	10–15	< 1	< 0.01
Survival (half-life in days)	21	5	6	3	2

*Monomeric form.

Table 2–3. Properties of the Immunoglobulins as Related to Blood Group Antibodies

Property	IgG	IgM	IgA
Placental transfer	Yes	No	No
Primary response	No	Yes	?
Secondary response	Yes	No	?
Activate complement	Yes	Yes	No
Agglutinate saline-suspended cells	Rarely	Yes	Yes
Hemolysis in vitro	No	Yes	No

Most circulating antibodies are of the IgG class. IgM is the antibody class traditionally associated with the early, or primary, response to antigenic stimulation (Table 2–3). Cold agglutinins and the blood group antibodies anti-A, anti-B, anti-P_1, and Lewis antibodies are often of the IgM class. The principal antibody in secretions is IgA, although some circulating antibodies (e.g., anti-A or anti-Rh) may be IgA. Secretory IgA consists of a dimer and an associated secretory piece. IgA antibodies do not activate complement. IgD is present in trace amounts in serum; its function is not known. IgE, or reaginic antibody, is also present in low concentration in serum, and is the antibody responsible for many types of antibody-mediated allergic and anaphylactoid reactions. IgE antibodies directed against IgA have been reported to cause transfusion reactions after transfusion of IgA-containing blood components into IgA-deficient persons [6].

CLASSIFICATION OF BLOOD GROUP ANTIBODIES BY SEROLOGIC BEHAVIOR

Blood group antibodies have been classified according to their serologic behavior, as well as by their specific physical and chemical properties (see Table 2–3). The serologic grouping, although less precise than the chemical one just outlined, continues to be used, since it is based on the reaction patterns observed in the blood bank laboratory. In addition, there is some correlation between the physicochemical properties and the serologic activity of most blood group antibodies.

Saline agglutinins, formerly called *complete* or *bivalent antibodies,* are blood group antibodies that agglutinate erythrocytes suspended in saline solution. Depending on specificity, these may be *cold antibodies,* acting best at 4°C, or *warm antibodies,* with a temperature optimum around 37°C. In either case, nothing but antibody and a saline suspension of appropriate cells is needed to produce agglutination. Nearly all IgM blood group antibodies are saline agglutinins. Anti-A, anti-B, anti-P_1, and Lewis antibodies, and especially anti-I and anti-i, are cold-reacting.

IgG antibodies of the Rh, Kell, and Duffy systems and others formerly called incomplete, univalent, or blocking antibodies, react with erythrocytes to cause sensitization, or antibody coating, but do not usually cause agglutination of erythrocytes. Cells coated (sensitized) with these antibodies agglutinate only when subjected to additional treatment such as the addition of albumin, polyvinylpyrrolidone, antiglobulin serum, or one of the proteolytic enzymes. All but a very few act best at 37°C. Nearly all of the antibodies detected after alloimmunization with blood group antigens are of the warm-reacting "incomplete" variety.

The Immune Response

The introduction of an antigen into a susceptible host sets off a complex set of reactions known as the *immune response*. This response involves at least four groups of cells—*macrophages, T lymphocytes, B lymphocytes,* and *plasma cells*—and leads either to antibody formation or to an alteration of the cellular immune response of the individual. For the most part, the *humoral response* i.e., that response leading to the production of circulating antibody, is of most interest and importance to blood bankers, for from it comes the antibodies that are involved with blood group incompatibility and transfusion reactions.

Macrophages

Macrophages are the cells involved in the first step of some immune responses, since they are responsible for the initial interaction with, and processing of, antigen. These cells ingest the antigen and through internal digestive processes convert it to a form in which it can be presented to the T lymphocytes of the immune system. In some cases, macrophage and T lymphocyte interaction requires shared HLA antigens of the Class II (DR) type (see Chap. 3). Macrophages are also important in the immune response because, after they react with T cells, they release interleukin-1, a chemical mediator that stimulates T cell multiplication.

T Lymphocytes

T, or thymus-dependent, lymphocytes are concerned primarily with cell-mediated immunity as exemplified by delayed hypersensitivity reactions, the rejection of transplanted organs or tissues, and the direct lysis of cells that are infected with various viral agents. They also have an important role in controlling immune responses by helping (*T-helper*) or suppressing (*T-suppressor*) other immunologically active cells. The various subsets of T cells can be identified by the presence of surface markers that are detected by reactions with highly specific monoclonal antibodies (Table 2–4).

B Lymphocytes

B lymphocytes are derived from bone marrow and are responsible for the secretion of antibody. Mature, actively secreting B lymphocytes are known as *plasma cells*. Antibody production follows a complex series of interactions in

Table 2-4. Surface Markers of Human T Lymphocytes as Determined by Selected Monoclonal Antibodies

Cluster Designation	Monoclonal Antibodies	Percentage of Peripheral Blood Lymphocytes	Functional Characteristics of T Cells
CD3	OKT3, Leu-4	70–80	Mature T cells, pan T cell marker
CD4	OKT4, Leu-3	35–55	Helper/inducer
CD8*	OKT8, Leu-2	20–35	Cytotoxic/suppressor
CD2	OKT11, Leu-5	80–85	E-rosette receptor-associated
CD1	OKT6, Leu-6	0	Thymic antigen

*Also present on natural killer (NK) cells.
Note: The term *cluster designation* (CD) has been introduced to standardize terminology without reference to a particular monoclonal antiserum.

which macrophage-processed antigen, along with signals from T helper lymphocytes, stimulates an appropriate B cell both to produce antibody and to multiply. The daughter cells that result from this multiplication are known as a *clone* and represent a group of cells derived from a single cell; they are committed to the production of a single antibody specificity. A portion of the cells from any such clone go on to become plasma cells and are, in this way, committed to continued antibody production. A second portion of the clone remains as B lymphocytes that are permanently programmed to respond to the original stimulating antigen by proliferation, plasma cell generation, and antibody formation. In this way, the phenomenon of *immunologic memory* becomes established, and provision is made for enhanced antibody formation (recall) at the time of subsequent contact with the antigen.

ANTIBODY FORMATION

The sequence of events beginning with the injection of antigen, its processing by macrophages, and the ultimate formation of circulating antibodies by B cells requires time. There is a lag of about 7 to 10 days, known as the *induction period,* during which only very sensitive tests occasionally detect minute amounts of circulating antibody. After about 10 days, circulating antibodies usually become evident if an immune response has occurred. At this time, the antibodies are predominantly IgM, and it has become popular to consider IgM to be the only kind of antibodies formed in a primary response. More probably, both IgM and IgG antibodies are formed, but only IgM can be demonstrated during the early stages of antibody production. In any event, the antibodies that continue to be produced are usually IgG. Depending on the animal immunized, the antigen itself, the amount of antigen used, and many other factors, the peak of antibody production will be reached in 10 to 30 days. In the case of blood group antigens, however, the response is often slower. If no additional antigen is injected, antibody production usually diminishes over about a year to a point where antibodies may no longer be detectable. For the blood group antigens, antibody production may continue for long periods with measurable amounts of antibody often present for years.

The first injection of antigen causes antibody-producing cells to develop a memory so that a second injection of the same or a related antigen is followed by a response different from the primary one. The lag, or induction, phase is shortened from 10 days to 1 day or even less. In addition, antibody production is enhanced so that high titers are reached rapidly. Finally, the antibodies produced by this second injection have better combining quality (high-affinity antibodies). This entire process is called an *anamnestic,* or *secondary, response*. At times, such a response may be seen after injection of an antigen that differs from the one used for the primary response if the two antigens are closely related. For example, a rise in the titer of typhoid antibody is usually seen when the secondary stimulus is a related antigen such as paratyphoid B.

Alloimmunization

Alloimmunization follows introduction of antigen from one individual into a different individual of the same species, for example, the injection of Rh-positive blood into an Rh-negative person. Since there are over 400 different blood group antigens on red cells, each time a transfusion is given antigens are transfused into a recipient who lacks them. The response, as measured by antibody production, will vary depending on factors involving both the antigen and the condition of the recipient at the time of injection. These factors act in unknown ways so that the incidence of alloimmunization after transfusion is low [7, 8].

IMMUNIZATION BY BLOOD GROUP ANTIGENS

Data on deliberate injection of erythrocytes to stimulate antibody formation are scanty and are limited to the Rh, Kell, and Duffy systems. Some of these experiments were done in the 1950s, and some more recently, but it is doubtful that additional research of this nature will be done, because of an increased awareness of the hazards of the injection of foreign blood. The experiments showed that of the common blood group antigens, D in the Rh blood group system was the most potent immunogen [9, 10]. Sixty percent of the Rh-negative persons tested produced anti-Rh after four injections of Rh-positive blood. The D antigen was more immunogenic than C, E, c, K, or Fy^a. ABO-compatible Rh-positive blood was more effective in stimulating Rh-negative recipients to produce Rh antibody than was ABO-incompatible blood. These experiments, plus evidence from clinical studies in Rh-negative mothers who gave birth to Rh-positive infants, suggest that the rapid removal of ABO-incompatible cells may be related to a striking diminution of their immunizing potential (see Chap. 9).

Blood group antigens other than D are weak immunogens, and immunization by them after transfusion is infrequent. In one study of 111 patients who had received a total of 376 units of blood, careful antibody detection tests were done every 5 days for a period of 35 days [11]. Sixty of the seventy-two patients who were still alive were tested again a year after transfusion. There was evidence of immunization in 3 percent of those studied. This figure is higher than the 1 percent predicted by Giblett [7], the 0.37 percent reported by Myhre and co-workers [12], or the 0.78 percent incidence seen by Spielmann and Seidl [13]. The important antibodies found most frequently after immunization to blood group antigens are anti-K, anti-E, and anti-c [14]. These data, plus a wealth of clinical observations, form the basis for the accepted and recommended practice of limiting pretransfusion blood grouping to ABO and D. There is no indication for further routine antigen testing, nor is there any reason to advise matching groups other than ABO and D, unless unexpected* blood group antibodies are present (see Chap. 5). Needless to say, once any clinically important antibody has been detected, only blood lacking the corresponding blood group antigen is acceptable for transfusion.

For years it had been recognized that the incidence of immunization to the K and c antigens differed when persons who had been immunized by transfusion were compared with those whose immunization resulted from pregnancy (transplacental hemorrhage or fetomaternal bleeding). Allen and Warshaw explained this seeming paradox by an ingenious mathematical analysis of the frequencies of K and c in the general population [15]. When a single transfusion is given, the opportunity for K incompatibility on a random basis is 8.2 percent, compared with a 15.3 percent chance for c incompatibility. At first glance, excluding differences in immunogenicity, it would seem that after transfusion, c immunization should be found more frequently than K immunization. This is the case for the first transfusion, but in a series of transfusions *each is from a different donor*. The chance of K incompatibility and the likelihood of subsequent immunization increase with each transfusion to a maximum of 91 percent (the frequency of K-negative persons in the population), but the maximum exposure to c can reach only 20 percent, that is, the frequency of c-negative persons. When the same reasoning is applied to pregnancy, it is modified by one important fact: the father is usually the same for each pregnancy. In this case, statistically speaking, the maximum exposure for any mother during repeated pregnancies is 16 percent for c, but only 8.2 percent for K. Thus, since each patient is transfused with blood from more than one donor, but each woman usually bears the children of one father, immunization to K should be

---

*Unexpected refers to blood group antibodies not normally found in unimmunized persons. The terms *irregular* and *atypical* have also been used.

more frequent than that to c after transfusion, but less frequent than that to c from pregnancy. And so it is.

Antigen-Antibody Reactions

Reactions between antigens and antibodies can take place in vivo or in vitro. T lymphocytes mediate those reactions that are in the province of cellular immunity. For the most part, these involve protection against viral or fungal infection, or the rejection of foreign tissue grafts. In vivo, B lymphocyte reactions are mediated by circulating antibodies, at times with associated factors such as the proteins in the complement system, and are known as humoral immunity. In autoimmune states, in vivo antigen-antibody reactions may actually cause diseases such as acquired hemolytic anemia or idiopathic thrombocytopenic purpura.

In Vitro Antibody-Mediated Reactions

The reactions between antigens and antibodies that occur in vitro are of great interest and importance to laboratory workers because it is through them that antigens or antibodies can be detected and studied. The specific nature of these reactions depends on a host of variables including the kind of antibody, the reaction conditions, and the particulate size of the antigen. There are, however, some general principles that apply to almost every antigen-antibody reaction:

1. The reaction is *specific;* that is, an antibody reacts with one, or at most with a few, closely related epitopes. This characteristic specificity is what makes antigen-antibody reactions unique. In antigen-antibody reactions, entire molecules react. There is no exchanging of pieces or fractions of molecules, and no new product is formed.
2. The union of antigen with antibody is *firm but reversible*. With proper conditions, the reaction can be reversed, and both antigen and antibody recovered relatively unchanged.
3. The antigen-antibody reaction is a *surface phenomenon* that does not alter the primary structure of either reactant.
4. The reactants *combine in varying proportions* depending on the conditions of the experiment. This is quite different from most chemical reactions, in which the ratio of one chemical or molecule to another is always the same.

Antigen-antibody reactions are usually rapid, often taking place in less than a minute, although exceptions are known.

Most antigen-antibody reactions occur in two stages. First, antigen combines with antibody; then, some change occurs so that the antigen-antibody complex becomes demonstrable either by eye or by measurement with laboratory instruments. The stages usually overlap in time, and the complex becomes evident while further combination is occurring. The formation of the antigen-antibody complex is, in all likelihood, an electrochemical event and related to the attraction between molecular forces that are positively and negatively charged.

The serologic manifestation of antigen-antibody combination is determined by the reaction conditions, the antigens and antibodies involved, and the size of the antigen. Antibodies are immunoglobulins and, as such, are soluble. Their molecular size, therefore, is of little importance in this regard. Antigens, on the other hand, may be relatively small or large, or, even more important, may be a part of comparatively huge structures such as erythrocytes, leukocytes, tissue cells, or bacteria. For this reason, the particulate size of the antigen is vitally important in determining the physical nature of the antigen-antibody complex.

PRECIPITATION

The mixing of enough *soluble* antigen with an antibody-containing solution is usually followed by the formation of a visible precipitate. This precipitate is an *antigen-antibody complex,* the proportions of antigen and antibody being determined by the concentration of each in the mixture. The quantitative aspects of precipitin reactions have been carefully studied and are similar for many kinds of precipitating antibodies and soluble antigens. To understand the events that occur during precipitation reactions, one must assume that the IgG antibody molecule has but two reactive sites (see Fig. 2–1), whereas antigens may have multiple sites (epitopes) that can react with a given antibody. Thus, when a relatively small amount of antigen is added to an excess of antibody, complexes that have much antibody and little antigen are formed. This is known as the *prozone* and is marked by little or no precipitate formation. As increasing amounts of antigen are added to the same quantity of antibody, the proportion of antigen to antibody changes until a stage of optimum proportions is reached. At this point, the *equivalence zone,* the antigen-antibody complexes contain about two molecules of antibody for each molecule of antigen. Addition of more antigen now shifts the reaction to a phase of antigen excess, *post-zone,* in which complexes contain a large amount of antigen and lesser amounts of antibody. Antigen-antibody complexes formed with too much antigen or too much antibody are more soluble than those formed with optimum concentrations of each reactant. The largest amount of precipitate, then, is always found at the equivalence zone. Tests of the supernate at this stage show neither antigen nor antibody. It should be evident from the above that precipitin tests for antigen or antibody may show false-negative results if too much of either reactant is used.

Precipitation reactions can be done in test tubes, in capillary tubes, or in semisolid substances like agar, agarose, or gels such as acrylamide.

AGGLUTINATION

The most important of the antigen-antibody reactions in blood group work is *agglutination*. In agglutination, antibodies react with antigens that are parts of large structures, such as erythrocytes or bacteria, to form gross clumps or *agglutinates*. In many ways, the agglutination reaction is similar to the precipitation reaction, and one conveniently thinks of agglutination as a precipitation reaction that takes place on the surface of cells or bacteria. It is often possible to coat large particles (e.g., erythrocytes, latex spheres, or starch granules) with soluble antigen so that the antigen can be studied more easily in the laboratory. In this way, simple slide tests of agglutination may be used to show the presence of antibodies to soluble antigens. For example, latex particles coated with cytomegalovirus antigens are used in one of the most commonly employed tests for antibodies to the virus.

Agglutination reactions may be inhibited by an excess of either antigen or antibody, and there is, as expected, a zone of optimum proportions at which the agglutination is maximal. It is common practice to refer to the inhibition of agglutination caused by antibody excess as the *prozone phenomenon*. This is occasionally seen in blood bank work, in which reactions by agglutinating antibodies of high titer, particularly anti-D, may be weak or negative when done with undiluted serum.

The clumping of red blood cells by antibodies takes place in two stages. The first—combination of antibody with antigen—is usually rapid. Visible agglutination does not necessarily occur when antibodies and red cells react; in fact, agglutination itself is the second stage of the reaction. Much information is available about the factors involved in agglutination, although a great deal remains to be learned [16].

Formation of Agglutinates

ZETA POTENTIAL THEORY. Erythrocytes have a net negative electrical charge that arises largely from the ionization of carboxyl groups of sialic acid residues on the cell surface. The charge is approximately equal on all erythrocytes and, because like charges repel, erythrocytes in suspension do not come in contact with one another. In solutions of electrolytes—sodium chloride, for example— the erythrocytes attract a surrounding cloud of ions. The intensity of the cloud varies, depending on the intrinsic charge of the erythrocyte and the ionic constitution of the suspending medium. The electrical activity of this ionic cloud is known as the *zeta potential*, one effect of which is to keep erythrocytes in isotonic solutions separated by a distance of about 300 Å. This force or distance must be overcome before agglutination can occur [16].

SURFACE HYDRATION THEORY. A second theory of agglutination suggests that cell separation is maintained in red cell suspensions by a layer of water bound to the red cell surfaces (*hydration shell*). Antibody combination with red cells decreases the hydration layer and renders the red cells more agglutinable [17, 18].

Neither theory has been proved, and in all probability, some aspects of each are important. In addition, other factors such as antigen site density, cell surface shape, osmotic influences, the presence of polyelectrolytes or dissolved polymers, and the ionic strength of the suspending medium also play a role in bringing about agglutination [16, 19].

NEUTRALIZATION

At times, neither precipitation nor agglutination occurs, even though antigen and antibody have reacted. In such cases, *neutralization* experiments may be helpful. In work with viral agents, particularly, neutralization is a useful technique. A dose of virus known to be lethal for a test animal is mixed with the serum to be tested for antibodies against the virus. The mixture is then injected and the test animal observed. Neutralizing antibodies in the test serum will be shown by the failure of the lethal dose of virus to kill the test animal. Another example of a neutralization reaction occurs when an individual who has been exposed to toxin (antigen)-producing bacteria is injected with antitoxin (antibody). Here the reaction between toxin and antitoxin, in vivo, protects the recipient by neutralization of the toxin.

ANTIBODY LABELING

Direct evidence of antigen-antibody combination is obtained when antibody molecules are labeled or tagged in such a way that they can be easily traced. This can be done with a radioisotope such as ^{125}I, which when coupled to an antibody, becomes an integral part of the antibody molecule. The antibodies, now radioactive, can be tested with various tissues and substances. Those that possess the corresponding antigen will react with the isotope-labeled antibodies and can be detected by counting the radioactivity. An almost identical approach can be used by binding the antibodies to a substance, such as fluorescein isothiocyanate, that glows with a bright green color when exposed to ultraviolet light. Various tissues or cells, after treatment with fluorescein-labeled antibody, can be studied with a fluorescence microscope to demonstrate the presence of antigen-antibody complexes. Antibodies can also be labeled with various enzymes and used in the enzyme-linked immunosorbent assay (ELISA or EIA) to detect antigens or antibodies [20]. The principle is similar to that employed in radiolabeling, except that a color change, rather than radioactivity, is detected as an endpoint.

IMMUNE HEMOLYSIS

Another serologic manifestation of the antigen-antibody reaction is *immune lysis*. The destruction of bacteria (*bacteriolysis*) or erythrocytes (*hemolysis*) by antibodies plays an important part in the immune defense mechanism of most animals and is, in addition, a valuable laboratory technique [21]. Lytic reactions, both in vivo and in vitro, require antibody, antigen, and a third group of reactants known collectively as *complement* [22]. The importance of complement was first suspected because immune lysis of red cells or bacteria required some unknown factor present only in fresh serum. In addition, the precipitate formed from known quantities of some antigens and antibodies weighed more when the reaction product was obtained using fresh, rather than stored or heated, serum. Fresh serum, it was reasoned, contained a substance, first called *alexin* but now known as complement, that actually became part of the antigen-antibody complex. Heating the serum to 56°C destroyed this material.

Certain antibodies lyse red cells or bacteria if fresh serum containing complement is present, but agglutinate the same cells if aged or heated serum is used. Complement, the material required for immune lysis, is not an antibody, since it does not result from antigenic stimulation but is present in all normal animals. Furthermore, the activity is nonspecific; complement from one species is effective in antigen-antibody reactions in many other species. Complement does, however, enter into many antigen-antibody reactions and, in so doing, will modify the serologic manifestation of these reactions.

The Complement System

Components of Complement

The complement system is a multimolecular self-assembling system constituting one of the primary humoral mediators of inflammation and tissue damage. In the *classical activation pathway* (Fig. 2–2), at least 11 different proteins act as enzymes or cofactors in a complex chain reaction. A related activation reaction, the *alternative pathway,* involves several additional components. There are also five different proteins that control activity or synthesis of the various complement components. One complement protein, C4, has been shown to carry the Chido and Rodgers antigens [23].

The various components of complement are designated C1, C2, C3, etc. Activated components are indicated by adding a bar over the numeral (C$\overline{1}$, C$\overline{4}$, C$\overline{2}$, C$\overline{3}$, etc.), whereas fragments of the various components are indicated by the addition of lowercase letters (e.g., C3a, C3b, etc.). The reaction sequence of antigen, antibody, and complement is shown in Fig. 2–2. Activation of one component leads to the activation of another component, usually by an enzymatic mechanism. All components are activated in appropriate numerical order except for C4, which is activated by C1 and, in turn, activates C2. During the sequence, some of the activated components become fixed to the cell membrane; others are cleaved and release fragments into the plasma.

Several of the polypeptides released into the plasma during in vivo complement activation are known to have important biologic activity (Table 2–5). C3a, or anaphylatoxin, causes smooth-muscle relaxation, erythema and edema of the skin, and histamine release. C5a acts as a major chemotactic factor of neutrophils, causes mast cell degranulation, and increases vascular permeabil-

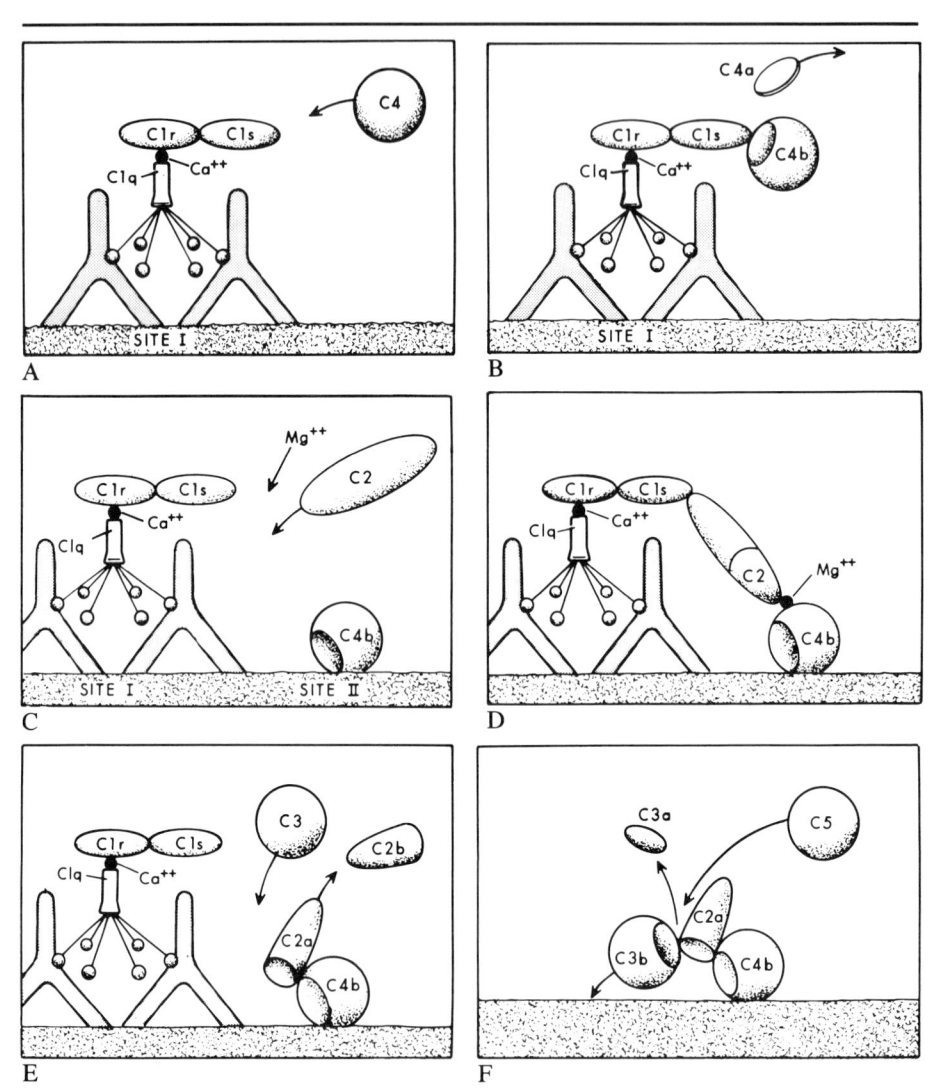

Figure 2–2
The classical pattern of complement attack on the red cell membrane. Sequential activation and fixation of C1 through C9 eventually lead to cell lysis. Note that after the stage of C4b,2a activation, the original antibody-cell interaction is no longer required. Thus, cells can be coated with complement and lysed even though antibody itself may elute. (Modified from M. M. Mayer, The complement system. *Sci Am* November 1973; 229:54–66. With permission.)

Figure 2-2 (Continued)

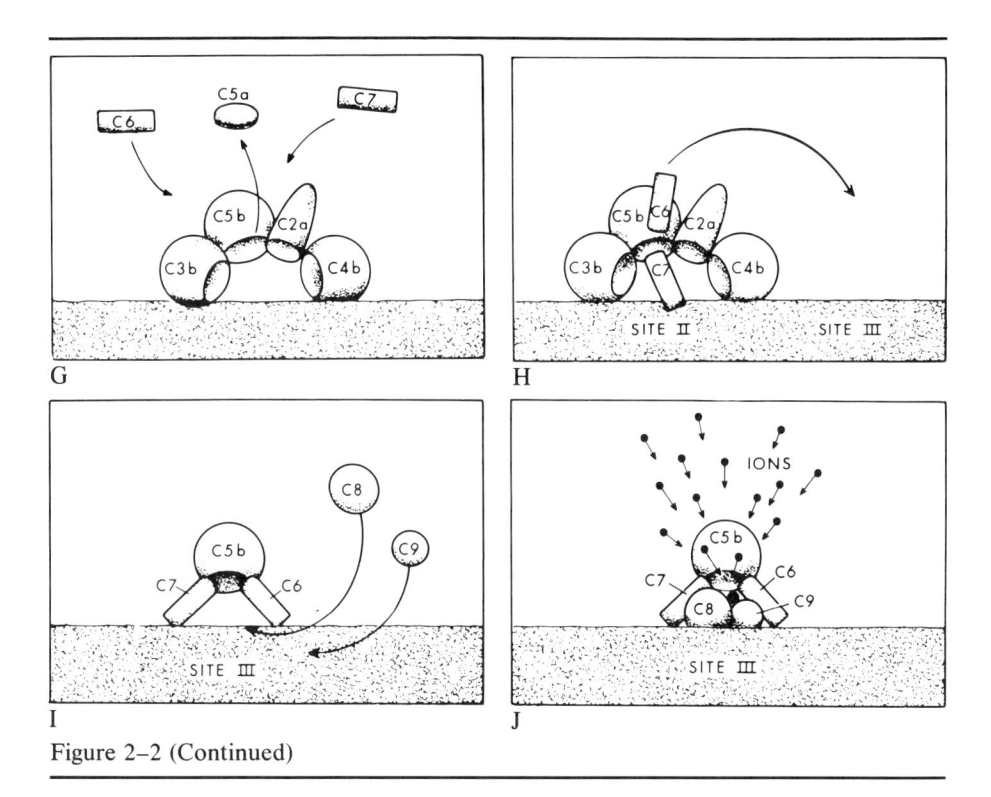

ity. It is more active than C3a on a molecular basis, but is released in smaller quantity. These polypeptides may be partly responsible for the signs and symptoms seen in some transfusion reactions. If the complement sequence proceeds to full activation, cell lysis ensues; however, the presence of specific serum inactivators can lead to a situation in which red cells may be coated (sensitized) with early complement components without proceeding to end-stage hemolysis.

The combination of C1 with cell-bound antibody initiates the sequence. Two adjacent complement-binding sites are required (see Fig. 2-2A). Since IgM is a pentamer, a single molecule bound to two adjacent antigen sites on the red cell membrane will be adequate for activation. For IgG, two *juxtaposed* antibody molecules are required. To bring this about, 800 to 1,000 molecules of IgG antibody must first react with the red cell, since most blood group antigen sites are evenly dispersed over the membrane. This explains why IgM is more efficient at complement activation than is IgG.

C1, the first component, is a macromolecule consisting of three fragments—C1q, C1r, and C1s—held together by calcium ions. In the presence of calcium-binding agents such as ethylenediaminetetraacetate (EDTA), this complex

Table 2-5. Some of the Complement Activation Polypeptides and Their Biologic Activities

---

C3a or anaphylatoxin
  Relaxes smooth muscles
  Contracts endothelial cells in postcapillary venules
  Causes skin erythema and edema
  Releases histamine from mast cells

C5a
  Causes chemotaxis of neutrophils
  Increases vascular permeability
  Activates neutrophils to release lysozyme
  Marginates leukocytes in the blood vessels
  Contracts smooth muscles
  Degranulates mast cells
  Induces leukotriene production, especially leukotriene-B4

C3b
  Mediates immune adherence and opsonization
  Releases immune complexes from leukocyte surface

---

tends to fall apart, and complement activation cannot occur. The C1 complex is heat-labile and will be destroyed by heating to 56°C, a procedure known as *inactivating* the serum.

The bound C1, particularly the C1s fragment, acts enzymatically on circulating C4 to produce two fragments: C4a and C4b. C4b has an active site and combines directly with the red cell membrane (see Fig. 2-2). Many C4 molecules can be activated and fixed by a single C1s complex. C2 is now acted upon by the cell-bound C4b in conjunction with C1s (see Fig. 2-2). Cell-bound C4b,2a has the potential for activating several thousand molecules of C3. The C4b,2a combination is itself unstable, and it must be regenerated constantly with new C2. When C2 is the complement component present in the lowest concentration, as it usually is, it becomes rate limiting, and complement-fixation tests measure C2 concentration.

The activation of C3 is the key step in the complement sequence. In vivo, C3 is the most important mediator of the immunologic defense mechanism. In vitro, C3 activation allows the continuation of the complement sequence to cell lysis. Once C3 has been attached to the red cell membrane, the original antigen-antibody complex is no longer required, and the antibody may dissociate from the cells, leaving them coated only with complement components. The action of C4b,2a on C3 splits C3 into two fragments: C3a, which is not bound to the red cell, and C3b, which is (see Fig. 2-2). A normal serum component, *C3b inactivator,* now splits the bound C3b into two new fragments, C3c and C3d; this step is not shown in Fig. 2–2. The C3c dissociates from the red cell, leaving cell-bound C3d. If C3b inactivator is present in excess, red cells will be coated with only C3d. If, on the other hand, the amount of C3b inactivator is limited or if the incubation time is short, both C3c and C3d will be present. The presence of C4b,2a,3b on the red cell activates the remaining complement components, C5 through C9, and thereby brings about membrane damage and cell lysis.

Complement in Blood Group Serology

Complement is essential in any blood group antibody test that depends on hemolysis of erythrocytes for an endpoint. For practical purposes, however, antibodies that lyse erythrocytes also agglutinate them. Immune anti-A and some antibodies of the Lewis, P, or Kidd systems may cause hemolysis in addition to agglutination, and complement may aid their identification and classification during blood group or crossmatching tests. In these cases, immune lysis of erythrocytes, with liberation of hemoglobin into the supernate, is a positive test that would appear as a negative one if plasma (which lacks Ca^{++} and Mg^{++}) or inactivated serum is used and hemolysis cannot occur. In blood bank work it is helpful to use fresh serums, and it is essential to look for any evidence of red cell destruction and record it as a positive test.

As was mentioned earlier, complement actually participates in, and becomes a part of, antigen-antibody complexes in some systems. When this occurs during the reaction of certain blood group antibodies with erythrocytes, the red cells become coated (or sensitized) with complement components as well as with specific antibody. The union between complement and the cell is, in some of these cases, more stable than that between antibody and erythrocyte. A test for complement coating may be, in those situations, a more reliable indicator of previous antigen-antibody reaction, and the antiglobulin test can be helpful, provided that the antiglobulin serum contains antibodies against C3 [24, 25].

There is a decline in complement activity as serum ages. This process is accelerated by heating, and a temperature of 56°C for 30 minutes will inactivate complement. On the other hand, serum frozen at −20 to −85°C retains complement activity for years. Thus, there is great variability, and Garratty has advised that normal serum be stored no longer than listed below if complement activity is important [26]:

Temperature	*Storage Time*
−55°C or lower	3 months
−20°C	2 months
4°C	2 weeks
Room temp.	36 hours
37°C	A few hours

Factors Affecting Blood Group Antigen-Antibody Reactions

Almost all blood grouping tests are antigen-antibody reactions with *hemagglutination* (agglutination of red cells) as the endpoint. Whether they are done in test tubes, in capillary tubes, on microscope slides, or by automated equipment, a positive result is almost always marked by the detectable erythrocyte clumps. As stated earlier, these agglutinates form in two stages. The reaction between the blood group antigen and antibody comes first and is followed by the actual formation of agglutinates. The many factors that affect the reactions will be discussed, with emphasis on those that are of practical importance in blood-grouping tests.

Red Blood Cell Antigens

Red cells for blood group determinations must be selected, preserved, and used in a manner that gives optimum reactivity during testing procedures. Erythrocytes that have been improperly selected or stored may give false-negative or false-positive reactions.

Dosage

Dosage is defined as a quantitative difference in reactivity between antigens controlled by genes in the homozygous and heterozygous state (see Chap. 3). The effects of dosage are not apparent with all blood group antigens, and even where dosage is present, selected serums may be needed to demonstrate it. Dosage can be shown by electron microscopy, by EIA, or by using radio-labeled antibodies [27–29]. It can also be seen, at times, when reaction strengths or titration endpoints are compared. In some cases, particularly with weak antiserums, the dosage phenomenon may cause negative reactions with cells having heterozygous expression of the antigen. Dosage is commonly seen with M, N, C, c, E, e, Jk^a, and Jk^b, but not with most other, blood group antigens.

Red Cell Genotype

The expression of certain blood group antigens, particularly in the ABO and Rh systems, is markedly influenced by *genotype*. The basis for this phenomenon is not fully understood, but the effect, seen in both homozygous and heterozygous states, is clearly different from that of dosage. Much information on effects of genotype has been obtained by the use of radiolabeled antibodies, which allow accurate quantitation of the amount of antibody bound by red blood cells of different genotypes. Decreased uptake of antibody goes hand in hand with weaker serologic reactions. For example, the Rh genotype of the person from whom the cells were drawn must be considered when results of serologic testing are evaluated. In particular, when antibody titers are compared, the titrations should be done using cells reflecting similar genotypes to minimize errors from this effect. In some cases, titration endpoints may vary three- or fourfold or more when cells reflecting different genotypes are used.

In the ABO system, there are well-recognized, weakly reacting variants of both A and B (see Chap. 3). In most families, these represent the gene products of additional alleles at the ABO locus and are inherited according to the expected mendelian pattern. In the Rh system, weak reactions may be due to inherited "weak" alleles or may be caused by a suppressor effect of one Rh factor on another (see Chap. 3).

Age of Cells

Many studies have shown that red cells stored in the commonly used blood bank anticoagulant solutions maintain their reactivity for at least 37 days, and even longer if the cells are stored in the solutions that are used for the commercial reagent red blood cells intended for typing and screening in the blood bank [30, 31]. Since the reactivity of the I,i blood group antigens is labile, fresh cells are needed for accurate results when testing for them.

Storage

Antigen reactivity is well preserved for years in red cells frozen and maintained at temperatures below $-30°C$. At refrigerator temperature, 2°C to 8°C, reactivity is adequate for at least 21 days, but higher temperatures may lead to rapid deterioration of antigen. All blood samples must be kept in the refrigerator unless they are actually being used. The habit of leaving cells on the laboratory bench for long periods of time should be discouraged.

Quantitative Aspects

Directions for most blood-grouping tests in tubes specify a 2 to 5 percent suspension of cells. Cell concentration is important, since more-concentrated cell suspensions generally cause weaker reactions (Table 2-6). A 2 percent suspension is best for tube tests, while a 35 to 45 percent suspension is needed for tests done on glass slides. Testing for hemolysins is similar, and weaker cell suspensions are desirable for the most sensitive reactions.

Blood Group Antibodies

In blood group work, variable reactions between antigens and antibodies frequently result from differences in antibodies themselves. Not all serums that contain antibodies of a single specificity—anti-A, for example—react in the same way. Even antibodies from one individual may react differently at different times so that reactions on one day may vary from those on another. Stored serums can lose some or all of their reactivity.

Table 2-6. Relation of Strength of Suspension of A_1 Cells to Titer of Anti-A Isoagglutinins in Group O Serum*

Strength of Suspension of A_1 Cells (%)	Dilution of Group O Serum					
	1:100	1:150	1:200	1:250	1:300	1:350
0.5	4+	4+	4+	4+	3+	2-3+
1.0	4+	4+	4+	4+	3+	1+
2.0	4+	4+	4+	2+	1+	0
3.0	4+	3+	1+	0	0	0
4.0	2-3+	1+	+vw**	0	0	0
5.0	1+	0	0	0	0	0

*From H. Chaplin, M. C. Wallace, E. Chang, *Am J Clin Pathol* 1956; 27:721. With permission.
**Very weak.

AVIDITY

The reaction between an antibody and its corresponding antigen is an equilibrium reaction:

Antigen + antibody ⇌ Antigen-antibody complex

In simple terms, this means that mixtures of antigens and antibodies always contain some of each reactant and some of the antigen-antibody complex. The speed with which a particular antibody combines with antigen and the stability of the resulting complex are measures of the *avidity* of the antibody. Avidity is not related to specificity, and antibodies of one specificity may have high or low avidity. In blood bank work, antibodies that have high avidity react quickly with appropriate red cells to give tight, easily seen agglutinates. Such antibodies are especially useful for the preparation of typing serums intended for slide testing.

In laboratory experiments, the first antibodies formed after the injection of an antigen are usually of low avidity and are highly specific for the antigen used. As the immunologic response progresses and as more antibodies are formed, particularly if booster injections are given, antibodies of higher avidity are produced. These antibodies often show a broadened specificity as well, in that they react with more and different epitopes than did the original antibodies. In clinical cases relating to blood group antibodies, an increase in avidity with continued immunization is known, but broadening of specificity is, as yet, unproven. The persistent positive direct antiglobulin test seen in some patients after a delayed hemolytic transfusion reaction may be an example of this phenomenon, but this is poorly understood [32, 33]. There is often a correlation between the titer (see under Titer, below) and the avidity of a given antibody, as shown by higher titer values in antibodies with greater avidity.

The terms *affinity* and *combining power* also describe the efficiency with which antibody combines with antigen, and these terms are used in immunology to describe such relationships, often using complex mathematical formulas.

Titer

As antibody-containing serums are diluted with increasing amounts of a nonreactive diluent, a point will be reached where the antibodies can no longer be detected by the test being used. This test for quantitation of antibodies is known as *titration,* and is discussed in Chapter 4.

Storage of Antibody-Containing Serums

Some antibody molecules, including many that are important in blood bank work, are labile and easily lose activity. Whenever possible, fresh serums should be used for all tests, and samples are best kept in the refrigerator when not in use, since higher temperatures generally lead to a rapid loss of antibody activity. Patient samples that need to be stored for a long time should be frozen, although antibody activity may be lost after freezing and thawing. Before use, serums that have been frozen must be *completely* thawed and thoroughly mixed. Repeated thawing and freezing will diminish reactivity in some cases. Antiserums that are prepared as reagents for commercial distribution often have added preservatives, and freezing of these may be deleterious. If they must be kept for unduly long periods, it is best to consult with the manufacturer about proper storage conditions.

Since it is well known that some antibodies lose their reactivity in transit, or even in the freezer, test results on fresh samples may not be the same as those obtained after storage or shipment of the serum. This is particularly troublesome when weak antibodies are mailed to reference laboratories for confirmation or further testing.

Reaction Conditions

The serologic properties of antigens and antibodies determine the conditions under which positive reactions are most easily detected. These are discussed in Chapter 4.

References

1. Hood LE, Weissman IL, Wood WB, Wilson JH. *Immunology,* 2nd ed. Redwood, CA: Benjamin/Cummings, 1984.
2. Roitt I. *Essential Immunology,* 5th ed. Oxford: Blackwell Sci, 1984.
3. Barrett JT. *Textbook of Immunology,* 4th ed. St. Louis: C. V. Mosby, 1983.

4. Tonegawa S. The molecules of the immune system. *Sci Am* 1985; October: 122–31.
5. Romans DG, Tilley CA, Crookston MC, et al. Conversion of incomplete antibodies to direct agglutinins by mild reduction: evidence for segmental flexibility within the Fc fragment of immunoglobulin G. *Proc Natl Acad Sci USA* 1977; 74:2531–5.
6. Burks AW, Sampson HA, Buckley RH. Anaphylactic reactions after gamma globulin administration in patients with hypogammaglobulinemia: detection of IgE antibodies to IgA. *N Engl J Med* 1986; 31:560–4.
7. Giblett E. A critique of the theoretical hazard of inter vs. intraracial transfusion. *Transfusion* 1961; 1:233–8.
8. Grobbelaar BG, Smart E. The incidence of isosensitization following blood transfusion. *Transfusion* 1967; 7:152–6.
9. Stern K, Davidsohn I, Masaitis L. Experimental studies on Rh immunization. *Am J Clin Pathol* 1956; 26:833–43.
10. Stern K, Goodman HS, Berger M. Experimental isoimmunization to hemoantigens in man. *J Immunol* 1961; 87:189–98.
11. Dowaliby JM II. Isoimmunization by transfusion. Yale University M.D. Thesis, 1967.
12. Myhre BA, Greenwalt JJ, Gajewski M. Incidence of irregular antibodies occurring in healthy donor sera. *Transfusion* 1965; 5:350–4.
13. Spielmann W, Seidl S. Prevalence of irregular red cell antibodies and their significance in blood transfusion and antenatal care. *Vox Sang* 1974; 26:551–9.
14. Lostumbo MM, Holland PV, Schmidt PJ. Isoimmunization after multiple transfusions. *N Engl J Med* 1966; 275:141–4.
15. Allen FH Jr, Warshaw AL. Blood group sensitization. A comparison of antigens K1 (Kell) and c (hr'). *Vox Sang* 1962; 7:222–7.
16. Steane EA. Red blood cell agglutination. In: Bell CA (ed). *Seminar on Antigen-Antibody Reactions Revisited*. Washington, DC: American Association of Blood Banks, 1982; 67–98.
17. Good W, Wood JE. The hydration effect of alkali metal and halide ions on the Rh-anti-Rh system. *Immunology* 1971; 20:37–42.
18. Voak D, Downie DM. The sensitivity of the Rh-anti-Rh system to ordered water of hydration. *Immunology* 1974; 26:673–5.
19. Van Oss CJ, Mohn JF, Cunningham RK. Influence of various physicochemical factors on hemagglutination. *Vox Sang* 1978; 34:351–61.
20. Yolken RH. ELISA: enzyme-linked immunosorbent assay. *Hosp Pract* 1978; 13:121–7.
21. Rosse WF. Correlation of in vivo and in vitro measurements of hemolysis in hemolytic anemia due to immune reactions. In: Brown EB (ed). *Progress in Hematology*, Vol. VIII. New York: Grune, 1973; 71–5.
22. Mayer MM. The complement system. *Sci Am* 1973; 229:54–66.
23. Tilley CA, Romano DG, Crookston MC. Localization of Chido and Rodgers determinants to the C4d fragment of human C4. *Nature* 1978; 276:713–5.
24. Howard JE, Winn LC, Gottlieb CE, et al. Clinical significance of the anti-complement component of antiglobulin antisera. *Transfusion* 1982; 22:269–72.
25. Wright MS, Issitt PD. Anticomplement and the indirect antiglobulin test. *Transfusion* 1979; 19:688–94.
26. Garratty G. The effects of storage and heparin on the activity of serum complement with particular reference to the detection of blood group antibodies. *Am J Clin Pathol* 1970; 54:531–8.
27. Hughes-Jones NC, Gardner B, Lincoln PJ. Observations of the number of available c, D, and E antigen sites on red cells. *Vox Sang* 1971; 21:210–6.

28. Caren LD, Bellavance R, Grumet FC. Demonstration of gene dosage effects on antigens in the Duffy, Ss, and Rh systems using an enzyme-linked immunosorbent assay. *Transfusion* 1982; 22:475–8.
29. Masouredis SP, Sudora E, Mahan L, Victoria EJ. Quantitative immunoferritin microscopy of Fy^a, Fy^b, Jk^a, U, and Di^b antigen site numbers on human red cells. *Blood* 1980; 56:969–77.
30. Snyder EL, Hezzey A, Joyner R, et al. Stability of red cell antigens during prolonged storage in citrate-phosphate-dextrose and a new preservative solution. *Transfusion* 1983; 23:165–6.
31. Myhre BA, Demaniew S, Nelson EJ. Preservation of red cell antigens during storage of blood with different anticoagulants. *Transfusion* 1984; 24:499–501.
32. Salama A, Mueller-Eckhardt C. Delayed hemolytic transfusion reactions; evidence for complement activation involving allogeneic and autologous red cells. *Transfusion* 1984; 24:188–93.
33. Chaplin H. The implication of red cell-bound complement in delayed hemolytic transfusion reactions. *Transfusion* 1984; 24:185–7 (editorial).

3. The Blood Groups

Serum from an animal of one species causes the red blood cells of another species to form clumps, as was first recognized in 1875 by Landois, who sacrificed an opportunity to become better known by not extending his research to tests between serum and cells from humans. It was left to Landsteiner to describe, in 1900, the first three phenotypes of the ABO blood group system, based on the observation that most human serums regularly contain agglutinating antibodies (agglutinins) directed at antigens on certain other human red blood cells.

Since then, some 400 blood group antigens have been recognized, and each new discovery came about through the detection of a specific antibody directed at the antigen in question. Most frequently, the antibody was found in a human serum, but in a few cases, it arose in animals after deliberate immunization. Sometimes the newly discovered antibody was, like the regularly occurring antibodies of the ABO blood group system, capable of agglutinating antigen-positive red blood cells suspended in physiologic saline. More often it was not a direct agglutinin, but required the application of an antiglobulin test (described in 1945) for its detection, which is one reason (but not the only one) that relatively few blood group antigens were discovered in the first half of the twentieth century. Table 3-1 lists the established blood group systems as defined by the International Society of Blood Transfusion (ISBT) Working Party on Terminology for Red Cell Surface Antigens [1].

Blood group antigens vary greatly in their *immunogenicity,* which is the term applied to describe the ability of an antigen to stimulate antibody production. The corresponding antibodies differ accordingly in the frequency with which they are encountered in routine blood bank work. Some are rare and are most often seen as components of antibody mixtures in serums from people who are prone to produce antibodies. Others occur in nearly all people exposed to the necessary immune stimuli, and still others arise without an obvious immunizing event and are usually seen as direct agglutinins, reactive in tests performed at or below room temperature against red cells suspended in saline.

Some Genetic Considerations

Blood group antigens are inherited characteristics, being transmitted from one generation to the next by means of genetic information contained in the nuclei of the two parental germ cells, which merge at the moment of fertilization to form the embryo. In humans, 23 pairs of *chromosomes* carry the necessary genetic material, one of each pair being derived from the male parent, the other from the female parent. The chromosomes of one pair, XX in females and XY in males, are called the sex chromosomes, since they determine the sex of the embryo. One red cell antigen, Xg^a, is coded for by genetic material borne on

Table 3–1. The Recognized Blood Group Systems

Name of System	No. of Antigens	Principal Antigens
ABO	5	A, B, AB, A_1, H
MN	30	M, N, S, s, U
P	2	P_1, P^k
Rh	46	D, C, E, c, e
Lutheran	15	Lu^a, Lu^b, Lu^{ab}
Kell	22	K, k, Kp^a, Kp^b, Js^a, Js^b
Lewis	2	Le^a, Le^b
Duffy	5	Fy^a, Fy^b, Fy3, Fy4, Fy5
Kidd	3	Jk^a, Jk^b, Jk^{ab}
Diego	2	Di^a, Di^b
Cartwright	2	Yt^a, Yt^b
Xg	1	Xg^a
Scianna	3	Sm (Sc1), Bu^a (Sc2), Sc3
Dombrock	2	Do^a, Do^b
Colton	3	Co^a, Co^b, Co^{ab}
Landsteiner/Wiener	3	LW^a, LW^{ab}, LW^b, (Ne^a)
Chido/Rogers	8	Ch1, Ch2, Ch3, Ch4, Ch5, Ch6, Rg1, Rg2

The systems and antigens listed in this table are as approved by the ISBT Working Party on Terminology for Red Cell Surface Antigens at a meeting held in Munich in 1984 [1], updated at a further meeting held in Sydney in 1986, the proceedings of which await publication at the time of writing.

the X chromosome. The genes for the others are carried on the *autosomes,* as the remaining 22 pairs of chromosomes are called.

GENETIC TERMINOLOGY

The basic units of heredity borne on the chromosomes are called *genes,* which are made up of coiled, ladder-like molecules of deoxyribonucleic acid (DNA). The mechanism of gene action is still not fully understood. Genetic information is coded into the complicated DNA molecule by the sequence in which four basic substances called *nucleotides* are arranged. This controls the sequence of amino acids in the protein synthesis governed by that particular DNA, which, in turn, determines the composition of the corresponding gene product. The gene that determines each specific characteristic occupies a predetermined position on the chromosome, called its *locus*. The same set of gene loci occurs on each of any pair of chromosomes, and in the same order; hence, there is a matched set of genes from each parent. The alternative genes that can occupy a given locus are called *alleles,* and in the course of normal inheritance, every person inherits one of any given pair from each parent. As an example, the three major alleles that determine the ABO groups are *A*, *B*, and *O*, of which any person may have only two. There are apparent exceptions to this rule, but for the moment, it is better to keep the discussion as simple as possible.

Zygosity, Genotypes, and Phenotypes

A person who inherits two identical genes at a given locus, such as *A* from each parent, is said to be *homozygous* for that gene. In this example, the *genotype* is *AA*, while the *phenotype*, which merely describes the observed reactions with available antiserums, is A. A person inheriting nonidentical alleles, such as *A* from one parent and *O* from the other, is *heterozygous* for both *A* and *O*, and the genotype is *AO*. Since there is no antiserum specific for the product of *O*, it is convenient to think of this gene as an *amorph*, although the mere fact that it does not yield a product we can demonstrate does not necessarily mean it *has* no product. In the absence of "anti-O," the phenotype in this case is still A, and the usual means by which we can determine whether a person of group A possesses two *A* genes rather than an *A* and an *O* is by being fortunate enough to obtain informative results in a family study. For example, the group A offspring of parents who are both group AB may be assumed to be *AA*, whereas if one parent were group O (indicating homozygosity for the amorph), the offspring would have to be *AO*. Similar considerations apply to *B*.

Not all family studies are as informative as in the examples chosen here, although in blood group systems where the principal alleles are simple pairs and antiserums exist that can recognize the products of both alleles, the genotype can be determined with greater precision. But it is always wise to make such interpretations with caution, as there may be rare variant alleles that can introduce error. A person whose phenotype in the Kell blood group system is K+k−, for example, is almost certainly of the genotype *KK*, whereas the phenotype K−k+ implies *kk*. This conclusion, however, does not consider the existence of a gene called K^0. Since this produces neither K nor k, a K+k− person could be KK^0. That possibility is remote, since K^0 is rare; but any K−k+ offspring of a KK^0 person has to be kK^0, which would seem to exclude parentage based on the more obvious interpretation of the child's genotype as *kk*.

By convention, italics are always used when denoting genes and genotypes, and phenotypes are rendered in ordinary roman type. By another convention, antigen designations using subscript characters become superscript in describing the corresponding genes, while those using superscript characters retain the superscript. Conventions do not have to make sense; they exist merely to facilitate communication and understanding.

In the case of characteristics determined by genes borne on the X chromosome, only females can be homozygous or heterozygous. Males, who owe their sex to the Y chromosome they inherited from their father, and who can therefore possess only one X chromosome, have room for only one allele of a given pair of X-borne alleles and are described as being *hemizygous* for any X-borne gene of which the product can be demonstrated to be present. Thus, while an Xg(a+) woman may be homozygous or heterozygous for Xg^a, an Xg(a+) man can only be hemizygous.

Dominance and Recessiveness

Blood group genes are almost all considered to be *codominant,* which is to say that the product of each allele is detectable whether the person concerned is homozygous or heterozygous for the gene in question. Some antigens show an effect called *dosage,* however, meaning that the strength of their reactivity is perceptibly stronger in the homozygote than in the heterozygote.

In genetics, the term *recessive* is normally applied when a characteristic is detectable only when present as a product of a gene inherited from both parents. In blood grouping work, however, it is commonly used more loosely in describing the situation in which either a gene is considered to be an amorph (because no antibody exists that can detect its product) or, alternatively, the gene product is merely assumed to be present in double dose because antigens known to be products of its alleles have not been detected. An example is group O in the ABO system, wherein homozygosity for *O* is assumed because products of *A* and *B* are demonstrably absent. At this point, it is useful to ponder the distinction between a gene product tangibly detectable and one assumed to be present. If there existed an antibody that was able to agglutinate only group O cells because they are representative of homozygosity for *O,* then we could regard *O* as being truly recessive. As things are, we do not know with certainty that group O people actually *are* homozygous for a single amorphic gene called *O*. There could just as easily be more than one *not-A-and-not-B* gene, any of which may determine an undetectable product.

Linkage and Synteny

In germ cell division (*meiosis*), when the cells containing only 23 single chromosomes are created, it is a matter of pure chance which of each pair of homologous chromosomes passes to each daughter germ cell. Moreover, each chromosome pair behaves independently of the other 22, so that the genes carried on each are inherited independently of all others. Genetic material is frequently exchanged between the chromosomes of each pair during meiosis, which results in the failure of genes on the same chromosome to be inherited together. This phenomenon, known as *crossing over,* occurs with a frequency that is dependent on the distance separating the loci concerned. Understandably, when genes occupy adjacent loci there is less likelihood of a crossover than when they occupy loci that are more distant from one another. When genes are so close that crossing over is rarely observed, the loci concerned are said to be *linked,* as in the case of the locus for *M* and *N* and that for *S* and *s* in the MNSs system. Linkage between these two loci was apparent through the observation, in 1947, that the newly recognized S antigen occurred more commonly with M than with N, an example of a state called *linkage disequilibrium.*

Sometimes blood group genes, although on the same chromosome, do not show measurable linkage. This is the case with the genes of the Rh and Duffy blood group systems, which are both controlled from loci on chromosome 1, the largest of the autosomes. Since linkage cannot be demonstrated between them, the loci concerned must be separated by a distance that enables them to *segregate independently* as often as not. The term used to describe the relationship between genes that are on the same chromosome but are not linked is *synteny.*

Related and Unrelated Antigens

Some blood group antigens have a genetic relationship with one another, and have accordingly been classified into blood group *systems*. The demonstration of a genetic relationship usually starts with evidence that two antigens are the product of an allelic pair of genes, as in the case of K and k of the Kell system. Blood group systems may expand in two ways. A newly recognized characteristic may prove to be the product of another allele at the original locus, or linkage may be confirmed between an established locus and that of some other gene or allelic pair. These relationships are most often confirmed through mathematical analysis, but an allelic relationship between two gene products may be suspected if, for example, the red cells of people who make the antibody directed at one are invariably positive for the other. Such a relationship is particularly convincing if family members who *must* possess any gene for which the propositus is homozygous (namely, parents or offspring, who are called *obligate heterozygotes*) are all positive for the relevant antigen.

Antigens of High and Low Frequency

Some antigens occur with a very high frequency while others are encountered very uncommonly, occasionally only in a single family. Those of high frequency are called *public antigens,* and those of low incidence have been referred to as *private antigens*. People whose red cells are negative for a high-frequency antigen may develop the corresponding antibody. Once that occurs, the provision of compatible blood for transfusion may require recourse to a registry of known rare donors.

The lack of a high-frequency antigen may imply homozygosity for a rare allele, the product of which—assuming it *has* a detectable product—could be a low-frequency characteristic; hence, there is a possibility that cells of such a phenotype will be found to possess a low-frequency antigen. Relatively few such *reciprocally related* pairs of antigens have been recognized, as it happens, but the investigation of an antibody appearing to be directed at a newly recognized high-frequency antigen would normally include testing of the antibody-maker's red cells for as many low-frequency factors as possible.

Polymorphism and Anthropology
Many of the blood group antigens that are important in blood transfusion are the products of allelic pairs, and if each of a given pair occurs with a significant frequency in any human population group, then the relevant antigens are examples of *polymorphism* in that population. Sometimes, these readily demonstrable inherited characteristics show markedly different frequencies in different populations. This is of interest in the field of anthropology, since a study of the frequencies in given populations may yield evidence about origins and early migration routes. As an example, the observed incidence of the Di^a (Diego) antigen among American Indians suggests an origin in Asia.

Some Additional Useful Genetic Terms
When linked genes are traveling together, as indicated by the fact that their products are always inherited together, they are said to be in *cis*. In the reverse situation, where the gene products are always passed on separately, the genes are in *trans*. To illustrate the point, the genotype of a person of the MNSs phenotype M + N + S + s + is more likely to be *MS/Ns* than *Ms/NS* because *S* travels more commonly with *M* than with *N*. Without a family study, however, it is impossible to know, in any given case, which genotype is actually correct. If such a study is informative, we can establish whether *S* is being inherited along with *M* or with *N*. If the former, then *M* and *S* are in *cis,* as are *N* and *s,* while *M* and *s* (and *N* and *S*) are in *trans*.

In any family study, the person possessing the characteristic that attracted our interest to the family in the first place is called the *propositus* if he happens to be male, the *proposita* if female. When it is necessary to use the plural, the appropriate word is supposedly *propositi,* even if the people concerned are all female, although *propositae* would be grammatically more correct in the latter context. The complexities associated with Latin endings can easily be shirked, however, by the simple ruse of adopting the term *proband,* which means the same as propositus and can be applied indiscriminately and unselfconsciously to either sex.

The Significance and Purpose of Blood Groups
The purpose for which blood groups exist has so far eluded explanation. Their biologic function is unknown. Some of them appear to be integral components of the red cell envelope, as cells lacking certain normal antigens possess membrane defects.

The ABO System

By studying the patterns of agglutination that occur when serum and red blood cells from different human bloods are mixed together, Landsteiner* recognized three distinct human blood groups. The limited number of bloods included in the study did not include the group we know today as AB, which it was left to von Decastello and Sturli,* students of Landsteiner, to describe in 1902, 2 years after Landsteiner's original report.

The essence of the discovery was that blood lacking A from the red cells invariably contains the agglutinin anti-A in the serum, and that lacking B invariably contains anti-B. This feature is called *Landsteiner's Law*. This is illustrated in Table 3–2, along with the observed frequencies of the four major groups in the U.S. population.

It was not at first realized that the blood groups A and B were inherited characteristics. In 1908, Epstein and Ottenberg* suggested that this may be the case, but offered no concrete evidence to support the idea. The first clear indication that the blood groups were under genetic control came in 1910 from von Dungern and Hirszfeld,* who later described the subgroups of A; but it was 1924 before a German mathematician named Bernstein* postulated the existence of three alleles, thereby presenting the manner in which the ABO blood groups are inherited as we understand it today.

The antigens A and B, which are not confined to the red cells but are also tissue antigens, are produced by a pair of alleles, *A* and *B*. A third gene, *O*, is considered to be an amorph because there is no antibody directed at any product it may have; hence, the O phenotype is taken to indicate homozygosity for *O*, since both A and B are absent, while the phenotype AB indicates the genotype *AB*. The genotype of persons belonging to groups A and B cannot be determined without a family study, as the lack of anti-O means that the phenotype is the same whether the genotype is *AA* or *AO*. This is also the case for *BB* or *BO*.

Some Pertinent Biochemistry

A detailed discussion of the ABO phenotypes must consider some biochemical aspects, if only at a superficial level, as a means of recognizing the relationships between the antigens and understanding why certain of the antibodies react in the way they do.

The antigens of the ABO system, being carbohydrates, cannot themselves be direct gene products. Moreover, the presence of A and B on the red cells, as

---

*The original reports were published in German; however, English translations of these papers have been published by the Blood Transfusion Division, U.S. Army: Camp FR Jr, Ellis FR, Conte NF. *Selected Contributions to the Literature of Blood Groups and Immunology.* (In 4 volumes.) Fort Knox, KY: U.S. Army Medical Research Laboratory, 1963–73.

Table 3-2. The ABO Blood Groups

Red Cell Reactions		Serum Reactions		Blood Group	Frequency (%)*	
Anti-A	Anti-B	A Cells	B Cells		Whites	Blacks
+	0	0	+	A	40	26
0	+	+	0	B	12	20
0	0	+	+	O	44	50
+	+	0	0	AB	4	4

*U.S. combined figures from Mourant et al. [2] and Chicago blood donors [3]; 85,240 white and 17,797 black.

well as on platelets, some leukocytes, and other tissue cells, depends on the product of another gene, *H*, which is inherited independently of the *ABO* locus. The genes *A* and *B*, and also *H*, code for specific enzymes called *glycosyltransferases*, which add sugars to a precursor substance on the red cells. The product of the *H* gene, L-fucosyltransferase, first attaches L-fucose to the precursor chain, making a new substance that is recognizable as the H antigen. If the *A* gene is also present, its product, using the newly added L-fucose as the substrate, adds a further sugar, *N*-acetylgalactosamine (GalNAc). This is responsible for A antigen specificity, while *B*, which codes for D-galactosyltransferase, causes the B-specific immunodominant sugar, D-galactose (Gal), to be added. In the absence of the genes for both A and B, L-fucose remains the terminal sugar, giving rise to the strong reactivity of group O cells with anti-H reagents.

Some residual H is detectable in some phenotypes, the least being when both A^1 and *B* genes are present, which accounts for the negative reactivity of A_1B cells with anti-H. Group A_1B cells are not quite devoid of H antigen, but what H remains requires anti-H of exceptional potency to show reactivity. Red cells of the A_1 phenotype are nonreactive with most examples of anti-H, too, although trace reactions may occur due to small amounts of residual H. B cells are usually agglutinated to some degree with anti-H, as the transferase produced by *B* converts fewer L-fucose receptors than that produced by *A*.

A, B, AND H AS SOLUBLE SUBSTANCES IN TISSUE SECRETIONS

Besides being present as surface antigens in the form of glycolipids on the red blood cells, A, B, and/or H may also be present in soluble form as glycoproteins in certain tissue secretions. The ability to secrete soluble ABH substance is controlled by a gene *Se*, which is inherited independently of *A*, *B*, and *H*. People who are either homozygous or heterozygous for *Se* are *secretors*, and have in certain of their body fluids soluble substance(s) corresponding to the ABH present on their red blood cells. Homozygosity for *se*, the allele of the secretor gene, occurs in approximately 22 percent of the population, who are therefore *nonsecretors*. Sometimes, the testing of body fluid (usually saliva) for soluble antigens provides information that aids in the determination of ABO blood group status in someone whose antigens are poorly expressed on the red cells, or in whom equivocal reactions have been obtained in normal ABO blood grouping tests.

THE SUBGROUPS OF A

The subdivision of group A into A_1 and A_2, and of group AB into A_1B and A_2B, was founded on the notion that the antibody in group B serum comprises two components. One is called anti-A and is capable of reacting with *all* group A and AB cells, the other is called anti-A_1 and reacts only with group A_1 and group A_1B cells. Thus, by absorbing group B serum with A_2 cells, the "anti-A" component may be removed, leaving behind the antibody that reacts only with cells of the A_1 and A_1B subgroups. Such *absorbed anti-A* reagents were used to distinguish between the A subgroups for many years before Bird identified a more consistently reliable anti-A_1 agglutinin (*lectin**) in an extract from the seeds of a plant called *Dolichos biflorus* [4], nowadays the source of almost all anti-A_1 reagents.

It is convenient to accept the conventional belief that there are two clearly separable antibody specificities in group B serum, and that the distinction between A_1 and A_2 is straightforward. This is an oversimplification. The existence of cells that give variable reactions with anti-A_1 reagents necessitates the recognition of a third subgroup, which has been called *A-intermediate*, sometimes written A_{int}, but that classification is not a straightforward one to make, either, as differences in the potency of anti-A_1 reagents used for subgrouping commonly cause difficulty in determining the demarcation point between A_1 and A_{int} and that between A_{int} and A_2.

The number of receptors varies with the phenotype. Group A_1B cells, for instance, possess more A receptors than A_2 cells and fewer than A_1 cells. There is also measurable variation in the number of receptors within subgroups. Hence, the priorities applied in determining the optimal final dilution of each lot of anti-A_1 lectin, which are influenced also by the strength of A antigen on the indicator cells available at the time of manufacture, may give rise to significant differences in the classification of some individual bloods by different reagents.

To put the situation in proper perspective, it is a matter of no great significance that a minority of group A bloods may be classified as A_1 on some occasions, as A_{int} on others, and as A_2 on others. The truth is that nobody really knows to which subgroup these cells properly belong, and nobody who gives it rational thought really cares. We must shake off the obsession to assign a

---

*In blood group serology, the term *lectin* usually means a plant protein that agglutinates red blood cells and may show blood group specificity.

distinct and unequivocal classification to every single blood specimen, and school ourselves not to feel threatened if someone else arrives at a different conclusion from ours. It is clear that, at a phenotypic level at least, the distinction between A_1 and A_2 is largely quantitative. This proposition is supported by the fact that absorption with A_2 red cells eventually removes all antibody reactivity from group B serum, even though it supposedly contains a component (anti-A_1) that does not agglutinate A_2 cells.

On most occasions, group A_2 red cells are reactive with anti-H because the transferase produced by the A^2 gene converts fewer L-fucose sites to A than that produced by A^1. Sometimes, however, the A_2 and A_2B phenotypes may reflect a deficiency of H, rather than A as a product of A^2. Voak and associates have reported that 1 in 169 of A_2s and as many as 1 in 13 of A_2Bs are of this origin, where the A^1 gene, though present, is unable to produce enough A sites to give rise to the A_1 phenotype because there are too few L-fucose receptors for its transferase to convert [5]. This demonstrates the fallibility of A subgrouping as an aid to the resolution of disputed parentage problems.

Approximately one-fifth of group A bloods belongs to the A_2 subgroup. A similar proportion of ABs are A_2B. Sometimes, anti-A_1 occurs as an unexpected alloantibody in persons whose A antigen is not A_1. Anti-A_1 may be present in some 2 percent of group A_2 and about 26 percent of A_2B bloods, but is usually an agglutinating antibody that may not be detected in the antibody detection procedure if testing at room temperature is not a part of that routine. On the rare occasions that an example of anti-A_1 appears to be clinically significant, compatible blood is easily selected by testing donors of the appropriate group (A or AB) with an anti-A_1 reagent. Providing the recipient's antibody has been correctly identified, bloods found to be nonreactive with a *Dolichos biflorus* lectin that is suitable for A subgrouping should prove to be compatible.

Just as the serum of a group A_2 (or an A_2B) person may contain anti-A_1, so may the serum of someone whose red cells possess very little H contain anti-H. Again, this is seldom detectable above room temperature, and may not be detected at all by current antibody-detection methods.

Weaker Subgroups of A

Although there are subgroups representative of even weaker expression of A than the A_1 and A_2 subgroups, their precise classification is made difficult by the expected heterogeneity within categories, as is equally true for A_1 and A_2. The matter is further complicated because reports by separate authors have sometimes concerned the same entity under different names. Most of the subgroups characterized by the weaker grades of reactivity are rare. They are only of academic interest. If a weak subgroup is encountered, it is usually no more important that it be precisely classified than was the case for A_1 and A_2. If unexpected antibodies active at 37°C are detected and a transfusion is needed,

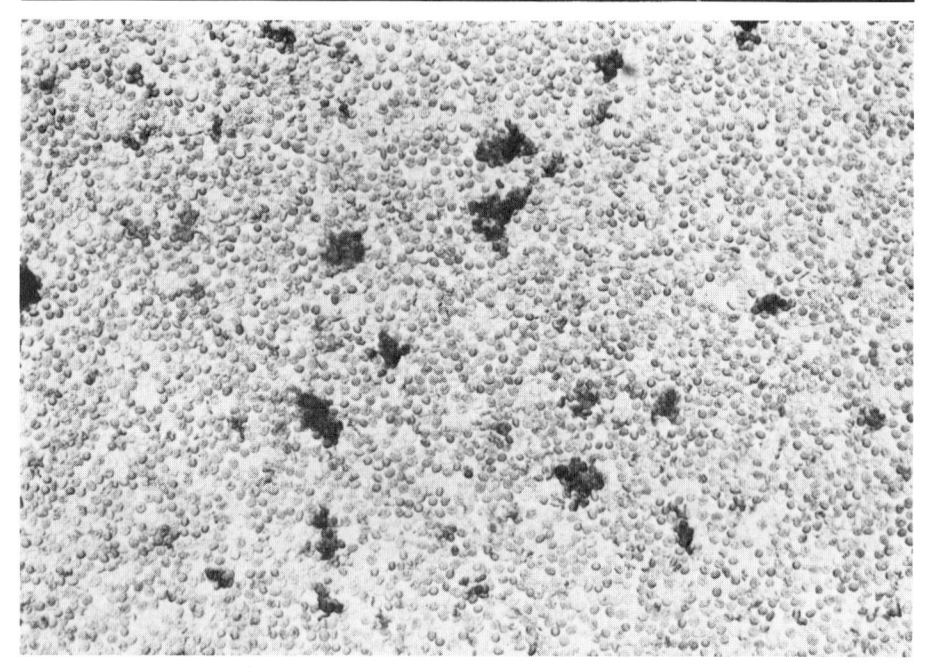

Figure 3-1
Photomicrograph showing mixed-field agglutination. Note that agglutinates stand out against a background of unagglutinated red cells.

donor blood is most appropriately selected on the basis of common sense and crossmatch compatibility.

A_3 red cells are generally recognized by *mixed-field* agglutination when tested with anti-A. The appearance of large and definite agglutinates against a background of unagglutinated cells is characteristic, and anti-A_1 may be detectable in the serum. Even lower on the scale of antigen strength is A_x, of which most examples do not react convincingly with anti-A serums at all, but are agglutinated by group O serum, i.e., anti-A,B. When grouping recipients, it is unnecessary to carry out the additional test with anti-A,B. The recognition of A_x is considered of more importance in donors because of a reported case, in 1959, of a transfusion reaction resulting from the administration of a unit of A_x donor blood to a group O recipient [6]. The reaction between anti-A,B and A_x cells is invariably weak, however, and may not be detected if the test is interpreted after immediate centrifugation and the tube is then discarded.

A licensed commercial anti-A reagent made from a blend of murine monoclonal antibodies became available in 1986. It gives spectacularly strong reactions with most A_x red cells, even in an immediate-spin test. Such impressive reactivity enables A_x cells to be detected without using anti-A,B serum. An accompanying disadvantage, however, is that the reagent occasionally appears to recognize the variable amount of A-specific sugar that has been reported to be present on group B red cells [7]. This leads to the possibility of falsely interpreting the ABO group of such samples to be $A_{subgroup}B$. This limitation can be overcome by retesting the cells of apparent group AB recipients with a conventional (polyclonal) anti-A reagent.

OTHER SUBGROUPS

Subgroups of B exist that correspond more or less to some of the subgroups of A, but are rarer. These feature variable expression of B antigen and, in some cases, the presence of a form of anti-B in the serum.

The *acquired B* phenotype, which may be mistaken for a subgroup, is more likely than most of the inherited B variants to be encountered in a hospital blood transfusion service. It is encountered most often in patients suffering from colorectal carcinoma or intestinal obstruction, and may be transient.

Acquired B resembles group AB, except that a form of anti-B is ordinarily present in the plasma, which will make the red cells of group AB donors incompatible. Testing the saliva for A and B substance may be an aid to resolving the problem. If the patient is a secretor, A substance will be present in the saliva, whereas B substance will not.

Two explanations have been offered for the acquired B phenomenon. One is that increased permeability of the intestinal wall enables a bacterial polysaccharide from *Escherichia coli*$_{86}$ to be adsorbed to the red cells; the other is that a bacterial enzyme converts the A-specific sugar to one specific for B. The latter mechanism would explain why acquired B is only seen in group A bloods.

THE BOMBAY PHENOTYPE (O_h)

An atypical ABO phenotype that is of definite clinical significance, although so rare that the average blood bank worker will never see it, is that known as *Bombay,* referring to the region of India in which it was first encountered [8]. This phenotype still occurs predominantly in people from the Indian subcontinent, but is not confined to them. In routine forward/reverse ABO grouping, it seems to be group O, since neither A nor B are present, and both anti-A and anti-B are found in the serum. Antibody screening will show that all group O cells are incompatible. This is due to the presence of anti-H, which may be as strong as the expected antibodies of the ABO system. Testing the cells with an anti-H reagent, such as a lectin made from an extract of *Ulex europaeus* seeds, will show that H, like A and B, is absent.

The Bombay type results from being homozygous for the gene *h,* an allele of *H* that does not produce the glycosyltransferase needed to place L-fucose on the cells (see p. 87). This accounts for the fact that the cells are nonreactive with anti-H, since they are devoid of H antigen. They cannot possess A or B

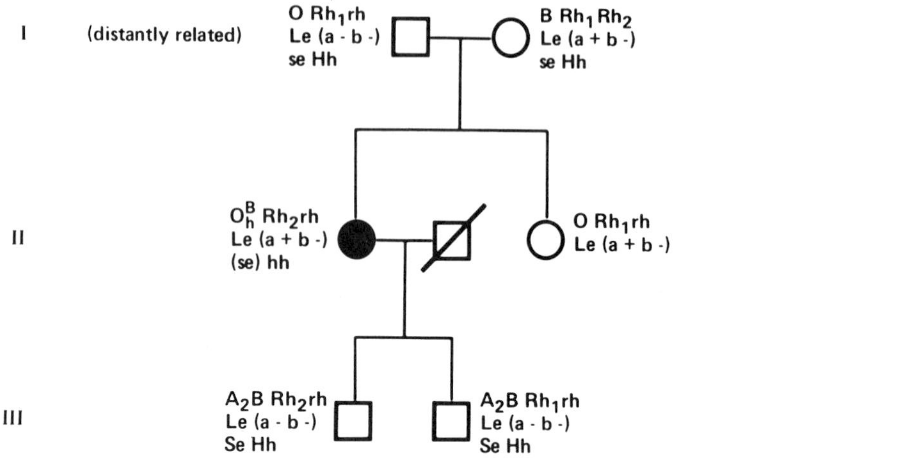

Figure 3-2
Pedigree of a family illustrating the inheritance of the O_h^B (Bombay) phenotype. Note that the proposita has passed a B gene to both of her sons, having inherited it from her mother. The lack of the H gene, however, has caused the expression of B in her own red cells to be suppressed. See text for explanation. (From M. Bergren and C. Moss, unpublished observations. This case was kindly referred to us by Mrs. Carol Moss, Riverview Hospital, Noblesville, IN.)

either, because the lack of the L-fucose receptor means that the immunodominant sugars associated with A and B cannot be added, even if the appropriate glycosyltransferases are present. The notation O_h is used for this phenotype, with a superscript added to denote the true genetic blood group of the person, if this is known from the results of a family study; for example, O_h^A or O_h^B. Figure 3-2 illustrates the mode of inheritance in a family in which the proband was O_h^B and was recognized when all group O blood was found to be incompatible.

People who belong to the O_h phenotype are nonsecretors of A, B, and H, as the H gene is required, along with Se, for the soluble substances to be present in the secretions. The presence of anti-H in the serums of Bombay bloods is merely an extension of Landsteiner's law: since H is absent from the cells, anti-H is regularly present in the serum. This may vary in potency, just as there is variation in the strength of anti-A and anti-B, but the anti-H has the same significance as any other ABO incompatibility. The only blood suitable for transfusion will be that of a donor who is also O_h.

Para-Bombay

A few bloods resembling O_h are found on closer study to belong to a similar phenotype having a different genetic origin, though the practical significance is the same. The red cells may show weak reactions with anti-A and/or anti-B, but

H is still absent from the red cells and anti-H is consequently present in the serum. The effect is believed to be caused by a modifying gene that allows H to be present in the secretions but not on the red cells.

The Rh System

The antigens of the Rh blood group system were not the next to be recognized after A and B, but the clinical importance of the antigen now known as D justifies a departure from chronological sequence. In 1940, Landsteiner and Wiener reported a hitherto unrecognized human blood group characteristic they called the *Rh factor,* which had been recognized by agglutinating antiserums produced in guinea pigs and rabbits immunized with the red cells of rhesus monkeys [9]. The significance of this discovery became clear when Wiener and Peters noted that human antibodies associated with three cases of hemolytic transfusion reaction appeared to be of the same specificity [10]. Such a case, in which a transfusion reaction occurred in a woman who had just given birth to a stillborn fetus and received a transfusion of her husband's blood, had been reported in 1939 by Levine and Stetson [11]. Since the red cells of the woman's husband were positive for the antigen in question, it was speculated at the time that the antibody had been produced in response to an antigen inherited by the fetus from the father. The relationship between Rh blood group incompatibility and the disease known as *erythroblastosis fetalis,* now more often called hemolytic disease of the newborn, was established by Levine and his associates in 1941 [12].

Subsequent events proved that the antigen recognized by the original animal anti-rhesus of Landsteiner and Wiener was not, after all, identical to the clinically important human antigen that had been called Rh_0, or D. By this time the Rh terminology had become firmly established, so at Levine's suggestion, the name LW was adopted for the original rhesus antigen, using the initials to honor Landsteiner and Wiener. Human examples of anti-LW have been found in people who were either D-positive or D-negative but LW-negative. Family studies showed that the LW antigen is inherited independently of Rh. It bears only a phenotypic relationship to the Rh system, in that adult D-positive cells are more strongly LW-positive than adult D-negative cells. The lack of linkage with Rh eventually led to LW being renamed and transferred to its own system, which is discussed on page 105.

As investigators in the early 1940s became increasingly aware of the need to test for antibodies to the Rh factor, particularly in obstetric practice, new specificities began to be recognized. These, though not the same as the original Rh antibody, bore an unmistakable relationship to it.

GENETICS AND TERMINOLOGY

Nomenclature in the Rh system was for many years the subject of vigorous and sometimes acrimonious debate between opposing schools of thought, one sup-

Table 3–3. The Principal Rh Phenotypes in the Different Systems of Notation

Reaction with Anti-					Phenotype			
D	C	E	c	e	Rh-Hr	CDE	Shorthand	Numerical
+	+	0	+	+	Rh_1rh	DCce	R_1r	Rh: 1, 2, −3, 4, 5
+	+	0	0	+	Rh_1Rh_1	DCe	R_1R_1	Rh: 1, 2, −3, −4, 5
+	0	+	+	+	Rh_2rh	DcEe	R_2r	Rh: 1, −2, 3, 4, 5
+	0	+	+	0	Rh_2Rh_2	DcE	R_2R_2	Rh: 1, −2, 3, 4, −5
+	+	+	+	+	Rh_z	DCcEe	R_1R_2	Rh: 1, 2, 3, 4, 5
+	0	0	+	+	Rh_0	Dce	R_0r	Rh: 1, −2, −3, 4, 5
0	0	0	+	+	rh	dce	rr	Rh: −1, −2, −3, 4, 5
0	+	0	+	+	rh'rh	dCce	r'r	Rh: −1, 2, −3, 4, 5
0	0	+	+	+	rh"rh	dcEe	r"r	Rh: −1, −2, 3, 4, 5
0	+	+	+	+	rh_yrh	dCcEe	r_yr	Rh: −1, 2, 3, 4, 5

porting the Rh-Hr system of Wiener, the other favoring notations based on the CDE concept of Fisher and Race. A third system devised by Rosenfield and associates is also employed in the literature, and in a few cases, may be the only one by which an antigen possesses a name [13]. This numerical method of notation was intended mainly as a method of conveying serological information without making genetic presumptions. Table 3–3 shows the principal Rh phenotypes expressed in the different systems of nomenclature.

The Reactivity of Rh Antibodies

Anti-D is almost always an immune antibody, even when it directly agglutinates red cells suspended in saline, which is usually a transient phenomenon. Enzyme techniques, or the use of macromolecular additives in various ways, may cause D-positive red cells to be agglutinated by anti-D. Otherwise, the antiglobulin test is the most reliable test procedure for detecting it. These remarks apply equally to immune examples of the other Rh specificities, but in some cases, the antibodies may have arisen in the serum without a red-cell–induced stimulus and may exist wholly or predominantly in the form of IgM. A few examples of anti-E, sometimes anti-c, and occasionally other Rh antibodies, may show better reactivity as direct agglutinins than at the antiglobulin phase of the test.

Variable and Variant Expression of D

The first indication that the D antigen can show variable reactivity was recognized by Stratton, who introduced the term D^u to describe the D antigen on cells that reacted with some anti-D serums and not others [14]. Stratton's study was carried out only with anti-D serums that were able to agglutinate saline-suspended D-positive cells, so the variability he observed and reported was not identical with the manifestations of diminished D expression most often referred to by the collective name D^u at the present time. The form of "D^u" recognized by Stratton came later to be called *high-grade* D^u, and the term *low-grade* D^u was adopted for a form of D recognized only by an indirect antiglobulin test with suitable anti-D serums. These classifications oversimplify the varying grades of D antigen expression, which at the other end of the scale, may include examples of stronger-than-normal reactivity [15, 16].

High-grade D^u can be due to the interaction of a *dCe* gene in *trans*, as originally observed and reported by Ceppelini and his co-workers, who noted the phenomenon in cells representative of the genotype *DCe/dCe* [17]. It may also occur in *Dce/dCe;* and somewhat similar weakened expression of D may accompany the presence of the Rh40 (Targett) antigen, a low-frequency characteristic belonging to the Rh system [18].

High-grade D^u, which many investigators prefer to classify with normal D, is usually recognized when a blood sample shows no reaction with a low-protein anti-D serum (or sometimes feeble agglutination), but a high-protein anti-D is strongly reactive. The difference in reactivity is due to the fact that a low-protein test system is inherently less sensitive than a high-protein one, rather than a difference in antibody potency.

Even within the classification of low-grade D^u, perceptible variation in antigen strength may be observed. In some cases, this is probably attributable to the gene interaction effect superimposed on a D antigen already so weakly expressed as to be called D^u. The genotype *dCe/D^uce* may be expected to lead to a more weakly expressed form of D^u than *D^uCe/dce,* for instance. Still weaker is the difficult-to-detect form of D that accompanies the Rh33 antigen [19], which may require an anti-D reagent of exceptional potency for its detection, even by the indirect antiglobulin test [20]. As in the interpretation of A subgrouping tests, the variable reactions seen in typing for D are most often due to differences in the properties of reagents used, or to subtle variations of technique. They are unavoidable and unimportant.

To the extent that the D^u phenotype is indicative of *quantitative* variability in the expression of D, its significance is minimal. Occasionally, however, the aberrant reactivity may be attributable to *qualitative* differences in the antigen, as suggested by the observation that persons of the D^u phenotype may, on occasion, produce a form of anti-D. Argall, Ball, and Trentelman are the investigators most often credited with being the first to make this observation in 1953 [21], but Shapiro had mentioned such a case some 2 years previously, in a passing aside in a paper reporting the results of a population study, which may explain why his priority has been overlooked [22]. Other cases were soon recognized, and in some, it was persons whose cells possessed an apparently normal strength of D that were observed to have produced anti-D. One explanation is that D is a mosaic comprising a number of individual components, one or more of which may be missing from some D-positive red cells [23, 24]. The absence of part of the D antigen enables the person concerned to make an antibody that would appear identical in specificity to anti-D, except that it would not be reactive with that person's own cells, nor with others of the same deviant D-positive phenotype.

Tippett and Sanger devised a system of classification based on six categories, which has since been extended to include further subdivisions of the original categories [25, 26]. These subdivisions of D have comparatively little importance from a clinical standpoint, although it is clear that persons possessing some variant kinds of D antigen can make anti-D if exposed to red cells having a normal D antigen. To keep matters in perspective, however, this kind of immune response is rarer than anti-E or anti-c in people lacking the relevant antigen and exposed to the necessary immune stimulus.

DETERMINATION OF GENOTYPE

When the serum of a pregnant patient contains an Rh antibody, it is useful, for prognostic purposes, to know whether the infant's father is homozygous or heterozygous for the gene that determines the corresponding antigen. If he is homozygous, all his offspring will possess the antigen, whereas if he is heterozygous, only half of them will have antigen-positive cells.

In the Rh system, each antigen may originate from several genes, so it is possible for a person to be heterozygous in the sense of having inherited a different Rh gene from each parent, yet be homozygous for D in the sense of possessing two genes that code for the production of D. This is equally true of the other Rh antigens, but in the case of C and c, and of E and e, the antiserums needed to identify the antigens resulting from allelic pairs of genes are available. Thus, zygosity for C/c and E/e can be determined with reasonable confidence. In the case of D, however, the lack of an antiserum to detect the product of d, if any, means that, unless a family study is possible and yields informative results, the genotype must be deduced on probability, based on the frequency with which the different Rh genes occur. For example, the phenotype D + C + E − c − e + (DCe) can derive from either of two genotypes, *DCe/DCe* or *DCe/dCe,* the former representing homozygosity for *D,* the latter, heterozygosity. There is no serologic way to determine the true genotype of a person whose blood belongs to this phenotype. However, since the gene *DCe* is, in round figures, 20 times more common in the population than *dCe,* the strongest probability is that the genotype is *DCe/DCe.*

A second example illustrates how the ethnic origin of the person concerned must be considered in making a presumption of genotype. The phenotype D + C + E − c + e + (DCce) usually means the genotype *DCe/dce* in a white person, because among whites, the gene *dce* has a much higher incidence than *Dce. Dce* is very common in blacks, however, so the genotype *DCe/Dce* is the most likely in them. The probability of homozygosity for *D* is always higher in

Table 3-4. Frequencies of the More Common Rh-Positive Genotypes

Phenotype		Genotype		Genotype Frequency in the Total Population (%)	Likelihood of Zygosity (%)*	
CDE	Rh	CDE	Rh		Homozygous	Heterozygous
DCce	Rh$_1$rh	*DCe/dce*	R^1r	32.0		
		DCe/Dce	R^1R^0	2.0	6	94
DCe	Rh$_1$Rh$_1$	*DCe/DCe*	R^1R^1	17.0		
		DCe/dCe	R^1r'	0.8	96	4
DcEe	Rh$_2$rh	*DcE/dce*	R^2r	11.0		
		DcE/Dce	R^2R^0	0.7	6	94
DcE	Rh$_2$Rh$_2$	*DcE/DcE*	R^2R^2	2.0		
		DcE/dcE	R^2r''	0.3	86	14
DCcEe	Rh$_z$	*DCe/DcE*	R^1R^2	12.0		
		DCe/dcE	R^1r''	1.0	89	11
		dCe/DcE	$r'R^2$	0.3		
		DCE/dce	R^zr	0.2		
Dce	Rh$_0$	*Dce/dce*	R^0r	2.0		
		Dce/Dce	R^0R^0	0.07	3	97

*The figures given are for the random white population. Among blacks, the *Dce* (R^0) gene is very much more common, which will greatly increase the probability of homozygosity, most particularly when the phenotype is DCce (Rh$_1$rh), DcEe (Rh$_2$rh), or Dce (Rh$_0$).

blacks than in whites when that probability depends on the difference in frequency between *dce* and *Dce*. Table 3-4 lists the more common Rh genotypes and gives their approximate frequencies in the general population of the United States.

Compound Antigens

In 1953, Rosenfield and his fellow workers reported an antibody directed at an Rh-related antigen they called f, which appeared to exist only as a product of the genes *dce, Dce,* and *D^{u}ce* [27]. Later, Rosenfield and Haber found that certain anti-C serums gave reactions suggesting they were directed not at C itself, but at a *compound antigen,* Ce (rh$_i$), a product of genes that produce both C and e (*DCe* and *dCe*) that is absent whenever C is inherited with E, as in the products of *DCE* or *dCE* [28]. The later observation suggested that f could also be a compound antigen, in this case, ce, present only when c and e are inherited together as products of the same gene.

With red cells representing the several genotypes that can give rise to the phenotype DCcEe, the antibodies anti-ce and anti-Ce give opposite reactions. Either or both antiserums enable the probable genotype to be determined with greater confidence. *DCe/DcE* is always the most likely genotype in this situation, although alternatives that must also be considered are *DCe/dcE, dCe/DcE, DCE/dce, DCE/Dce,* and *dCE/Dce*. The last three are ruled out if the cells are found to be reactive with anti-Ce and nonreactive with anti-ce, but these are the only possibilities if the reverse reactions are obtained.

A matter of practical significance in the use of Rh phenotyping serums is that most examples of anti-C in Rh-positive persons are *predominantly* anti-Ce. This means they react more strongly with cells possessing C as a product of *DCe* or *dCe* than those having C as the product of *DCE* or *dCE*. In some cases, the difference in reactivity may be so marked that the weaker reaction is mistakenly interpreted as negative, especially since red cells chosen for a positive control test are almost invariably Ce-positive as well as C-positive, and therefore strongly reactive. Compound antigens CE and cE also exist, but antibodies to them are rare.

OTHER RH ANTIGENS

Table 3–5 lists more than 40 antigens having a proven relationship with the Rh system. Most are of limited significance to the average worker in a blood serology laboratory. There is, however, some practical importance to being aware of these antigens, as their presence (or absence) may lead to unexpected reactions with the standard phenotyping reagents.

Alleles of the Principal Genes

The earliest evidence of a gene allelic to any of Fisher's postulated CDE pairs came when a newly discovered antigen named C^w was considered to be a product of the C/c locus. A further antigen, C^x, is considered to be produced by a fourth allele at the same locus. The behavior of both C^w-positive and C^x-positive cells does not always appear to support the allelic relationship. Most examples of anti-C, for instance, react with red cells from almost all bloods belonging to the C^wc or the C^xc phenotypes, though this appears to suggest the simultaneous presence of products from three allelic genes. It has been suggested that most anti-C serums, although produced in an immune response to C alone, contain inseparable anti-C^w and anti-C^x components. This explanation sounds believable, but does not altogether fit the facts. For instance, the supposed anti-CC^wC^x serums are nonreactive with some C^w-positive cells, notably those in which C^w and c can be demonstrated by family study to be products of the same gene [29].

The Antigen G

An observation that perplexed early investigators was that "anti-C + D" was sometimes found in serums from women whose only exposure to an immune stimulus had been pregnancy, and whose husbands were D-positive but C-negative. A possible cause of this effect was suggested by Allen and Tippett in

Table 3–5. Equivalent Systems of Notation for the Antigens of the Rh System

Numerical	CDE	Rh-Hr	Other	Numerical	CDE	Rh-Hr	Other
Rh1	D	Rh_0		Rh25*			
Rh2	C	rh'		Rh26	c-like	hr^A	Deal
Rh3	E	rh''		Rh27	cE	rh_{ii}	
Rh4	c	hr'		Rh28		hr^H	Hernandez
Rh5	e	hr''		Rh29			Total Rh
Rh6	ce	hr	f	Rh30	D^{Cor}		Go^a
Rh7	Ce	rh_i		Rh31		hr^B	
Rh8	C^w	rh^{w1}		Rh32		$\overline{\overline{R}}^N$	Troll
Rh9	C^x	rh^x		Rh33		R_0^{Har}	Hill
Rh10	ce^s	hr^v	V	Rh34		Hr^B	Bastiaan
Rh11	E^w	rh^{w2}		Rh35			1114
Rh12	G	rh^G		Rh36			Be^a
Rh13		Rh^A		Rh37			Evans
Rh14		Rh^B		Rh38			Duclos
Rh15		Rh^C		Rh39	C-like		
Rh16		Rh^D		Rh40			Targett
Rh17		Hr_0		Rh41	Ce-like		
Rh18		Hr		Rh42	Ce^s	rh_i^s	Thornton
Rh19		hr^S		Rh43			Crawford
Rh20	e^s		VS	Rh44			Nou
Rh21	C^G			Rh45			Riv
Rh22	CE	rh	Jarvis	Rh46			Secka
Rh23	D^w		Wiel	Rh47			Dav
Rh24	E^T						

*Rh25 was formerly assigned to the LW antigen, now divided into LW^a and LW^{ab} and part of a blood group system in its own right. It is inherited independently of the Rh locus, and the association with the Rh antigens is purely phenotypic; hence, it has been formally dropped from the Rh system. The number Rh25 accordingly becomes redundant. One or two other antigens on the list are candidates to be dropped from the system at some time in the future.

1958, after they had encountered a previously unrecognized phenotype in a Boston blood donor, Mrs. Crosby. Her red cells were D-negative and C-negative, but were quite strongly agglutinated by serums containing anti-CD. Furthermore, after being incubated with anti-CD serums, the cells yielded an eluate that reacted with both D-positive-C-negative and D-negative-C-positive cells. The explanation suggested was that a previously unrecognized Rh antigen, G, is a product of any gene that produces either C or D. This can mean that the immune response to D-positive-C-negative (G-positive) red cells in a D-negative-C-negative (G-negative) person may include an anti-G component

[30]. The products of the responsible gene were later found to include a rather weak C antigen.

Later, with the recognition of other examples, came the realization that the r^G phenotype is heterogeneous. When it occurs in blacks, the G antigen associated with it is perceptibly weaker than when it occurs in whites. This is also true of the G antigen produced by the r''^G gene.

None of the phenotypes mentioned has any practical significance in blood transfusion.

Variant Antigens in Blacks

Among blacks, antigens thought to be variants of e are of several kinds, and occur quite commonly. The antigens hr^S and hr^B, for which there are no equivalent CDE names, spring to most minds as examples, which is unfortunate because these have not been reported as Rh antigens that occur predominantly in blacks. They are supposedly components of e that may be *missing* from the e antigen possessed by some blacks. The subject is too complex to be treated here; it is sufficient for most practical purposes to know that bloods reacting weakly with anti-e serums are common among blacks, and that these may be falsely interpreted as e-negative, even with anti-e serums that are of acceptable potency.

DEPRESSIONS, SUPPRESSIONS, AND DELETIONS

Partial Deletion

A blood lacking any C, c, E, or e antigens, but with unusually strong expression of D, was reported in 1950 by Race, Sanger, and Selwyn [31]. The phenotype resulted from homozygosity for a gene the authors called *D--*. A stronger-than-normal D antigen is also a feature of cells from heterozygotes (*D--/DCe, D--/DcE*, etc.). Most reported examples of the *D--* phenotype have been recognized in people who produced an antibody directed at a high-frequency antigen of the Rh system, anti-Rh17. This antibody may appear to contain a separable component, most often anti-e, but extended absorption with e-negative cells usually removes all activity.

The genetic background of *D--* is believed to be a partial deletion of genetic material from the chromosome, resulting in a loss of the *C/c* and *E/e* loci. Other partial deletions include D··, DC^w-, DC-, Dc-, and $D^{IV}(C)-$, D(C)(e), D(c)(E), and d(c)(e), each of which is heterogeneous. Parenthesized characters are used in these notations to indicate an antigen of diminished strength.

Rh_{null} and Rh_{mod}

Rare though it is, the Rh_{null} phenotype deserves brief mention, if only because of the abnormal red cell morphology associated with it and the accompanying hemolytic syndrome. The first example of a blood without detectable Rh antigens was described in 1961 by Vos and associates, who had found it in a population study involving Australian aborigines [32]. The phenotype was called ---/---, in the belief that it resulted from a total deletion of the Rh locus.

Later studies revealed, however, that Rh_{null} is most often due to the absence of a regulator gene called X^0r, which is unrelated to the Rh system. This type of Rh_{null} is called the *regulator type*. The other type results from being homozygous for an amorph at the Rh locus ($\bar{r}$). Both kinds of Rh_{null} are accompanied by a hemolytic syndrome that is usually well-enough compensated that the anemia, if any, is mild. Bizarre red cell morphology is also common to both, and the antigens of the LW system are absent.

A person with either form of Rh_{null} may make an antibody to a high-frequency antigen if exposed to red cells possessing normal Rh antigens. Apparently separable components, such as anti-e, may be present, but the specificity is most commonly that known as anti-Rh29, which is considered to be "whole Rh."

The Rh_{mod} phenotype was first reported in 1971 by Chown and his co-workers [33]. Another regulator gene, X^Qr, has been postulated as the cause of Rh_{mod}, but in reality, the difference between this phenotype and the regulator kind of Rh_{null} appears to be one of degree. The atypical red cell morphology is the same, as is the accompanying hemolytic syndrome, but with Rh_{mod} cells, the presence of markedly suppressed Rh antigens can be demonstrated by careful serologic testing, providing sufficiently potent antiserums are available. Commercial reagents are not always suitable, as minimum-potency requirements for U.S. licensure are not designed to detect such feebly expressed antigens.

The Kell System

The founding antigen of the Kell blood group system, K, was the first "new" antigen to be recognized through the application in blood group serology of the antiglobulin test, a technique originally described by Moreschi in 1908 [34], which was reported as a method to detect Rh antibodies in 1945 [35, 36].

K is considered to be next in immunogenicity to D, but immunogenicity is not the only property that influences the frequency with which the antibody to a particular antigen is encountered. In the case of anti-K, a factor to be taken into account is the relative infrequency of the K antigen, which occurs in only about 9 percent of the white population and a somewhat lesser percentage of blacks.

Within a few years, new antigens were encountered that appeared to be related to K, one of them apparently the product of a gene allelic to the one responsible for K, which was accordingly called k [37]. Another pair of reciprocally related antigens, Kp^a and Kp^b, were considered to be products of a linked locus [38, 39], and another phenotype emerged that was not only K-negative and k-negative, but also Kp(a−b−). This was called K_0 [40]. The K_0

Table 3-6. The Principal Antigens of the Kell Blood Group System and Their Frequencies

Reactions with Anti-								Frequency (%)	
K (K1)	k (K2)	Kp^a (K3)	Kp^b (K4)	Js^a (K6)	Js^b (K7)	Ku (K5)	Phenotype*	Whites	Blacks
+	0					+	K+k−	0.2	Rare
+	+					+	K+k+	8.8	2
0	+					+	K−k+	91.0	98
		+	0			+	Kp(a+b−)	Rare	0
		+	+			+	Kp(a+b+)	2.3	Rare
		0	+			+	Kp(a−b+)	97.7	100
				+	0	+	Js(a+b−)	0	1
				+	+	+	Js(a+b+)	Rare	19
				0	+	+	Js(a−b+)	100	80
0	0	0	0	0	0	0	K$_0$	Exceedingly rare	

*Note that not all the theoretically possible Kell phenotypes have been recognized. The type K+Kp(a+b−), for example, has never been found, as *K* and *Kp^a* do not travel together on the same chromosome. Moreover, since Kp^a is a predominantly white antigen, and Js^a is predominantly black, it has been simpler to present the phenotypes in the form shown here than to attempt to represent all possible combinations of antigens.

phenotype is exceedingly rare, and although it does not possess any of the formed Kell system antigens, it is nevertheless rich in K_x, an antigen thought to be a precursor substance that is present in trace amounts on cells of the other Kell system phenotypes. There is one exception; red cells of the McLeod phenotype [41], which features weakly expressed antigens of the Kell system, lack K_x altogether and are morphologically abnormal. The McLeod phenotype is seen in patients with one form of chronic granulomatous disease [42].

A numerical scheme of notation similar to that used for the Rh system has been devised [43]. It recognizes 22 antigens numbered up to K24, the antigens assigned to K8 and K9 having been dropped from the system.

Table 3-6 presents the reaction patterns of the first seven antibodies of the Kell system to be recognized, with the frequencies of the relevant phenotypes in the U.S. population.

ANTIBODIES OF THE KELL SYSTEM

Kell system antibodies are most likely to be detected by the indirect antiglobulin test, although occasional examples may react as direct agglutinins. This may be a transient phenomenon, dependent on the application of a careful technique and the use of fresh indicator cells. The inconsistent behavior of anti-K as an agglutinin appears to have been the origin of a belief, once widely held, that the

K antigen is unstable in storage. Such has not been our experience using the antiglobulin test. We have consistently found the K antigen to be detectable on commercial screening cells 6 weeks or more after they were drawn from the donor, even when we were testing serums containing anti-K of feeble potency.

Another popular belief about the behavior of anti-K (and, perhaps by association, antibodies directed at the other antigens of the system) is that the antiserum may be nonreactive in a low–ionic strength test system. While it appears that individual examples of anti-K have been observed to have weak reactivity after incubation in a low–ionic strength environment, this is not true of all examples, nor perhaps even of the majority.

The MNSs System

Anti-M was recognized in 1927, after a series of animal immunization experiments by Landsteiner and Levine [44]. The existence of N (and also of the unrelated antigen we now call P_1) was reported shortly afterward [45].

M and N are products of an allelic pair of genes, *M* and *N*, that give rise to three possible genotypes—*MM, MN,* and *NN*—with three corresponding phenotypes—M, MN, and N. The discovery of anti-S in 1947, with the realization that this antibody was directed at an antigen related to M and N, was the beginning of increasing complexity now rivaling that of the Rh system [46]. *S,* the gene that produces S, appeared to belong to a second allelic pair, closely linked to the first, which was established conclusively with the discovery of s a few years later [47]. As is the case with the Rh system, the antigens determined by one locus may be seen in any combination with those determined by the other, although once any combination is observed to be traveling together, crossing-over is extremely unlikely. The combinations occur with variable frequency; *Ns* is the most common, followed by *Ms* and *MS*, with *NS* by far the least common. Among blacks, a third allele of *S* and *s* called S^u produces no S or s [48]. Nor does it produce U, a high-frequency antigen defined by an antibody first reported in 1953 as the cause of a fatal hemolytic transfusion reaction [49]. Not all S-negative-s-negative red cells are U-negative; some examples possess a weakly expressed U antigen that may not react directly with all examples of anti-U, although the presence of U may be demonstrated by adsorption/elution. Table 3–7 shows the principal phenotypes of the MNSs system, and lists their frequencies in the U.S. population.

OTHER ANTIGENS OF THE MNSs SYSTEM

Numerous additional antigens have been assigned to the MNSs system, most of them being low-frequency characteristics that have little practical significance in the blood transfusion laboratory. Some of these low-frequency antigens are related to one another as members of the *Miltenberger subsystem;* one, M^g, is the product of an allele at the *M/N* locus and is not detected by anti-M or anti-N.

Table 3-7. The Principal Phenotypes of the MNSs Blood Group System

Reactions with Anti-						Frequency (%)	
M	N	S	s	U	Phenotype	Whites	Blacks
+	0				M	28	26
+	+				MN	50	44
0	+				N	22	30
		+	0	+	S	11	3
		+	+	+	Ss	44	28
		0	+	+	s	45	69
		0	0	0	S^u	0	<1
		0	0	(+)	U^{wk}	0	Rare

Glycophorin A and Glycophorin B

The sialoglycoproteins (SGPs) of the red cell membrane—their sequences of amino acids and variety of attached carbohydrate side chains—contribute to some of the differences in reactivity detected in serologic tests. The SGP present in greatest amount on human red cells is glycophorin A, a structure that penetrates the membrane and extends into the cytoplasm. The antigens M or N reside at the end of the external portion of the structure, which is why an alternative name for glycophorin A is MN SGP. Approximately 500,000 copies of the MN SGP are believed to be on each red cell, while in the case of glycophorin B, the Ss SGP, there are only 100,000 copies. This lesser sialoglycoprotein, which is believed to carry the U antigen, as well as S and s, has as its first 26 amino acids from the terminal a region identical to that occupying the same position on glycophorin A when the N antigen is present. Thus, an N-like antigen called 'N' exists on N-negative red cells, which explains the cross-reactivity that commonly occurs with anti-N. The 'N' antigen is absent from U-negative cells, since these are believed to reflect the *absence* of glycophorin B; but the detectability of 'N' is enhanced in any phenotype that derives from an increased amount of glycophorin B, which may cause the cells to be mistyped as N-positive. As an example, red cells possessing the low-frequency antigen Dantu, which is associated with a hybrid sialoglycoprotein, carry a substantially increased amount of 'N' antigen [50].

ANTIBODIES OF THE MNSs SYSTEM

Anti-M and anti-N may both occur in human serums without an obvious immune stimulus, with anti-M being the more common. Both are most commonly direct agglutinins, active at temperatures below 37°C, and both may show dosage. Weak examples may react convincingly only with cells having homozygous expression of the particular antigen.

Anti-S and anti-s are more often of immune origin, usually being detected by the indirect antiglobulin test. Treatment of the red cells with proteases cleaves the SGPs at various points (depending on the particular enzyme), so many of the antibodies of this system become undetectable in an enzyme test system. M and N appear to be destroyed, and reports about S and s are contradictory. This is probably because of a lack of uniformity among enzyme tests used by different investigators. The position occupied by the U antigen, however, is between the enzyme cleavage points and the membrane surface, so anti-U remains reactive when enzyme test procedures are used.

The P System

Approximately 79 percent of whites and 96 percent of blacks have on their red cells an antigen called P_1, which was called P when it was first recognized by Landsteiner and Levine [45]. Red cells that lack P_1 are called P_2. The P_1 antigen shows considerable variability in the strength of its expression, ranging from being strong enough to recognize anti-P_1 in virtually any P_2 serum to being so weak as to be detectable only with the most potent examples of the specific antibody.

The p phenotype results from the absence of a high-frequency antigen called P, which was called Tj^a when first described [51], and is present on both P_1 and P_2 red cells. A further antigen, P^k, is substituted for P on rare occasions.

ANTIBODIES OF THE P SYSTEM

Anti-P_1 occurs very commonly in serums from persons of the P_2 phenotype, but is seldom detectable above room temperature. Mollison has suggested that anti-P_1 may be capable of shortening the survival of transfused cells through its ability to bind complement [52], but this seldom seems to produce clinically recognizable adverse effects. However, the detection of an example of the antibody in a 37°C test, or at the antiglobulin phase, would be grounds to select P_2 blood for transfusion.

Serums from p persons regularly contain an antibody that was originally called anti-Tj^a, but is now considered to be anti-PP_1P^k; and anti-P occurs regularly in P^k serums. These two antibodies commonly show hemolysis of antigen-positive red cells when tested in vitro, and both are clinically significant. The biphasic hemolysin of paroxysmal cold hemoglobinuria (PCH) is often but not invariably, of anti-P specificity.

The LW System

The antigen detected on human red cells by the immune animal antiserums of Landsteiner and Wiener was renamed LW on the discovery that it was not identical with D [53]. The opportunity to study human examples of anti-LW, moreover, led to the realization that LW is present on D-negative red cells, but in substantially lesser amounts than on D-positive cells. Hence, although LW is not linked genetically to the Rh system, there is a phenotypic relationship with D, in that adult D-positive red cells show a significantly stronger reaction with anti-LW serums than adult D-negative cells do. This is not the case with red cells from umbilical cord blood specimens, which react strongly with anti-LW regardless of their D antigen status.

In 1981, a hitherto unknown blood group antigen, Ne^a, was recognized and shown to have a frequency of approximately 5 percent in Finland, although a considerably lower frequency in other European populations [54]. Sistonen later noted that anti-Ne^a showed similar behavior to anti-LW in giving stronger reactions with Ne(a+) cells if they were D-positive than if they were D-negative [55]. This observation led to a study in which 11 unrelated LW-negative persons, as well as obligate heterozygotes in their families, were all found to be Ne(a+), thereby confirming that LW and Ne^a are the products of allelic genes [56]. The principal antigens were thus renamed as LW^a and LW^b, respectively, and the former LW-negative phenotype became LW(a−b+). The red cells of one LW-negative person, Mrs. Big., were found to be LW(a−b−), and the potent example of "anti-LW" she had earlier been reported to have made in pregnancy [57], which was already known to agglutinate other LW-negative cells, was deduced to be anti-LW^{ab}.

ANTIBODIES OF THE LW SYSTEM

The reactivity of LW antibodies is similar to that of immune Rh antibodies. Bovine albumin at a sufficient concentration in the test mixture may produce direct agglutination, but reactions are consistently detectable by the antiglobulin technique, and reactivity is usually enhanced in an enzyme test system. Anti-LW^{ab} has been known to occur transiently, occasionally as an obvious autoantibody, but sometimes less obviously because the strength of the LW^a antigen on the cells is transiently diminished to the point where it seems to be absent [58, 59]. The direct antiglobulin test is usually positive in these cases, but may not be strongly so if the LW^a antigen itself has become only weakly detectable.

The Lewis System

The Lewis antigens, Le^a and Le^b, bear a complex relationship with the ABO system and with secretor status. Neither is a true red cell antigen. Both occur as soluble substances in the body fluids, including the plasma, that attach themselves secondarily to the red cells. The Le^a and Le^b antigens originate from a gene called *Le,* which produces a glycosyltransferase that converts a precursor substance to Le^a. The ultimate product, however, depends on whether or not the *Se* gene is present. In ABH nonsecretors (*se/se*), there is no further conversion of Le^a, and the red cell phenotype is Le(a+b−), whereas in secretors (*Se/Se* or *Se/se*), most of Le^a is converted to Le^b, and the phenotype

Table 3–8. The Phenotypes of the Lewis Blood Group System

Reactions with Anti-			Frequency (%)	
Le^a	Le^b	Phenotype	Whites	Blacks
+	0	Le(a+b−)	22	23
0	+	Le(a−b+)	72	55
0	0	Le(a−b−)	6	22

The frequencies listed refer to adult blood samples. It is common for the red cells to be nonreactive with both anti-Le^a and anti-Le^b at birth, but weak reactions may be seen with serums that agglutinate both Le(a+b−) and Le(a−b+) adult red cells.

is Le(a−b+). The Le(a−b−) phenotype results from the absence of the *Le* gene, regardless of secretor status.

The phenotypes of the Lewis system, with their frequencies in the U.S. population, are shown in Table 3–8.

ANTIBODIES OF THE LEWIS SYSTEM

The Lewis antibodies occur commonly, usually without an obvious immune stimulus, almost exclusively in persons of the Le(a−b−) phenotype. Most often, agglutination is detected in tests using saline-suspended cells at temperatures below 37°C. Anti-Le^a is the most common, but anti-Le^b may be present in addition or on its own. Anti-Le^a, in particular, may show hemolysis of antigen-positive cells, especially in an enzyme test, and is sometimes reactive at the antiglobulin phase, providing an anti–human globulin serum containing an anti–complement component is used. Most examples of the Lewis antibodies are harmless. The detection of hemolysis, however, or of definite agglutination at the 37°C or antiglobulin phases, would justify the selection of donor blood negative for the antigen.

The Duffy System

The Fy^a and Fy^b antigens were recognized within a year of each other and established to be the products of allelic genes *Fy^a* and *Fy^b* [60, 61]. A third allele, *Fy,* which produces no Fy^a or Fy^b, was postulated to exist in 1955 and to occur with such a frequency in blacks that would explain why 70 percent of that population group belongs to the Fy(a−b−) phenotype [62], although this is almost unknown in most other populations so far tested. Curiously, it was a white person of the Fy(a−b−) phenotype in Australia whose serum was found to contain the first example of anti-Fy3, which is directed at an antigen present on all cells except those of the Fy(a−b−) phenotype [63].

Two additional antibodies have been recognized: anti-Fy4, which is believed

Table 3–9. The Phenotypes of the Duffy Blood Group System

Reactions with Anti-		Phenotype	Frequency (%)	
Fy^a	Fy^b		Whites	Blacks
+	0	Fy(a+b−)	19	8
+	+	Fy(a+b+)	48	2
0	+	Fy(a−b+)	33	22
0	0	Fy(a−b−)	Rare	68

(but not all that convincingly proved) to be directed at a product of the *Fy* gene that occurs so commonly in blacks [64], and anti-Fy5, which appears to define a product of some interaction between the *Fy* and *Rh* loci, since Fy(a−b−) cells of normal Rh phenotypes and Rh$_{null}$ cells of normal Duffy phenotypes are the only cells found to be nonreactive [65].

A variant gene, *Fy^x*, has been reported as the source of a weakened form of the Fy^b antigen that may not always be reactive with anti-Fy^b serums of otherwise acceptable potency [66].

The phenotypes of the Duffy system, and their frequencies in the U.S. population, are listed in Table 3–9.

ANTIBODIES OF THE DUFFY SYSTEM
When anti-Fy^a or anti-Fy^b are present in a serum, they are for all practical purposes always the result of an immune response, and are reactive by the indirect antiglobulin test. Enzymes inactivate Fy^a and Fy^b, but not Fy3, Fy4, or Fy5.

The Kidd System

The two principal antigens of the Kidd blood group system, Jk^a and Jk^b, were first recognized in 1951 and 1953, respectively, and were determined to be the products of a further allelic pair of genes, unrelated to any other blood group system [67, 68]. The phenotype Jk(a−b−) was recognized a few years later [69], and was subsequently found to be common in certain Pacific Island populations. People whose cells are Jk(a−b−) may make an antibody that reacts with all cells possessing either Jk^a or Jk^b. This is considered to be directed at a separate antigen, Jk^{ab}, rather than being simply an inseparable mixture of anti-Jk^a and anti-Jk^b. Jk^{ab} is sometimes called Jk3.

As a point of interest, screening for red cells of the Jk(a−b−) phenotype can be accomplished economically by a nonserologic method, thanks to a serendipitous discovery by Heaton and McLoughlin, who were attempting to do a platelet count on a Samoan patient using the Technicon Platelet Autocounter II. An unexpectedly high count led to the realization that the patient's red cells

Table 3–10. The Phenotypes of the Kidd Blood Group System

Reactions with Anti-		Phenotype	Frequency (%)	
Jk^a	Jk^b		Whites	Blacks
+	0	Jk(a+b−)	28	57
+	+	Jk(a+b+)	49	34
0	+	Jk(a−b+)	23	9
0	0	Jk(a−b−)	Not reported*	

*The phenotype Jk(a−b−) has a significant frequency among certain Pacific Island population groups.

were unusually resistant to lysis by the 2 M urea solution used to dilute the test sample, presumably due to some membrane abnormality. The fact that certain unusual phenotypes are associated with irregularities of the red cell membrane (notably Rh$_{null}$ in the Rh system and the McLeod phenotype of the Kell system), combined with the knowledge that Samoans belong to a population group in which the Jk(a−b−) phenotype is relatively common, led to the patient's red cells being appropriately tested and confirmed to be of that phenotype. Other red cell samples known to be Jk(a−b−) were then demonstrated to show similar resistance to lysis by urea; hence, it is possible to screen for the Jk(a−b−) phenotype by simply suspending the red cells in 2 M urea and examining for resistance to lysis [70]. Cells showing such resistance are then tested with anti-Jk^a and anti-Jk^b.

The phenotypes of the Kidd system are listed in Table 3–10, along with their frequencies in the U.S. population.

ANTIBODIES OF THE KIDD SYSTEM

Anti-Jk^a and anti-Jk^b are usually detected by the antiglobulin test, but may react as direct agglutinins in an enzyme test procedure, and they show considerable enhancement in an enzyme antiglobulin test. Occasionally, these antibodies may even agglutinate untreated antigen-positive cells in a saline test procedure, but this property is quickly lost on storage of the serum. Both antibodies bind complement strongly, and are sometimes seen to hemolyze cells possessing the appropriate antigen during incubation at 37°C. Their detectability may be enhanced by using an antiglobulin reagent containing an anti-complement component. Weak examples of either may go through a stage of being reliably detectable only with cells having homozygous expression of the specific antigen, reflecting the strong propensity of both antibodies to show dosage. Anti-Jk^a and anti-Jk^b both have a deserved reputation for abruptly becoming undetectable over a short time period, and for causing delayed hemolytic transfusion reactions. Such reactions, which are occasionally severe, occur when the antibodies go undetected in pretransfusion testing, but gain potency rapidly when the administration of unsuspectedly incompatible blood causes a secondary immune response. Persons of the Jk(a−b−) phenotype may make anti-Jk^{ab} (anti-Jk3).

Other Blood Group Systems

Except in special circumstances, such as when a clinically significant antibody has been detected in a recipient's serum, only the ABO group and the D antigen status need to be considered in selecting blood for transfusion. The other antigens of the Rh system, and those of certain other blood group systems, have been reviewed in some detail in the foregoing pages because antibodies to them are sometimes found in the course of routine transfusion practice.

The phenotype frequencies of most of the remaining blood group systems are listed in Table 3–11. Xg^a requires special treatment because of the different frequencies according to sex. These are listed in Table 3–12. In both tables, only the frequencies in the white population are given, as there are no reliable data concerning the phenotype frequencies in blacks or other ethnic groups.

THE LUTHERAN SYSTEM

The Lutheran system began, like many others, with the discovery of antibodies defining the products of an allelic pair of genes. The Lu(a−b−) phenotype came to light when Dr. Mary Crawford tested her own cells and found she belonged to it, and then realized in the course of a family study that she had inherited a lack of Lutheran antigens from her father as a dominant characteristic [71]. An alternative form of Lu(a−b−) results from being homozygous for an amorphic allele *Lu*, but the dominant form is more common, and is an effect caused by an unlinked inhibitor gene called *InLu* (from *Inhibitor*Lutheran), a name that has been challenged on the grounds that the gene also suppresses expression of antigens belonging to other blood group systems. Among others, the i, P$_1$, and Au^a antigens are suppressed. The Lutheran system presently comprises 15 antigens, but the corresponding antibodies are seldom powerfully reactive and usually not clinically important. Reactions are most often seen by the antiglobulin test, but anti-Lu^a and anti-Lu^b are sometimes seen as direct agglutinins, often showing characteristic mixed-field agglutination.

THE SEX-LINKED ANTIGEN

A unique feature of an X-borne characteristic is that women are more likely to have it than men, since they have two X chromosomes, whereas men have only one. Men never inherit it from their fathers, as they receive their single X chromosome from their mothers, while the daughters (and the mothers) of men who have it must also have it. These features all apply to the X-borne blood group antigen Xg^a. Anti-Xg^a is a rare antibody. It most often reacts only by the antiglobulin technique, but has occasionally been encountered as a direct ag-

Table 3–11. Phenotypes of the Cartwright, Colton, Diego, Dombrock, Lutheran, and Scianna Blood Group Systems

System	Reactions with Anti-		Phenotype	Frequency (%)
Cartwright	Yt^a	Yt^b		
	+	0	Yt(a+b−)	91.9
	+	+	Yt(a+b+)	7.9
	0	+	Yt(a−b+)	0.2
Colton	Co^a	Co^b		
	+	0	Co(a+b−)	89.4
	+	+	Co(a+b+)	10.4
	0	+	Co(a−b+)	0.2
	0	0	Co(a−b−)	Very rare
Diego	Di^a	Di^b		
	+	0	Di(a+b−)	0*
	+	+	Di(a+b+)	Rare*
	0	+	Di(a−b+)	100
Dombrock	Do^a	Do^b		
	+	0	Do(a+b−)	17.2
	+	+	Do(a+b+)	49.5
	0	+	Do(a−b+)	33.3
Lutheran	Lu^a	Lu^b		
	+	0	Lu(a+b−)	0.15
	+	+	Lu(a+b+)	7.5
	0	+	Lu(a−b+)	92.35
	0	0	Lu(a−b−)	Rare
Scianna	Sc^1	Sc^2		
	+	0	Sc: 1, −2	99.7
	+	+	Sc: 1, 2	0.3
	0	+	Sc: −1, 2	Very rare
	0	0	Sc: −1, −2	0†

*The Di^a antigen has a much higher frequency in populations of Mongolian origin, including American Indians.
†The Sc: −1, −2 phenotype is not as rare in certain Pacific Island populations.

Table 3–12. Frequencies of the Xg(a+) Phenotype in White Males and Females

Reactions with Anti-Xg^a	Phenotype	Frequency (%)	
		Males	Females
+	Xg(a+)	64	88
0	Xg(a−)	36	12

glutinin in a person without a history of exposure to a red cell–induced stimulus. It binds complement and becomes nonreactive in an enzyme test system.

High-Frequency and Low-Frequency Antigens

The high- and low-frequency blood group characteristics presently known, counting only those formally reported in the literature but not acknowledged to belong to any of the approved blood group systems, are listed in Table 3–13. There is no purpose in dwelling on them individually, because for the purposes of this book, we can cover in a few general remarks most of the rare problems they are likely to present.

Low-Frequency Antigens

Antibodies directed at antigens of low frequency occur commonly in serums from nonimmunized persons, sometimes with multiple specificities in a single serum. It is not unusual for some of these antibodies to belong to the IgG class of immunoglobulin, despite their nonimmune origin. Such multiple specificities are most common in the serums of patients with autoimmune hemolytic anemia, but we know of normal, healthy donors whose serum contains 20 or more separable specificities.

Sometimes antibodies directed at low-frequency antigens may be stimulated by pregnancy when the woman's husband is positive for the antigen. Several of those known have been reported to cause hemolytic disease of the newborn. This is a point to remember if a newborn infant presents with jaundice and a positive direct antiglobulin test yet the mother's serum appears to contain no detectable antibodies.

The unsuspected presence of one or more of these ubiquitous antibodies in reagent antiserums may, on rare occasions, be the cause of false-positive test results. This is an inherent source of error in performing red cell phenotyping tests. It is beyond the control of both licensed manufacturers and the licensing authority, and should be remembered when interpreting the results of such tests, particularly when making genetic presumptions that may have far-reaching consequences. It should also be realized that licensed manufacturers of blood grouping serums draw their raw material from common sources. Antiserums of the same specificity purchased from two or more commercial sources may have been manufactured from the plasma of the same donor, and may therefore contain the same unsuspected contaminant. For some reason, anti-S serums are especially prone to contain these serologic contaminants. In a 1970 report, Sturgeon and his co-workers presented the circumstances surrounding a false exclusion of paternity and their subsequent recognition that five anti-S reagents from separate commercial sources, both in the United States and in Europe, were all manufactured from the same donor's plasma, and that, in

Table 3–13. High-Frequency and Low-Frequency Blood Group Antigens Not Belonging to the Established Blood Group Systems

High-Frequency Antigens		Low-Frequency Antigens	
Vel		Wr^a	(Wright)
Ge	(Gerbich)	By	(Batty)
Lan	(Langereis)	Chr^a	(Christiansen)
Cs^a	(Cost)	Sw^a	(Swann)
Gy^a	(Gregory)	Bi	(Biles)
At^a	(Augustine)	Bx^a	(Box)
Yk^a	(York)	Ls^a	(Lewis II)
Kn^a	(Knops)	Tr^a	(Traversu)
Jo^a	(Joseph)	Wb	(Webb)
Hy	(Holley)	Bp^a	(Bishop)
Jr^a	(Jacobs)	Or	(Orriss)
Cr	(Cromer)	Gf	(Griffiths)
McC^a	(McCoy)	Wu	(Wulfsberg)
Ok^a		Jn^a	
Sl^a		Rd	(Radin)
JMH		Heibel	
Er^a		To^a	(Torkildsen)
Tc^a		Pt^a	(Peters)
Dr		Re^a	(Reid)
Es		An^a	(Ahonen)
In^b	(Salis)	Je^a	(Jensen)
Fritz		Mo^a	(Moen)
P		Hey	
I		Rl^a	(Rosenlund)
i		In^a	(Indian)
*Emm		Fr^a	(Froese)
*Lke		Rb^a	(Redelberger)
*AnWj		Li^a	(Livesey)
*Ge2		Vg^a	(Van Vugt)
*Ge3		Wd^a	(Waldner)
		Dh^a	(Duch)
		Pollio	
		Os^a	
		Hg^a	(Hughes)
		Tc^b	
		Tc^c	
		Nfld	
		Hor	
		*Milne	
		*Rasm	
		*Sw (Class I)	
		*Wes	

The list of antigens is as approved by the ISBT Working Party on Terminology for Red Cell Surface Antigens at its meeting in Munich in 1984 [1], with the antigens marked * being additions at a further meeting in Sydney in 1986. Lke is a transfer from the P system, and AnWj was earlier assigned to the Lutheran system.

consequence, all gave the same false-positive test results in a Chinese family in whom a low-frequency antigen of the MNSs system was present [72].

HIGH-FREQUENCY ANTIGENS

To be negative for a high-frequency antigen may imply homozygosity for a rare gene, whether that gene has a demonstrable product or not. This means that if such a person makes an antibody to the high-frequency antigen that is absent from his cells, it is among ABO-compatible brothers and sisters that potentially suitable donors are most readily to be found. Not considering ABO compatibility, the likelihood that the red cells of any brother or sister will be of the same rare phenotype as the patient is one in four.

Among high-frequency antigens to which numerous examples of the corresponding antibody have been found are Vel, Ge, and Yt^a. Anti-Vel is often an IgM antibody and binds complement. Fresh serums containing anti-Vel commonly lyse Vel-positive red cells. Anti-Ge is more often seen at the antiglobulin phase, although it may also occur as a direct agglutinin. Anti-Vel is certainly clinically significant, and anti-Ge is probably so, unlike anti-Yt^a, another specificity most often reactive by the antiglobulin test.

Fortunately, people having red cells that lack a high-frequency antigen are rare, so the possibility is remote that an antibody to such an antigen will be detected. If one is encountered, however, the rarity of the phenotype will make it difficult to find blood for transfusion. If the patient has no ABO-compatible siblings with the required antigen characteristics, it may be necessary to enlist the aid of an agency that maintains a file of known rare donors.

Miscellaneous Red Cell Antigens and Antibodies

Besides the antigens and antibodies mentioned, certain others exist that may cause problems with in-vitro testing, thereby necessitating investigation and possibly delaying the selection of blood for transfusion, while not themselves being of proven clinical significance.

THE I ANTIGEN AND ITS RELATIVES

The I antigen occurs on the red cells of almost all human adults, but is poorly developed at birth. In persons of the rare i_{adult} phenotype, anti-I occurs in the serum regularly as an alloantibody; otherwise, it is most often seen as a comparatively weak cold autoagglutinin in serums from people who do have I on their red cells. Most often, the antibody does not cause detectable agglutination above the temperature range from 4 to 10°C, and only rarely is it encountered at a sufficient level of potency to be clinically significant as the cause of cold hemagglutinin disease. The thermal range at which anti-I reacts is sometimes broad enough to interfere with serologic tests carried out at room temperature or even higher, however, or even occasionally in the antiglobulin phase after incubation at 37°C. This is because of its ability to bind complement at room temperature, even if it does not have a sufficiently broad thermal range to agglutinate cells at 37°C. It is in this way that anti-I is most often seen as a cause of difficulty in the interpretation of serologic tests.

Testing the serum against a cell suspension made from pooled umbilical cord bloods may help in the resolution of problems caused by examples of anti-I reactive at temperatures above that of the refrigerator, but the results should be interpreted with caution. I is not the only antigen that is poorly developed at birth; and especially potent examples of anti-I may require dilution before showing the expected reactions of anti-I.

Some examples of anti-I are not of straightforward specificity, being directed at antigens considered to be products of gene interaction. The most common example is anti-IH, which agglutinates only cells possessing both the I and the H antigens, and is considered to be specific for some product generated through interaction between the *H* and *I* genes.

On relatively uncommon occasions, a cold-reactive agglutinin is recognized that reacts *more strongly* with cord cells than with adult cells. This is a feature strongly indicative of anti-i specificity, or of an LW system antigen, as discussed on page 106. Curiously, anti-i is often the specificity of the cold autoagglutinin seen in association with infectious mononucleosis.

THE BG ANTIGENS

Among the more tiresome complications that sometimes arise in the course of testing human serums for blood group antibodies is the need to evaluate reactions that are normally perplexing, feeble, poorly reproducible, and hardly ever give a comprehensive pattern of reactions by which the antibody causing them can be identified. Such reactions are usually associated with one or more of the Bg antibodies. They are most commonly seen in the antiglobulin phase of the test, but may react as direct agglutinins if they are potent and the corresponding antigen is expressed with sufficient strength on the cells being tested. These antigens are called Bg^a, Bg^b, and Bg^c, when present on the red cells, and appear to correspond to the HLA antigens HLA-B7, HLA-B17, and HLA-A28, respectively. The Bg antigens are expressed with variable strength on red cells, not only among different antigen-positive persons, but commonly on different occasions on the *same* person's cells.

The Bg antibodies are difficult to identify with confidence because of their variable reactivity, the likelihood of multiple specificity, and the vastly variable expression on red cells of their corresponding antigens. They have limited clinical significance, however, being innocent of any association with hemolytic transfusion reactions. Whether the various forms of anti-Bg are merely separate properties of the anti-HLA specificities with which they are associated, or whether they are distinct antibodies that commonly go together, their presence in a recipient's serum may be a sign that could predict febrile reactions in the event of a transfusion, and provide an indication to administer leukocyte-poor red cells.

Histocompatibility Antigens

THE HLA SYSTEM

Most of the blood group antigens already described (e.g., Rh-Hr, Kell, Duffy) belong exclusively to red cells, although the ABO system is common to almost all body cells. Similarly, there are some antigens found only on granulocytes [73], and others only on platelets [74, 75]. However, a single, highly complex, polymorphic system called *HLA* is responsible for most of the antigenic factors possessed by platelets, leukocytes, and other tissue cells. *HLA* originally stood for *human leukocyte locus A*, but is now usually thought of as *human leukocyte antigen*.

HLA is the most complex immunogenetic system presently known in man. It is controlled by a major histocompatibility complex, or *supergene*, which includes several loci closely linked on the short arm of chromosome 6 [76, 77]. Each of these loci involves numerous alleles that control the production of their corresponding antigens. The antigens, in turn, are found on all nucleated cells in the body, and in some nonnucleated cells and body fluids as well. Some groups of these antigens exhibit cross-reacting characteristics that further increase the complexity of the system.

Immunogenetics

Genetic analysis of antigens determined by serologic testing of blood mononuclear cells (predominantly T lymphocytes) revealed that these antigens are the products of three major gene loci, each having multiple alleles. This genetic background has gradually become clearer over the years, although it has passed through bewildering changes of terminology. The World Health Organization standardized nomenclature so that serologic results from different laboratories could be compared (see Table 3–14 for the older names and numbers corresponding to the present ones).

The three principal loci are now designated A, B, and C, and their respective antigens are numbered 1, 2, 3, etc. As it happened, the antigens controlled by A and B loci were numbered before their genetic control had become apparent. To avoid confusion, those numbers were kept as newer terminology developed. Thus the A and B numbers do not duplicate each other: we have A1, A2, A3, A9, A10, A11, etc., and B5, B7, B8, B12, etc. In the case of the C and other loci, the numbers for each series start with 1 and continue in order. Insertion of a "w" before the antigen number indicates that it is a *workshop*, or tentative, designation, yet to be fully confirmed as an entity; thus, HLA-A3, but HLA-Aw33; HLA-B7, but HLA-Bw22. Some of the original antigens have been

Table 3-14. A Guide to Some Older HLA Antigen Designations[a]

Current	Older	Current	Older
HLA-A ["LA" (1st) Series]			
1	HL-A1, LA1	28	W-28, Ba*, Da15
2	HL-A2, LA2, Mac	29	W-19.1, W-29
3	HL-A3, LA3	30	W-19.2, W-30
9	HL-A9	31	W-19.3, W-31
10	HL-A10, Te12, To13	32	W-19.4, W-32
11	HL-A11, 1LN	w33	W-19.5, W-33
w19	W19, Li, Te19	w34	Malay 2
23	HL-A9.1, w23	w36	Mo*
24	HL-A9.2, w24	w43	BK
25	HL-A10.1, w25, To31	w66	LN
26	HL-A10.2, w26, To40		
HLA-B ["Four" (2nd) Series]			
w4	4a	40	W-10, BB
w6	4b	w41	Sabell
5	HL-A5, 4c, MH	w42	MWA
7	HL-A7, 4d	44	HL-A12 (not TT*)
8	HL-A8	45	TT*
12	HL-A12, Te9, Da4	w46	HS, SIN2
13	HL-A13, HN, To21	w47	407*, MO66, CAS, Bw40C
14	HL-14, MaKi, Te14	w48	KSO, JA, Bw40.3
15	W-15, LND, Te15	49	Bw21.1. SL-ET
16	W-16, U18	w50	Bw21.2, ET*
17	W-17, MaPi, SL, Te17	51	B5.1
18	W-18, CM*, Te18	w52	B5.2
21	W-21, ET	w53	HR
22	W-22, AA	w54	Bw22j, SAP1, J1, SN1
27	W-27, FJH	w67	SN2, Te90, 8w57
35	W-5, R*, Te5	w70	8w59, BU+SV
37	TY	w71	BU
38	W-16.1	w72	SV
39	W-16.2	w73	KA, 1EH

Please note that the asterisks in this table are part of the antigenic designations; they do not indicate a footnote.

[a]This table may help orient those reading literature written before official HLA designations were assigned (1977). Not all designations are included.

"split" into two or more distinct, but related, serologic specificities; for example, the broad specificity HLA-A10 includes the splits A25, A26, and Aw34. Table 3–15 gives the current list of loci and antigens.

The A, B, and C series antigens are also referred to as Class I antigens, or serologically defined, as distinct from the Class II antigens [77]. The latter are defined largely by the interaction of cells themselves (see below).

The ABC, or Class I, antigens are expressed on the surfaces of all nucleated cells in the body, with the possible exception of the nervous system. Biochemically, their molecules consist of two moieties, a beta-2-microglobulin, which is extracellular and invariant regardless of specificity, and a heavy chain with a molecular weight of 44,000. The latter has several "domains," including an intracellular portion and a distal hypervariable region that carries the antigenic specificity. Parts of the molecule are homologous in structure and sequence to immunoglobulins [77].

HAPLOTYPES AND PHENOTYPES. With respect to the A and B antigenic series, since a person has a chromosome from each parent, there will be four possible antigens, one for each locus from each parental chromosome. The two (one A and one B) are contributed as a set from one parent and constitute a *haplotype*. Sometimes typing detects only two or three antigens, instead of four. This usually means that the subject is homozygous for the gene controlling one or the other or both determinants. A phenotype A2,B8,B44, for example, probably means that the person has the haplotypes A2-B8 and A2-B44. That phenotype is usually written A2,x/B8,44, with "x" indicating the missing specificity. The notation "y" is used for a missing B series antigen, e.g., A2,A3/B7,y. The phenotype A2,x/B8,y most likely indicates a person homozygous for the A2-B8 haplotype. Of course, it is also possible that an antigen may appear to be lacking when in fact the subject has a low-frequency antigen for which the typing tray lacked the corresponding antiserum, an occurrence that is not rare when typing members of some ethnic groups.

A great deal of international collaboration continues in this field, with a series of workshops every two or three years. The proceedings of the international workshops are published in book form by a variety of publishers, under the title *Histocompatibility Testing 19--*. The latest such workshop manual is an exhaustive and detailed compendium of the current "official" status of all the accepted HLA antigens and antibodies [78].

HLA Typing
HLA Class I antigens and antibodies are determined by several techniques, the dominant and most reproducible one being the *lymphocyte microcytotoxicity* method [79]. In this technique, living lymphocyte suspensions from peripheral blood or lymphatic tissue are exposed to antiserums and complement. In the presence of the corresponding antigen, complement is fixed and the cells are

Table 3–15. HLA Specificities, 1984

A	B	C	D	DR
A1	B5	Cw1	Dw1	DR1
A2	B7	Cw2	Dw2	DR2
A3	B8	Cw3	Dw3	DR3
A9	B12	Cw4	Dw4	DR4
A10	B13	Cw5	Dw5	DR5
A11	B14	Cw6	Dw6	DRw6
Aw19	B15	Cw7	Dw7	DR7
A23(9)	B16	Cw8	Dw8	DRw8
A24(9)	B17		Dw9	DRw9
A25(10)	B18		Dw10	DRw10
A26(10)	B21		Dw11(w7)	DRw11(5),LB5
A28	Bw22		Dw12	DRw12(5)
A29(w19)	B27		Dw13	DRw13(w6),6.6,6.1,6Z
A30(w19)	B35		Dw14	DRw14(w6),6.9,6.3
A31(w19)	B37		Dw15	
A32(w19)	B38(16)		Dw16	DRw52(MT2)
Aw33(w19)	B39(16)		Dw17(w7)	DRw53(MT3)
Aw34(10)	B40		Dw18(w6)	
Aw36	Bw41		Dw19(w6)	
Aw43	Bw42			
Aw66(10)	B44(12)			
Aw68(28)	B45(12)			
Aw69(28)	Bw46		DQ	
	Bw47		DQw1(MT1, DC1, MB1)	
	Bw48		DQw2(MB2, Te24, DC3)	
	B49(21)		DQw2(MT4, MB3, DC4)	
	Bw50(21)			
	B51(5)			
	Bw52(5)			
	Bw53			
	Bw54(w22)		DP(SB)	
	Bw55(w22)		DPw1	
	Bw56(w22)		DPw2	
	Bw57(17)		DPw3	
	Bw58(17)		DPw4	
	Bw59		DPw5	
	Bw60(40)		DPw6	
	Bw61(40)			
	Bw62(15)			
	Bw63(15)			
	Bw64(14)			
	Bw65(14)			
	Bw67			
	Bw70			
	Bw71(w70)			
	Bw72(w70)			
	Bw73			
	Bw4			
	Bw6			

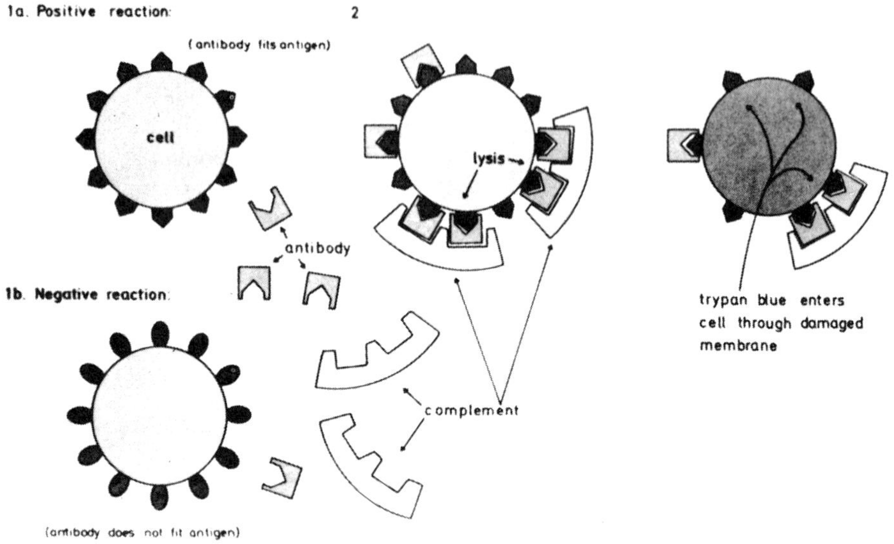

Figure 3-3
Principle of the lymphocytotoxicity test. A cell having the appropriate antigen reacts with a specific antibody and complement. As a result, trypan blue enters the cell through the damaged membrane and indicates that the cell surface antigen has been recognized by a specific antibody. (From F. Vogel, A. G. Motulsky, *Human Genetics*. New York: Springer Verlag, 1979. With permission.)

killed. Cell death is determined by a stain (either trypan blue or eosin), which penetrates the dead cells, but not any remaining living ones. Unaffected cells remain brilliantly refractile to microscopic observation (Fig. 3–3). Fluorescent indicators are also used. Other methods include leukocyte agglutination, and complement fixation on platelets in suspension.

The importance of Class I antigens in transplantation is that they are targets for the recipient's humoral antibody response, particularly when cytotoxic antibodies already exist in the host. In that case, the transplanted organ must lack the corresponding antigens, and must be serologically compatible to prevent accelerated rejection.

Reagent antiserums used in HLA typing are obtained, for the most part, by screening the serums of multiparous blood donors against panels of test lymphocytes of known antigenic phenotypes. Monoclonal HLA antiserums are beginning to appear, but their place in routine HLA typing is as yet uncertain.

The results of HLA typing are by no means as straightforward as those of red cell typing. Two major difficulties are the cross-reactivity of certain antigens and the multispecificity of antiserums. Thus, unlike red cell typing, accurate and reproducible results require the use of several antiserums of each major specificity. A satisfactory panel of test serums may include 60 to 100, or even more. Commercially available trays preloaded with HLA typing serums are convenient and reliable. They usually consist of a basic tray of 60 to 72 serums, and separate "extended" trays to identify splits and other narrower specificities, if needed (see p. 118).

Bw4 AND Bw6. Although they may appear to add complexity, some of the broad cross-reactive antiserums are actually useful in practice. For example, in the B series, anti-Bw4 and -Bw6 each recognizes a large group of mutually exclusive antigens and can be helpful in identifying splits of many complex antigens (Table 3–16). Also, incompatibility for Bw4 or Bw6 may influence the outcome of platelet transfusions in patients with alloimmunization caused by multiple transfusion exposures (see Chap. 8).

C SERIES ANTIGENS. The C antigens do not seem to be very important in either transplantation or transfusion, although they may be helpful in tracing the immunogenetic relationships within a family. There appears to be only one C locus, so a person will have one or two antigens, or none at all; blanks are fairly common.

B Lymphocyte Antigens (Class II)

In addition to the A, B, and C *serologically* defined segregant series, there are antigens defined by *lymphocyte interaction* in tissue culture, that is, by the *mixed lymphocyte culture* (MLC) *technique* (see below). The MLC antigens are apparently controlled by one locus, HLA-D, still within the major histocompatibility complex. Serologic typing of B lymphocytes has revealed yet another complicated series of antigens, closely associated with D, called DR (R for related), as well as some broad specificities called DQ (formerly MB), and another as yet little-understood group called DP. Exactly how these are related to the D (MLC) antigens remains uncertain.

MLC is an elegant and sensitive—though laborious—technique, which unfortunately requires several days to complete [79]. It entails incubation of living recipient lymphocytes with donor lymphocytes inactivated by treatment with mitomycin C, a substance that blocks DNA synthesis. If the donor cells are incompatible, the recipient's lymphocytes respond to the challenge by undergoing a blast transformation. This response, or stimulation, is quantitatively proportional to the degree of incompatibility, and it can be measured by the uptake of tritiated thymidine into the responding cells (Fig. 3–4). This is a *one-way* MLC. The test can also be done with living donor lymphocytes and inactivated recipient cells to complete a *two-way* procedure. MLC can be used to

Table 3–16. The Bw4 and Bw6 Antigenic Groupings*

Bw4	Bw6
5	7
13	8
17	14
27	18
37	w22
38 (16)	35
44 (12)	39 (16)
w47	40
49 (21)	w41
51 (5)	w42
w52 (5)	45 (12)
w53	w46
w57 (17)	w48
w58 (17)	w50 (21)
w59	w54 (w22)
w63	w55 (w22)
	w56 (w22)
	w60 (40)
	w61 (40)
	w62 (15)
	w64 (14)
	w65 (14)
	w67
	w70
	w71 (w70)
	w72 (w70)
	w73

*These are the antigens recognized respectively by anti-Bw4 and anti-Bw6. Bw4 and Bw6 reactivity can be used to help identify some of the splits of the B series of HLA antigens. The numbers in parentheses are the broader antigens, of which the others are splits.

select bone marrow and kidney donors from among a patient's relatives or other living donors, but is not applicable to cadaver transplants because of the time involved.

DR SERIES ANTIGENS. Serologic testing for the antigens of the DR and other B cell series requires a purified suspension of B lymphocytes, the separation of which from mixed peripheral blood lymphocytes seems as much art as science. T cells may be separated by rosetting with sheep red cells, or B cells may be

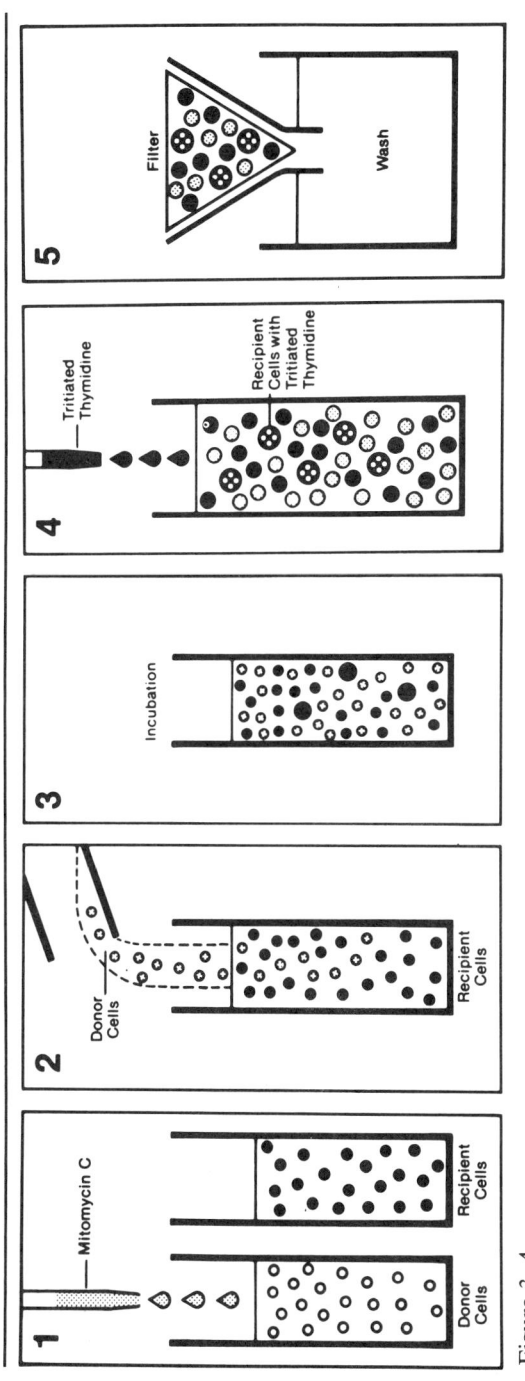

Figure 3–4
Mixed lymphocyte culture. (1) Donor lymphocytes are treated with mitomycin C, which prevents DNA synthesis but does not alter the cellular antigens. (2) The inactivated donor lymphocytes are mixed with the recipient's lymphocytes, which are not so treated. (3) The mixed cells are incubated together for 3 days. (4) Tritiated thymidine is added, and will be incorporated into the DNA of the recipient's cells if these have been stimulated by the donor cells, i.e., if the donor cells have antigens foreign to the recipient. (5) After a time, the cells are washed and filtered out. Radioactivity in the sediment remaining on the filter is proportional to the thymidine uptake by the recipient's cells.

trapped by nylon wool fibers. Alternatively, highly effective commercial separation mediums are available. Satisfactory DR typing trays resembling ABC typing trays are also commercially available. As with ABC typing, there are many serums of mixed and cross-reacting specificities, and the panels must include several of each specificity to assure accurate and reproducible results.

There seems to be only one genetic DR locus, so that each person has one or two antigens. But the absence of detectable DR antigens is rare; most of the time such an observation is probably caused by hyporeactivity of the lymphocytes being tested.

The importance of the Class II (D and DR) antigens in transplantation is that of selecting organs that will have the closest similarity possible to the host's own tissues, so that the transplant will not be recognized as foreign and rejected by the host's *cellular* immune system.

Biochemically, the Class II antigens consist of two associated chains, having molecular weights of 34,000 and 28,000, respectively, each with an intracellular and an extracellular portion. The antigenic specificity lies in the distal hypervariable regions. Again, as in the Class I molecules, there is an extensive homology with immunoglobulins, an intriguing and puzzling phenomenon. Class II antigens are much more restricted in distribution, being limited to macrophages, B lymphocytes, Langerhans cells of the skin, and activated T lymphocytes. The antigens seem to function in the presentation of foreign antigen by macrophages to T lymphocytes [77]. Perhaps the Class I antigens are the principal targets for antibody and killer lymphocytes, whereas Class II antigens are the determinants of immunogenicity.

Crossmatching

In addition to antigen matching, as in blood transfusion, histocompatibility is assayed by an antibody screening test and a "crossmatch." The antibody screen tests the patient's serum for cytotoxicity against a panel of test lymphocytes. The latter may range in number from about 20 samples, if carefully selected to include all the major HLA ABC antigens, to as many as 100 samples, if taken at random. The crossmatch, or *compatibility test,* is with the patient's serum against the prospective donor's lymphocytes by cytotoxicity. The substrate lymphocytes may be prepared from peripheral blood, or in the case of a cadaver donor, from a lymph node or a piece of spleen. Conventional microcytotoxicity is used for these antibody-detection tests in most laboratories, although fluorescent methods and antiglobulin procedures are being applied in some.

Screening and crossmatching are carried out generally at room temperature by techniques designed to detect the HLA ABC type of incompatibility, because that is the type that leads to acute graft rejection. Techniques to detect DR antibodies are also used in some laboratories, but are considered an optional extra procedure because serologic incompatibility of this type is of uncertain significance in graft survival.

HLA and Transplantation

The suitability of a tissue transplantation donor for a particular patient is based first on ABO compatibility with the patient's serum (except in the case of bone marrow), then on an attempt to match them by HLA antigens. Since the Rh antigens exist only on red cells, they are of no importance in transplantation. The several series of HLA antigens have a different significance in the various organ transplant situations.

Kidney Transplantation

The significance of HLA matching has become clearer in the case of renal allografting. Here, the best correlation is shown with living, related donors and recipients, where closer AB and DR matches result in better graft survival [77, 80]. As might be expected, the very best results are seen when the donor and recipient have identical AB and DR antigens. The C antigens seem to have little significance in transplantation.

With cadaveric transplants, the difference in survival between grafts that are well matched for HLA A and B and those that are poorly matched amounts to only 10 to 30 percent. DR matching may be more relevant to success, and in the past few years, preference has been given to DR matching over AB. Two-antigen DR-matched cadaveric renal transplants have about the same graft survival outcome as fully matched living-related donor transplants [81].

Transfusions, too, improve the survival of transplanted kidneys (see Chap. 6). The effect of HLA matching in transfused kidney recipients is much less pronounced than is the case with untransfused recipients. The same observation extends to the use of the immunosuppressive drug *cyclosporin A* [82]. Nevertheless, it is still considered good practice to select the best HLA match possible, both with living-related and cadaveric donors, as this undoubtedly reduces posttransplant complications and lessens the dose of immunosuppressive drugs needed [80].

THE EFFECTS OF THE LEWIS ANTIGENS. Lewis antigens are present on tubular epithelial cells in the kidneys of Lewis-positive persons [83], and some data have been presented to show that Lewis-positive kidney grafts do not survive as well in Lewis-negative recipients [84]. Lewis antibodies can be identified when Lewis-incompatible kidneys are rejected [85]. But the data are as yet incomplete, and are complicated by the fact that patients under dialysis therapy may lose the Lewis antigens from their red cells, thus being falsely typed as Le(a−b−) [84]. Presently in most centers, kidney donors are not typed for the Lewis factors, but that could change if more convincing data were presented.

CROSSMATCH AND MLC TESTS. In the case of living kidney donors (usually relatives of the recipient), the ABC and DR typing and T cell crossmatch are supplemented by an MLC test to determine compatibility of donor lymphocytes with the host's *cellular* immune system. MLC nonreactivity usually assures a good posttransplant survival of the graft. Since this test requires several days to complete, it is not useful in cadaveric transplants.

ORGAN PROCUREMENT AGENCIES. With the increasing national and international coordination of organ procurement facilities, it is becoming common practice to distribute serums of transplant candidates among various program coordinators to increase the likelihood of finding a compatible kidney. This is particularly the case for patients who are difficult to match, such as those with preexisting cytotoxic antibodies having a high frequency of reactivity.

Bone Marrow Transplantation

Marrow transplantation, while still a formidable procedure, has become widely accepted for an increasing variety of clinical conditions [86, 87, 88]. Because of the risks of the procedure, including that of graft-versus-host disease, most transplants have been from HLA-identical related donors (usually siblings of the patient), compatible by both cytotoxicity and mixed lymphocyte culture. Because many marrow transplant candidates lack an HLA-identical sibling, increasing numbers of transplants are now being successfully achieved from nonsibling blood relatives [89] and also from *un*related HLA-identical, MLC-compatible volunteers [90].

A side-issue of the use of unrelated donors has been the occasional well-publicized search for blood donors of a specified HLA type as possible candidates for bone marrow donation for a particular patient. Before we allow this kind of approach to be made directly to HLA-typed blood donors, we should think a little. Blood donors have volunteered to give blood and its components, and have been HLA typed mostly for platelet donation for patients refractory to regular platelet concentrates. They know what is involved in blood and component donation, and expect to be called on from time to time. But they do not know what is involved in marrow donation (e.g., time loss, possible travel to another city, a surgical procedure under anesthesia, possible complications). Until such donors have been educated as to the realities of marrow donation, without any pressure on them to donate, and have then volunteered to do so, it is not proper, in our opinion, to allow them to be approached as possible marrow donors for a particular patient.

A cluster of articles in *Transfusion* discussed the recruitment of HLA-typed marrow donors unrelated to potential recipients [91, 92, 93]. All agreed that ethical considerations in such a program are paramount. Two of the institutions used essentially the approach outlined above, namely, education of potential

Table 3-17. Principles of Operation of a Bone Marrow Donor Program*

1. A program of education and information is provided to potential donors describing the need for donors, the process of bone marrow donation, and transplantation.
2. A registry of potential donors is established after they have received the educational material and have given their permission for listing in the registry.
3. An organizational working agreement is established between the bone marrow donor program and the transplant center, which includes a description of
   a. the kinds of diseases and clinical situations to be treated by bone marrow transplantation from unrelated donors
   b. the nature of matching to define a suitable donor-recipient pair
   c. the nature of medical evaluation and care that the donor would receive
   d. the consent form for bone marrow donation
4. The donor registry is searched only on request of transplant physicians in the bone marrow transplant program affiliated with the donor program.
5. Results of all laboratory testing and medical examination of the potential donor are provided only to the bone marrow donor program and released to the staff only on consent of the donor.
6. Upon identification of a potential donor, the donor program staff provides sufficient information that the potential donor can make a decision about intent to donate.
7. A donor advocate is available for each potential donor matched to a patient.
8. Potential bone marrow donors receive a physical examination by a third-party physician before making the final decision of intent to donate.
9. The donor's identity is known only to the bone marrow donor program until intent to donate is declared. Then the donor's name is provided only to the transplant center physician.
10. The bone marrow donor program does not provide financial support to donors, but is willing to act in their behalf with employers or other parties to secure support for expenses encountered.

*Modified slightly from J. McCullough, G. Rogers, R. Dahl, et al. Development and operation of a program to obtain volunteer bone marrow donors unrelated to the patient. *Transfusion* 1986; 315-23. With permission.

donors about marrow donation, then obtaining their consent to be entered into a pool of available donors before approaching them for a specific patient [92, 93]. Table 3-17 gives the operating principles of the Minnesota group [92]. The third institution approaches donors only after receiving a request for marrow donors of a specified phenotype [91]. In this case, the potential donors are told that they are in a group of donors that may be compatible with a patient, and are given the opportunity to volunteer or not. Although the last authors stress the importance of exerting no pressure on the donor, we believe that the donor's knowledge that he may match a patient awaiting transplantation willy-nilly creates a coercive atmosphere.

Heart and Liver Transplantation

The value of HLA-matching for these procedures is not yet established. Recipients and donors are usually HLA-typed, but this does not enter into the selection process. Preliminary cytotoxic antibody screening, and compatibility testing with the prospective donor, are usually done. A positive antibody screen restricts the selection of a suitable donor organ, and raises formidable obstacles to transplantation in direct relation to the proportion of incompatibility against a donor population. A test indicating incompatibility with a particular donor is generally taken to exclude that donor because of the likelihood of acute rejection. With a negative antibody screening test, it is usually considered safe to transplant without awaiting the result of a compatibility test.

HLA AND TRANSFUSION

Platelets

HLA matching by lymphocyte typing for the A and B antigens is widely used in the selection of platelet donors for thrombocytopenic recipients who have become refractory to conventional platelet transfusions, presumably as a result of alloimmunization (see Chap. 8).

In view of the enormous number of HLA phenotypes, selection of matched platelets might seem impractical unless closely related donors were available. However, some phenotypes are relatively common, and furthermore, a good deal of cross-reactivity exists among HLA antigens. Within groups of cross-reacting antigens (CREGs), mutual immunogenicity is lower than would be the case between the antigens of different groups (Fig. 3–5). In other words, the patient's immune system may not recognize cross-reacting antigens as foreign. By taking advantage of this phenomenon and using platelet apheresis for platelet collection, alloimmunized recipients can achieve good platelet transfusion results from carefully selected donors without the need for an enormous panel of typed donors [94, 95].

In addition to HLA, which is by no means the final word in the success or failure of platelet transfusions, there are other antigens on platelets, some apparently specific to the platelet itself, others less well defined (Table 3–18). See Chapter 8 for a discussion of platelet refractoriness in general.

Granulocytes

There is much conflicting literature on the effects of HLA compatibility on the outcome of granulocyte transfusions. Cytotoxic antibodies (e.g., HLA) can affect transfused granulocytes, as is also true of other types of antibodies apparently more directly specific for granulocytes [73, 96]. In vivo effects of these can be detected, but the significance of such findings with respect to the outcome of clinical granulocyte transfusions is debatable. HLA selection is not

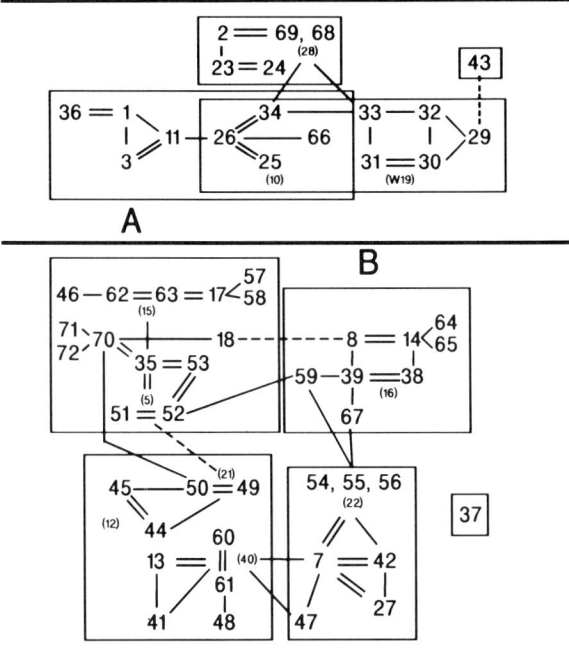

Figure 3-5
Cross-reactive groups of HLA antigens (CREGs). The enclosed areas include mutually cross-reactive antigens. Double lines connecting antigens indicate strong cross-reactivity, single lines less strong, and dashed lines weak. Smaller numbers in parentheses are the older, broader specificities. The "w" prefixes are omitted.

Table 3-18. Platelet-Specific Antigens (White Population)*

Group	Antigens	Frequency (%)	Remarks
PL^A	PL^{A1}	97	Posttransfusion purpura
	PL^{A2}	26	Neonatal thrombocytopenia
Ko	Ko^a	16	
	Ko^b	99	
PL^E	PL^{E1}	99+	Inadequate data as to clinical significance
	PL^{E2}	5	
Bak	Bak^a	91	

*Data from Décary [75].

generally considered necessary for unimmunized patients, although it may be essential for immunized recipients, particularly those who experience respiratory distress or other severe reactions to granulocyte transfusions.

OTHER HLA APPLICATIONS

The association of HLA types with certain diseases, e.g., that of HLA B27 with ankylosing spondylitis, continues to arouse a great deal of interest [97]. The connection exists presumably because of the close proximity of the HLA gene loci to those for immune responsiveness. The topic, however, is unrelated to transfusion, and will not be discussed further. The same applies to the widespread use of HLA typing in cases of disputed parentage, where HLA analysis can not only exclude parentage, but even allow a statistical estimate of the positive likelihood of parentage [98].

References

1. Lewis M. ISBT working party on terminology for red cell surface antigens: Munich report. *Vox Sang* 1985; 49:171–175.
2. Mourant AE, Kopéc, AC, Domaniewska-Sobczak K. *The Distribution of the Human Blood Groups and Other Biochemical Polymorphisms,* 2nd ed. New York: Oxford U Pr, 1976.
3. Huestis DW, Bove JR, Busch S. *Practical Blood Transfusion,* 3rd ed. Boston: Little, Brown 1981; 124.
4. Bird GWG. Specific agglutinating activity for human red blood corpuscles in extracts of *Dolichos biflorus. Curr Sci* 1951; 20:298–99.
5. Voak D, Lodge TW, Stapleton RR, et al. The incidence of H-deficient A_2 and A_2B bloods and family studies on the AH/ABH status of an A_{int} and some new variant blood types. *Vox Sang* 1970; 19:73–84.
6. Schmidt PJ, Nancarrow JF, Morrison EG, Chase G. A hemolytic reaction due to the transfusion of A_x blood. *J Lab Clin Med* 1958; 54:38–41.
7. Yates AD, Feeney J, Donald ASR, Watkins WM. Characterisation of a blood group A-active tetrasaccharide synthesised by the blood-group B gene-specified glycosyltransferase. *Carbohydr Res* 1984; 130:251–60.
8. Bhende YM, Deshpande CK, Bhatia HM, et al. A "new" blood-group character related to the ABO system. *Lancet* 1952; 1:903–4.
9. Landsteiner K, Wiener AS. An agglutinable factor in human blood recognized by immune sera for rhesus blood. *Proc Soc Exp Biol Med NY* 1940; 43:223.
10. Wiener AS, Peters HR. Hemolytic reactions following transfusion of blood of the homologous group, with three cases in which the same agglutinogen was responsible. *Ann Intern Med* 1940; 13:2306–22.
11. Levine P, Stetson RE. An unusual case of intragroup agglutination. *JAMA* 1939; 113:126–7.
12. Levine P, Burnham L, Katzin EM, Vogel P. The role of isoimmunization in the pathogenesis of erythroblastosis fetalis. *Am J Obstet Gynecol* 1941; 42:925–37.
13. Rosenfield RE, Allen FH Jr, Swisher SN, Kochwa S. A review of Rh serology and presentation of a new terminology. *Transfusion* 1962; 2:287–312.
14. Stratton F. A new Rh allelomorph. *Nature* 1946; 158:25.

15. Renton PH, Hancock JA. An individual of unusual Rh type. *Vox Sang (Old Series)* 1955; 5:135–42.
16. Renton PH, Hancock JA. Variability of the Rhesus antigen D. *Br J Haematol* 1956; 2:295–304.
17. Ceppelini R, Dunn LC, Turri M. An interaction between alleles at the Rh locus in man which weakens the reactivity of the Rh_0 factor (D^u). *Proc Nat Acad Sci USA* 1955; 41:283–8.
18. Lewis M, Kaita H, Allerdice RW, et al. Assignment of the red cell antigen Targett (Rh40) to the Rh blood group system. *Am J Hum Genet* 1979; 31:630–3.
19. Giles CM, Crossland JD, Haggas WK, Longster G. An Rh gene complex which results in a "new" antigen detectable by a specific antibody, anti-Rh33. *Vox Sang* 1971; 21:289–301.
20. Issitt PD, Wilkinson-Kroovand S, Pavone BG. Observations on detection of the D antigen made by R^{0Har} gene. *Afr J Clin Exp Immunol* 1980; 1:95–102.
21. Argall CI, Ball JM, Trentelman E. Presence of anti-D antibody in the serum of a D^u patient. *J Lab Clin Med* 1953; 41:895–8.
22. Shapiro M. The ABO, MN, P and Rh blood group systems in South African Bantu: a genetic study. *South Afr Med J* 1951; 25:187–92.
23. Wiener AS, Unger LJ. Rh factors related to the Rh_0 factor as a source of clinical problems. *JAMA* 1959; 169:696–9.
24. Wiener AS, Unger LJ. Further observations on the blood factors Rh^A, Rh^B, Rh^C and Rh^D. *Transfusion* 1962; 2:230–3.
25. Tippett P, Sanger R. Observations on subdivisions on the Rh antigen D. *Vox Sang* 1962; 7:9–13.
26. Tippett P, Sanger R. Further observations on subdivisions of the Rh antigen D. *Ärtzt Lab* 1977; 23:476–80.
27. Rosenfield RE, Vogel P, Gibbel N, et al. A "new" Rh antibody, anti-f. *Br Med J* 1953; 1:975.
28. Rosenfield RE, Haber GV. An Rh blood factor, rh_i (Ce), and its relationship to hr (ce). *Am J Hum Genet* 1958; 10:474–80.
29. Sachs HW, Reuter W, Tippett P, Gavin J. An Rh gene complex producing both C^w and c antigens. *Vox Sang* 1978; 35:272–4.
30. Allen FH Jr, Tippett PA. A new Rh blood type which reveals the antigen G. *Vox Sang* 1958; 3:321–30.
31. Race RR, Sanger R. Selwyn JG. A probable deletion in the human Rh chromosome. *Nature* 1950; 166:520.
32. Vos GH, Vos D, Kirk RL, Sanger R. A sample of blood with no detectable Rh antigens. *Lancet* 1961; 1:14–5.
33. Chown B, Lewis M, Kaita H, Lowen B. A new cause of haemolytic anaemia? *Lancet* 1971; 1:396.
34. Moreschi C. Neue Tatsachen über die Blutkörperschen Agglutinationen. *Zentralbl Bakteriol* 1908; 46:49, 456.
35. Coombs RRA, Mourant AE, Race RR. In-vivo iso-sensitization of red cells in babies with haemolytic disease. *Lancet* 1946; 1:264–6.
36. Coombs RRA, Mourant AE, Race RR. A new test for the detection of weak and incomplete Rh agglutinins. *Br J Exp Pathol* 1945;26:255–66.
37. Levine P, Backer M, Wigod M, Ponder R. A new human hereditary blood property (Cellano) present in 99.8% of all bloods. *Science* 1949; 109:464–6.
38. Allen FH, Lewis SJ. Kp^a (Penney) a new antigen in the Kell blood group system. *Vox Sang* 1957; 2:81–7.

39. Allen FH, Lewis SJ, Fudenberg H. Studies of anti-Kp^b, new antibody in the Kell blood group system. *Vox Sang* 1958; 3:1–13.
40. Chown B, Lewis M, Kaita H. A "new" Kell blood group phenotype. *Nature* 1957; 180:711.
41. Allen FH, Krabbe SMR, Corcoran PA. A new phenotype (McLeod) in the Kell blood group system. *Vox Sang* 1961: 6:555–60.
42. Giblett ER, Klebanoff SJ, Pincus SH, et al. Kell phenotypes in chronic granulomatous disease: a potential transfusion hazard. *Lancet* 1971; 1:1235–6.
43. Allen FH, Rosenfield RE. Notation for the Kell blood group system. *Transfusion* 1961; 1:305–7.
44. Landsteiner K, Levine P. A new agglutinable factor differentiating individual human bloods. *Proc Soc Exp Biol Med NY* 1927; 24:600–2.
45. Landsteiner K, Levine P. Further observations on individual differences of human blood. *Proc Soc Exp Biol Med NY* 1927; 24:941–2.
46. Walsh RJ, Montgomery C. A new human isoagglutinin subdividing the MN blood groups. *Nature* 1947; 60:504.
47. Levine P, Kuhmichel AB, Wigod M, Koch E. A new blood factor, s, allelic to S. *Proc Soc Exp Biol Med NY* 1951; 78:218–20.
48. Greenwalt TJ, Sasaki T, Sanger R, et al. An allele of the S(s) blood group genes. *Proc Nat Acad Sci USA* 1954; 40:1126–9.
49. Wiener AS, Unger J, Gordon EB. Fatal hemolytic transfusion reaction caused by sensitization to a new blood group factor, U. *Science* 1953; 119:734–5.
50. Contreras M, Green C, Humphreys J, et al. Serology and genetics of an MNSs-associated antigen, Dantu. *Vox Sang* 1984; 46:377–86.
51. Levine P, Bobbitt OB, Waller RK, Kuhmichel A. Isoimmunization by a new blood group factor in tumor cells. *Proc. Soc Exp Biol Med NY* 1951; 77:403–5.
52. Mollison PE. *Blood Transfusion in Clinical Medicine,* 6th ed. Oxford: Blackwell Sci, 1979, 496.
53. Levine P, Celano MJ, Wallace J, Sanger R. A human "D-like" antibody. *Nature* 1963; 198:596–7.
54. Sistonen P, Nevanlinna HR, Virtaranta-Knowles K, et al. Ne^a, a new blood group antigen in Finland. *Vox Sang* 1981; 40:352–7.
55. Sistonen P. A phenotypic association between the blood group antigen Ne^a and the Rh antigen D. *Med Biol* 1981; 59:230–3.
56. De Veber LL, Clark GW, Hunking M, Stroup M. Maternal anti-LW. *Transfusion* 1971; 11:33–5.
57. Sistonen P, Tippett P. A 'new' allele giving further insight into the LW blood group system. *Vox Sang* 1982; 42:252–5.
58. Giles CM, Lundsgaard A. A complex serological investigation involving LW. *Vox Sang* 1967; 13:406–17.
59. Chown B, Kaita H, Lewis M. Transient production of anti-LW by LW-positive people. *Transfusion* 1971; 11:220–2.
60. Cutbush M, Mollison PL, Parkin DM. A new human blood group. *Nature* 1950; 165:188.
61. Ikin EW, Mourant AE, Pettenkofer HJ, Blumenthal G. Discovery of the expected haemagglutinin, anti-Fy^b. *Nature* 1951; 168:1077.
62. Sanger R, Race RR, Jack J. The Duffy blood groups of New York negroes: the phenotype Fy(a−b−). *Br J Haematol* 1955; 1:370–4.
63. Albrey JA, Vincent EER, Hutchinson J, et al. A new antibody, anti-Fy3, in the Duffy blood group system. *Vox Sang* 1971; 20:29–35.

64. Behzad O, Lee CL, Gavin J, Marsh WL. A new anti-erythrocyte antibody in the Duffy system, anti-Fy4. *Vox Sang* 1973; 24:337–42.
65. Colledge KI, Pezzulich M, Marsh WL. Anti-Fy5, an antibody disclosing a probable association between the Rhesus and Duffy blood group genes. *Vox Sang* 1973; 24:193–9.
66. Chown B, Lewis M, Kaita H. The Duffy blood group in Caucasians: Evidence for a new allele. *Am J Hum Genet* 1965; 17:384–9.
67. Allen FH, Diamond LK, Niedziela B. A new blood group antigen. *Nature* 1951; 167:482.
68. Plaut G, Ikin EW, Mourant AE, et al. A new blood group antibody, anti-Jk^b. *Nature* 1953; 171:431.
69. Pinkerton FJ, Mermond LE, Liles BA, et al. The phenotype Jk(a–b–) in the Kidd blood group system. *Vox Sang* 1959; 4:155–60.
70. Heaton DC, McLoughlin K. Jk(a–b–) red blood cells resist urea lysis. *Transfusion* 1982; 22:70–1.
71. Crawford MN, Greenwalt TJ, Sasaki T, et al. The phenotype Lu(a–b–) together with unconventional Kidd groups in one family. *Transfusion* 1961; 1:228–32.
72. Sturgeon P, Metaxas-Bühler M, Metaxas M, et al. An erroneous exclusion of paternity in a Chinese family exhibiting the rare MNSs gene complexes M^k and Ms^{III}. *Vox Sang* 1970; 18:395–406.
73. McCullough J. Granulocyte antigen systems and antibodies and their clinical significance. *Hum Pathol* 1983; 14:228.
74. Moore SB. Immune thrombocytopenias and platelet antibodies. *Mayo Clin Proc* 1982; 57:778–80.
75. Decary F. Platelet antigens. *Plasma Ther Transfus Technol* 1982; 3:251–8.
76. Bach FH, van Rood JJ. The major histocompatibility complex—genetics and biology. *N Engl J Med* 1976; 295:806–13, 872–8, 927–36.
77. Carpenter CB, Strom TB. Transplantation: immunogenetic and clinical aspects—part I. *Hosp pract* 1982; 17 (Dec.):125–34.
78. Albert Ed, Bauer MP, Mayr WR. *Histocompatibility Testing 1984*. Berlin: Springer, 1984.
79. Miller WV, Rodey G. *HLA without Tears*. Chicago: Am Soc Clinical, 1981.
80. Sanfilippo F, Vaughn WK, Spees EK, et al. Benefits of HLA-A and HLA-B matching on graft and patient outcome after cadaveric-donor renal transplantation. *N Engl J Med* 1984; 311:358–64.
81. Goeken NE, Thompson JS, Corry RJ. A 2-year trial of prospective HLA-DR matching: effects on renal allograft survival and rate of transplantation. *Transplantation* 1981; 32:522–7.
82. Lundgren G, Groth CG, Albrechtsen D, et al. HLA-matching and pretransplant blood transfusions in cadaveric renal transplantation—a changing picture with cyclosporin. *Lancet* 1986; 2:66–9.
83. Oriol R, Cartron JP, Cartron J, Mulet C. Biosynthesis of ABH and Lewis antigens in normal and transplanted kidneys. *Transplantation* 1980; 29:184–8.
84. Wick MR, Moore SB. The role of the Lewis antigen system in renal transplantation and allograft rejection. *Mayo Clin Proc* 1984; 59:423–8.
85. Spitalnik S, Pfaff W, Cowles J, et al. Correlation of humoral immunity to Lewis blood group antigens with renal transplant rejection. *Transplantation* 1984; 37:265–8.
86. O'Reilly RJ. Allogeneic bone marrow transplantation: current status and future directions. *Blood* 1983; 62:941–64.

87. Thomas ED. Overview of marrow transplantation. *West J Med* 1985; 143:143–7.
88. McGlave PB. The status of bone marrow transplantation for leukemia. *Hosp Pract* 1985; 20 (Nov.):97–110.
89. Beatty PG, Clift RA, Mickelson EM, et al. Marrow transplantation from related donors other than HLA-identical siblings. *N Engl J Med* 1985; 313:765–71.
90. Hows JM, Yin JL, Marsh J, et al. Histocompatible unrelated volunteer donors in marrow transplantation for aplastic anemia and leukemia. *Blood* 1986; 68:1322–8.
91. McElligott MC, Menitove JE, Aster RH. Recruitment of unrelated persons as bone marrow donors. A preliminary experience. *Transfusion* 1986; 26:309–14.
92. McCullough J, Rogers G, Dahl R, et al. Development and operation of a program to obtain volunteer bone marrow donors unrelated to the patient. *Transfusion* 1986; 26:315–23.
93. Briggs NC, Piliavin JA, Lorenzen D, Becker GA. On willingness to be a bone marrow donor. *Transfusion* 1986; 26:324–30.
94. Duquesnoy RJ, Filip DJ, Rodey GE, et al. Successful transfusion of platelets "mismatched" for HLA antigens to alloimmunized thrombocytopenic patients. *Am J Hematol* 1977; 2:219–26.
95. Dahlke MB, Weiss KL. Platelet transfusion from donors mismatched for cross-reactive HLA antigens. *Transfusion* 1984; 24:299–302.
96. McCullough J, Clay M, Hurd D, et al. Effect of leukocyte antibodies and HLA matching and the intravascular recovery, survival, and tissue localization of 111-Indium granulocytes. *Blood* 1986; 67:522–8.
97. McDevitt HO. The HLA system and its relation to disease. *Hosp Prac* 1985; 20 (July):57–72.
98. Bryant NJ. *Disputed Paternity*. New York: Thieme-Stratton, 1980, 110–8.

4. Testing of Donor Blood

Every time a donor is bled, certain testing of the blood is mandatory, regardless of how often the donor may have given blood previously, and however detailed and complete any previous records on the donor may be. The required tests on both new and established donors include verification of ABO and Rh groups, screening for unexpected antibodies if the donor has a history of possible exposure to an immune stimulus (either as a transfusion recipient or through pregnancy), and tests to exclude transmissible disease.

Besides the tests mentioned, others may be carried out on a selective basis. Tests for antibodies to cytomegalovirus (CMV), for example, may be done on a proportion of donors. The object of such testing is to enable serologically negative donor blood to be selected for recipients most likely to be at risk of being infected by the virus (see Chap. 7).

All donor testing, along with interpretations of test results, the labeling and documentation of each donor blood component, and its storage in readiness for issue, are covered by the collective term *blood processing*.

Methods of Testing for Blood Group Antigens and Antibodies

Reactions between blood group antigens and their corresponding antibodies are most often detected by hemagglutination tests, involving the incubation of serum (as the source of antibody) with red blood cells (as the source of antigen). Some antigen-antibody reactions are detected through *direct* agglutination of the red cells by an antibody, while others require an antiglobulin test to demonstrate that the red cells have become coated with antibody during incubation. In either case, the test procedure is essentially the same, whether its purpose is to determine the antigen status of a sample of red cells using a known source of antibody or whether red cells known to possess a given antigen are being used to detect the corresponding antibody in an unknown serum. The mechanisms of hemagglutination are dealt with in Chapter 2.

Direct Agglutination in a Saline Medium

Antibodies capable of producing direct agglutination of antigen-positive cells in a saline test medium most often belong to the IgM class of immunoglobulin. The IgM molecule is large enough to span the distance between red cells suspended in saline, since it consists of five basic immunoglobulin units joined in a circular configuration. Each immunoglobulin unit possesses two antigen-combining sites; hence, there are ten such sites in the whole IgM molecule. Most antibodies that occur without a red cell–induced stimulus belong to the IgM class, as do those that occur in the early stage of a primary immune response. Most naturally-occurring antibodies react optimally at cool temperatures, but the best reactions of most immune antibodies are seen at 37°C. The

IgM form of anti-D, for instance, occurring most probably as a transient phenomenon in a primary immune response, is likely to agglutinate best at 37°C, while anti-P_1 or anti-Le^b, which are natural agglutinins, are not likely to react at 37°C. In most cases, the nonimmune antibodies mentioned react best at 4°C, although they may be detectable in tests carried out at room temperature. The same is true of the natural forms of anti-A and anti-B, which occur regularly in bloods lacking the corresponding antigen(s), but sometimes develop immune characteristics through pregnancy, or through exposure to the A and B antigens—or to substances very like them—in the environment (see Chap. 2).

HEMOLYSIS

Hemolysis of antigen-positive red cells by an antibody indicates the binding of complement by the antibody and must be taken as indicating a positive test result. It is therefore an important feature of all antibody detection tests that the test mixture is examined for hemolysis as well as agglutination after centrifugation. Hemolysis occurs more often with IgM than with IgG antibodies, because IgM is more efficient at fixing complement than IgG (see Chap. 2).

SO-CALLED INCOMPLETE ANTIBODIES

When the earliest investigators of Rh immunization found that Rh antibodies were not always capable of agglutinating Rh-positive red cells directly in a traditional saline test medium, they supposed that Rh antibodies could exist in two forms. The first form was adjudged to be *complete* in the sense of possessing the two antigen-combining sites needed to form the bridges between red cells required to produce agglutination; while the second form was called *incomplete,* based on the premise that each molecule of antibody possessed only one antigen-combining site and could therefore attach only to one red cell at a time. Later knowledge established that complete antibodies were those of the IgM class, and those called *incomplete* were IgG. The term *incomplete antibody* has persisted, even though it is apparent that the IgG molecule does possess the two antigen-combining sites needed to cause agglutination under appropriate test conditions. The failure of most IgG antibodies to agglutinate red cells directly is attributable to the size of the IgG molecule in relation to the intercellular distance in a saline test medium. By reducing that distance in some way, or by increasing the flexibility of the antibody molecule itself, some IgG antibodies can be made to agglutinate antigen-positive red cells in saline suspension.

BOVINE ALBUMIN AS A POTENTIATOR OF DIRECT AGGLUTINATION

The expectation that some "immune" antibodies will show direct agglutination of antigen-positive cells at 37°C in a medium that includes bovine albumin owes much to history. It reminds us of the experience of the mid-1940s, when the use of human or bovine albumin at an appropriate concentration was the only means whereby "incomplete" Rh antibodies could be detected directly. Bovine albumin is seldom used nowadays at a concentration comparable with that employed in the early testing, which explains why comparatively few IgG antibodies, even those of the Rh system, show agglutination before the antiglobulin phase.

The technique most commonly used to potentiate agglutination is to add two drops of bovine albumin to a mixture that comprises two drops of serum and one drop of a red cell suspension in an aqueous medium. This procedure, though widely accepted for its convenience, is accompanied by a significant loss of sensitivity in terms of the ability to detect Rh antibodies as direct agglutinins. In the above test system, using the 22 percent bovine albumin preferred in most laboratories, the final protein concentration barely exceeds 11 percent, whereas with 30 percent albumin, it will be a little above 14 percent. On the other hand, if the cells are actually *suspended* in 22 percent bovine albumin and mixed in equal proportions with the serum being tested, the protein concentration will be 14 percent, and 18 percent if 30 percent bovine albumin is substituted as the suspending medium, as in the historic screening tests of the 1940s.

Polymerized bovine albumin (usually at a concentration around 24 percent) is more effective in potentiating direct agglutination by IgG antibodies than ordinary albumin solutions, since the larger polymers act in much the same way as macromolecular additives, overcoming the disadvantage of a relatively low-protein concentration in the test mixture [1].

THE ANTIGLOBULIN TEST

By far the most consistently dependable method of detecting immune blood group antibodies is the indirect antiglobulin test, in which a reagent made from serums of animals (usually rabbits) immunized with human immunoglobulins is used to detect antibody coated to the test cells after incubation with a serum. Since this method detects antibody bound during the first stage of agglutination, the distance separating the cells in suspension is not a factor.

In preparing anti-human globulin by animal immunization, the purified human proteins are generally injected into separate colonies of rabbits. For example, human IgG is given to one set of animals, while human complement in the form of C3 is given to a separate set. When the desired immune response has been obtained, blood is drawn from the animals and allowed to clot. The serum is then separated for detailed testing against suitably coated human red cells. If necessary, the raw rabbit serum is absorbed with uncoated human red cells to remove species agglutinins, then appropriately diluted for use. In the case of a polyspecific antiglobulin serum (namely, one that contains both anti-IgG and anti-C3), the final reagent is prepared by blending optimal proportions of the different animal antibodies.

Table 4–1. Some Causes of a Positive Direct Antiglobulin Test with the Usual Pattern of Anti-Human Globulin Reactivity

Condition	Usual Protein Coating
Hemolytic disease of the newborn	IgG
Delayed hemolytic transfusion reaction	IgG
Warm autoimmune hemolytic anemia	IgG or C3 (or both)
Cold autoimmune hemolytic anemia	C3
Collagen vascular disease	C3 (reactions usually weak)
Various drug-induced phenomena	IgG or IgG and C3

Direct Antiglobulin Tests

In the direct antiglobulin test, anti-human globulin is used to detect antibody (or complement) bound to the red cells in vivo. In certain disease states, as listed in Table 4–1, IgG or C3 (or both) may be bound to the red cells, resulting in a positive direct antiglobulin test. This may be a helpful diagnostic aid in diseases like autoimmune hemolytic anemia and hemolytic disease of the newborn.

When C3 binds to circulating red cells, enzymes usually cleave the molecule to leave only the C3d component attached to the cells. Hence, a polyspecific anti-human globulin designed for direct antiglobulin testing is required to contain antibody to C3d, as well as anti-IgG. The anti-C3d component is always adjusted to a substantially lower potency level than the anti-IgG, because it is impossible to achieve a high level of anti-C3d potency without some degree of specificity. Also, since small amounts of C3d exist on human red cells even in a healthy person, an antiglobulin serum containing too much anti-C3d would be useless because it would agglutinate virtually all human red cells. Opinions differ as to whether the presence of an anti-C4 component in an anti-human globulin reagent is the main source of nonspecific reactivity, supposedly because it readily detects complement bound by cold autoagglutinins. Although it is true that an anti-C4 component does not generally contribute to the usefulness of an anti-human globulin reagent, most manufacturers do not go to the trouble and expense of absorbing anti-C4 from their products before release, unless it is observed to be giving nonspecific reactions during quality control testing.

Indirect Antiglobulin Testing

The indirect antiglobulin test is used to detect bound antibody after serum and red cells have been incubated together for an appropriate time in vitro. The principle may be applied either using red cell suspensions possessing known antigens to detect antibodies in unknown serums or using serums containing known antibodies to detect the corresponding antigens on unknown red cells.

In either case, the first step is to incubate serum and cells together for an appropriate time, during which any antibody present in the serum becomes attached to the red cells if they are positive for the appropriate antigen. Unbound human protein is then washed away by successive changes of clean saline followed by centrifugation, and the washed cells are then tested with anti-human globulin.

Whether it is necessary, in the indirect antiglobulin test, to use an antiglobulin reagent capable of detecting C3 on the cell is still a subject for debate. A few antibodies (e.g., some examples of anti-Jk^a) have been detectable only with antiglobulin reagents containing anti-C3. This leads to a perception that a polyspecific anti-human globulin is essential to the reliable detection of all clinically significant blood group antibodies. However, the presence of enough anti-C3 to meet this purpose means that some antibodies that are *not* clinically significant may bind sufficient complement to be detected, thereby delaying transfusion and necessitating an investigation that would have been avoided had anti-IgG been used for the test. Notwithstanding a theoretical possibility that anti-IgG may fail to detect an antibody that could cause a potentially serious transfusion reaction, many laboratories use anti-IgG exclusively and have not encountered serious problems. We agree with this approach. The decision is plainly one that has to be made by the physician in charge of the blood bank.

Bovine albumin, though largely discredited as a potentiator when used by the usual antibody detection test procedure, has nevertheless been reported to enhance the sensitivity of the indirect antiglobulin test [2]. This observation has not been consistently confirmed by other workers. The discrepant findings of different groups of investigators may be attributable to unsuspected but significant variability in ionic strength between the different bovine albumin reagents they used [3]. Polymerized bovine albumin, which is acknowledged to show improved ability as a potentiator of direct agglutination, has not been noted to provide any advantage over regular bovine albumin at the antiglobulin phase of the test. All things considered, we see no advantage in using bovine albumin in tests for antibody detection.

Sources of Error in Antiglobulin Testing

Since even a very small amount of unattached human globulin can neutralize the anti-human globulin, the washing phase of the test is the most critical. Failure to wash adequately, or recontamination of the washed cells with human globulin, are the most common sources of error. The procedure of adding IgG-coated cells to all antiglobulin tests interpreted as negative is an effective means to recognize this source of error, but only if the control cells are *weakly* coated with IgG (see Chap. 5). In attempting to detect complement bound to the cells, the antiglobulin test is most reliable if there is a brief period of incubation at room temperature between the addition of antiglobulin reagent to the washed cells and centrifugation. At the direction of the FDA, anti-human

Table 4-2. Causes of False Antiglobulin Tests

False Negative Tests	False Positive Tests
Failure to add anti-human globulin	Overzealous reading
Inadequate washing of the cells, or re-contamination with IgG	Detection of complement bound by non-significant antibodies
Dirty or IgG-contaminated glassware	Overcentrifugation, causing difficulty in resuspending the cells
Inadequately potent or inadvertently neutralized anti-human globulin	Bacterial contamination of reagents
Fibrin clot in test serum (which can impair the efficacy of washing by entrapping human protein)	Colloidal silica (rare nowadays)

globulin manufacturers uniformly stipulate a 5-minute period of incubation at room temperature to carry out the direct antiglobulin test in this context. It is best, however, if the test is spun and read immediately and *then* incubated for the required period before being spun and read a second time for the detection of complement, as delay may impair the reaction with IgG. This is probably because immediate centrifugation forestalls the potential neutralization of the anti-IgG by traces of unattached human IgG remaining in contact with the cells due to imperfect washing, whereas any delay allows time for some neutralization to take place. The potential causes of false antiglobulin reactions are summarized in Table 4-2.

FACTORS INFLUENCING THE SENSITIVITY OF ANTIBODY DETECTION TESTS

Incubation Time

The formation of antigen-antibody complexes from mixtures of antigen with antibodies takes time, hence some incubation period—often an extremely short one—is required in blood grouping tests. Nearly all kinetic studies show that in the common blood group reactions, most antibody binding occurs rapidly (Fig. 4-1). On the other hand, attainment of equilibrium (the point at which the amount of complex formed is equal to the amount dissociating) takes longer. As expected, the time required for an equivalent amount of antibody binding varies with the antigen and with the antibody, and is one measure of avidity. Attempts to study the kinetics of these reactions with routine blood bank methods have been disappointing, and most data have been obtained from experiments with radioactive antibody or with sensitive quantitative hemagglutination systems. In one case, for example, uptake of antibody was rapid—80 percent within 10 minutes—and reached equilibrium within an hour (see Fig. 4-1).

Reactions between anti-A and A_1 cells are even faster, but reactions with weaker subgroups of A take longer to reach equilibrium. These data suggest

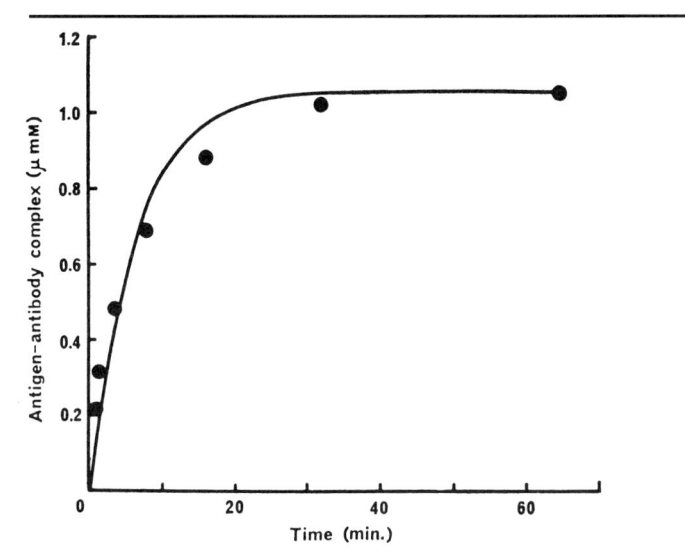

Figure 4–1
Rate of reaction between anti-c and c-positive red cells at 37°C. Note that most of the interaction takes place within the first few minutes of the incubation period. (From N. C. Hughes-Jones, *Br Med Bull* 1963; 19:174. With permission.)

that an incubation period of 15 to 60 minutes is adequate for the demonstration of most blood group antibodies. At least one clinical study has borne this out [4]. Shorter incubation periods may allow as much antibody binding as longer ones if the cells are suspended in some enhancing medium, such as low–ionic strength saline (see p. 144).

Incubation Temperature

For each blood grouping reaction, there is an optimal temperature range: (1) cold (4°C), (2) room temperature,* or (3) warm (37°C).

Almost all normal human serums contain some cold-reacting antibodies, and often all tests at 4°C are positive, making identification of specific blood-group antibodies difficult. At times, reactions that appear stronger at room temperature than at 37°C are even better in the cold, but the widespread occurrence of "nonspecific" cold autoagglutinins makes it more practical to detect some cold-agglutinating antibodies (such as anti-A, anti-Le^a and -Le^b, anti-M, and anti-P_1) at room temperature. This allows separation and identification of cold-reacting antibodies having a broader temperature range of reactivity.

Blood group antibodies that react best at body temperature (37°C) are impor-

---

*Room temperature varies from place to place, but as used by us it means 18 to 22°C. For precise work, a controlled temperature incubator may be required to maintain this range.

tant because they are usually the unexpected ones responsible for hemolytic transfusion reactions. Tests for these antibodies are essential, and require that serum-cell mixtures be incubated at 37°C. Few data are available on the optimum temperature for such reactions, but incubators must be above 35°C and below 39°C for best results.

Centrifugation

Centrifugation must be sufficient to produce a well-delineated cell button with a clear supernate, but must not pack the erythrocytes so tightly that they are difficult to dislodge and resuspend. Centrifuging at too high a speed, or for too long a time, will cause a cell button that is hard to shake out and read. This could lead equally to either a false-positive or a false-negative result.

Instructions supplied with antiserums should be followed carefully, and centrifugation times and speeds should be as recommended. We are convinced that the fixed-speed centrifuges so widely used are reliable and accurate, and that *complex routines of timer and speed calibration are an exercise in futility*. New equipment should be checked to see that it functions as expected. Thereafter, cell buttons should be looked at critically every time a test is run; and technologists should be constantly aware of the way the cells dislodge during reading. No quality control program can replace constant attention to the work at hand. The repetitive calibration of centrifuges contributes nothing to the reliability of test results.

Ratio of Antigen to Antibody

Nearly all the serologic reactions used in blood bank work depend on the principle of hemagglutination, which is very sensitive at some optimal ratio of antigen to antibody. As described in the section of Chapter 2 devoted to the prozone phenomenon, too much antibody may inhibit agglutination. This is a relatively infrequent phenomenon, however; more often, there is too little, rather than too much, antibody.

In antibody detection tests, it is common practice to mix one drop of a 2 to 5 percent red cell suspension with two drops of serum. These proportions are such that sensitivity and reactivity are adequate in almost every case, although some workers advocate as much as ten volumes of serum to one volume of cell suspension. Moore and his fellow workers, for example, have shown that increasing the ratio of serum to cells improved the detectability of some antibodies [5]. This may be an option worth considering in problem cases, but the use of large volumes of serum may not be practicable in routine work.

When typing with most commercial antiserums, it is more common to use one drop of serum instead of two to one drop of cell suspension, since in this situation the antibody is of known potency and the antiserum has been shown to be reliable by the manufacturer's recommended method of use.

For best results, the cell suspension should be closer to 2 percent than to 5

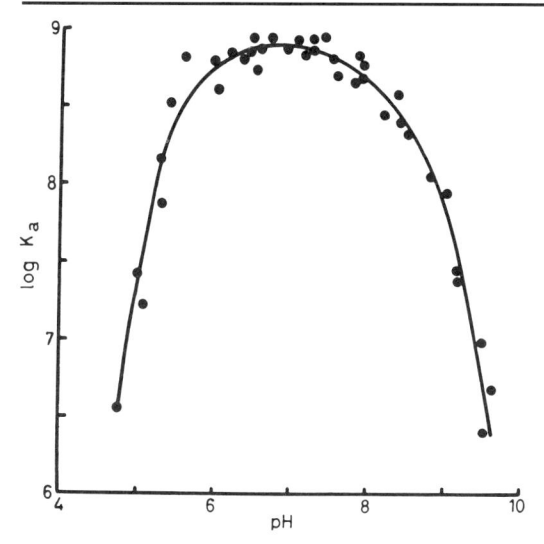

Figure 4–2
Relationship between pH and antibody uptake (expressed as the affinity constant K_a). The reaction is optimal at physiologic pH. Both high and low pH values show decreased uptake of antibody. (From N. C. Hughes-Jones, B. Garden, R. Telford, *Immunology* 1964; 7:75. With permission.)

percent. Cell suspensions of too high a concentration may lead to weak reactions or to false-negative results. We advise occasionally checking to be sure that 2 percent suspensions prepared by eye are close to their estimated concentration. Cell suspensions lower than 2 percent are not advised for routine work, although in experienced hands, a weaker suspension may improve the detectability of weak antibodies.

Where hemolysis is the endpoint, similar considerations apply. Cell suspensions that are too heavy may cause false-negative reactions.

Hydrogen Ion Concentration

The normal blood pH is about 7.42. This is close to neutral (7.0), and blood bank testing is almost always done at values near this. Even the plasma from blood in adenine-supplemented citrate-phosphate-dextrose solution, pH 6.9 to 7.2, is not too acid, and tests with it are satisfactory. At values above 8.0 or below 6.0, there is usually a loss of reactivity (Fig. 4–2). Occasional antibodies, particularly some cold-reacting ones and some examples of anti-M, react better in an acid medium [6]. Some abnormal erythrocytes, particularly those from patients with paroxysmal nocturnal hemoglobinuria, are prone to hemolysis at a low pH. This is also true when normal cells are treated with trypsin and then tested with some cold agglutinins, including autoagglutinins.

Ionic Strength of the Test Mixture

The first studies demonstrating increased antibody uptake when the test mixture is incubated in a low–ionic strength environment were published in 1964 [7–9]. The earliest practical application of that principle to enable the incubation time of antibody detection tests to be substantially shortened without compromising sensitivity did not appear until 1974. In that year, Löw and Messeter presented a report describing a new low–ionic strength solution (LISS) intended as a suspending medium for the red cells in antibody detection tests, and reducing the incubation time to only 5 minutes [10]. The low–ionic strength solution reported by these investigators contained sodium chloride at 0.03 M, with sodium glycinate at a sufficient concentration to make it iso-osmotic, enabling an ionic strength equal to 0.1 M sodium chloride to be attained in an incubating test mixture comprising one drop of serum and one drop of a 4 percent suspension of the indicator cells in LISS.

In the following years, numerous authors presented evidence supporting the use of a low–ionic strength test procedure as a means of improving antibody detectability. Some even claimed superior sensitivity for the low–ionic strength procedure, based on comparisons with conventional procedures. A more likely interpretation of these findings is that the incubation times commonly used in conventional test procedures had been too short for acceptable sensitivity all along, and that the opportunity for comparison merely exposed the deficiency. A low–ionic strength technique simply enhances antibody uptake and enables the duration of incubation to be substantially reduced while maintaining the original sensitivity.

LOW–IONIC STRENGTH ADDITIVES. The low–ionic strength test procedure described by Löw and Messeter was laborious, in that the indicator cells had first to be washed free of the medium in which they were originally suspended, then washed one further time in LISS before being resuspended to the appropriate concentration in the LISS solution. This procedure has to be repeated daily, since reagent red cells must not be *stored* in the low–ionic strength solution, and is wasteful if too many cells are prepared on any day. The technique was nevertheless adopted by many workers, sometimes with the modification that the concentration of red cells in LISS was adjusted to 2 percent, in order to allow the use of two drops of serum and two drops of cells, improving the ratio of serum to cells without affecting the ionic strength achieved in the original method. Resourceful commercial manufacturers soon provided the remedy to the inconvenience involved in having to prepare special suspensions of cells each day for antibody screening. A variety of low–ionic strength additive solutions soon became available, all formulated to achieve the desired ionic strength when used as an additive to a conventional test mixture comprising two drops of serum and one drop of cell suspension.

Some such additives contained, in addition, macromolecular substances capable of potentiating direct agglutination by some IgG antibodies. The others, being simply low ionic, did not potentiate agglutination, since one effect of lowering ionic strength is to *increase* the distance separating red cells in suspension, thereby diminishing the likelihood of agglutination.

POLYCATIONS IN THE DETECTION OF ANTIBODIES

When positively charged molecules like those of Polybrene® (hexadimethrine bromide) or protamine sulfate are added to a suspension of human red cells under appropriate conditions, the effect is to cause the cells to form rapidly into massive aggregates. The principle has been applied in automated hemagglutination tests for many years, where polycation aggregation substitutes for centrifugation as a means of bringing red cells coated with antibody into sufficiently close proximity for agglutination to take place. The same principle appears to have been applied to manual testing during the early 1950s in Germany, but it was several more years before manual adaptations of the automated polycation procedure were reported in the United States.

The low–ionic polycation (LIP) test for augmentation of hemagglutination was described by Rosenfield and his associates in 1979 [11], and a similar method was reported in the following year by Lalezari and Jiang [12]. These substantially similar methods are more cumbersome than most other manual test procedures, and call for skills that may deter all but the most adventurous and dexterous technologists. They are not easy to master, but are sensitive and require a minimum of incubation time.

Either test commences with incubation at low ionic strength, followed by centrifugation and replacement of the supernate with a solution of protamine or Polybrene, either of which immediately causes the red cells to aggregate. After a brief delay, the polycation solution is, in turn, removed and replaced by a solution that causes the aggregated cells to dissociate, which enables red cells that did not adsorb antibody during the initial incubation phase, as in a negative test, to be evenly resuspended, while those that became coated with antibody remain aggregated because of intercellular bridging that took place while the red cells were in very close proximity during the aggregation phase.

There are slight differences in the way in which the two methods are carried out, but the mechanism is essentially the same in either case. Both offer enhanced sensitivity for the detection of IgG antibodies as direct agglutinins. Even antibodies of the Duffy system, and others normally detected only by the antiglobulin technique, can show strong direct agglutination, after minimal incubation. For some reason, however, the methods are inconsistent in their ability to detect some antibodies, particularly anti-K. This limitation necessitates the retention of an antiglobulin test, which as normally applied is simply a conversion of the Polybrene test to an antiglobulin phase. This may not compensate for the deficiency in all cases. One study found an LISS antiglobulin test superior to a Polybrene antiglobulin test for compatibility testing, while another found that seven of forty examples of anti-K and two of twenty-two examples of anti-Fy^a were readily detected by a standard antiglobulin test, but not by a Polybrene antiglobulin test [13, 14]. All things considered, we recommend the low–ionic strength antiglobulin test as being the most consistently reliable method of detecting significant unexpected antibodies.

ENZYME TECHNIQUES IN SEROLOGIC TESTING

Proteolytic enzymes modify the red cell membrane in such a way as to make the cells agglutinable in a low-protein test system by certain IgG antibodies, especially those of the Rh system. The phenomenon is mostly attributable to enzymatic removal of sialic acid, which reduces the negative surface charge. Papain and ficin are the enzymes most commonly used, and the principle may be put into practice either in a one-stage or in a two-stage test. The former is the most convenient, as it merely necessitates the addition of the chosen enzyme, suitably buffered, to a conventional mixture of serum and cells. The fact that both serum and enzyme are present together in the test mixture compromises the sensitivity of the procedure because human serum possesses properties that inhibit enzyme action. For this reason, enzyme reagents intended for a one-stage test method usually contain an excess of the enzyme; but this, too, is a disadvantage, as enzymes tend to destroy the ability of immunoglobulin to agglutinate cells carrying the corresponding antigen by cleaving the IgG molecule in the vicinity of the hinge region.

In a two-stage enzyme test procedure, the indicator red cells are pretreated with a solution of the chosen enzyme, usually at about one-tenth the concentration needed for a one-stage test. The enzyme is then washed away with saline, and the treated cells are resuspended to the desired concentration in saline or some other iso-osmotic suspending medium. If this is done under aseptic conditions, the useful shelf life of the treated cells is no shorter than that of untreated cells, but such preparation is impracticable outside a commercial manufacturing environment.

A two-stage enzyme technique is readily applicable in the context of tests with screening cells or panels, as the number of individual cell suspensions to be prepared is limited, and it is no less convenient to prepare a large volume than that merely sufficient for a single test. It is not convenient, however, in the crossmatching situation, where the cells of each donor selected would have to be individually prepared.

In carrying out a two-stage enzyme test procedure, the serum is simply mixed with the suspension of enzyme-treated red cells, and the test is incubated at 37°C for at least 15 minutes (immediate spin and room temperature are superfluous with enzymes). After incubation, the cells will have settled into a gravity button and the tubes may be examined for agglutination *without* centrifugation. Centrifugation may be used following 10 to 15 minutes of incubation, but this results in cooling the mixture and enhances the reactivity of certain cold agglutinins like anti-I, anti-P_1, and the Lewis antibodies, all of which are likely to show increased reactivity in a centrifuged enzyme test. To limit the extent of enzyme treatment would overcome this disadvantage, but at the cost of diminished sensitivity, which would therefore be self-defeating.

After being examined for direct agglutination, the test mixtures may be taken to the antiglobulin phase, if required. This may occasionally result in the detection of reactions not recognized by any other means (e.g., weaker antibodies of the Kidd system). Rare instances have been noted in which an antibody showed its strongest reactivity by an enzyme-antiglobulin reaction [15]. However, some Rh antibodies detectable as direct agglutinins in an enzyme test procedure may become undetectable when the same test mixture is taken to the antiglobulin phase. In using an enzyme technique, the examination for direct agglutination is its most important aspect.

The biggest disadvantage of an enzyme technique is that certain antigens are destroyed or become nonreactive following the enzyme treatment. Since the principle of the test involves cleavage of the sialoglycoproteins, it is not surprising that antigens such as M and N do not react after the treatment, since these are borne on glycophorin A, the major sialoglycoprotein. S and s are also glycoprotein antigens, but reports vary as to the reactivity of anti-S and anti-s with enzyme-treated cells, possibly reflecting differences in the enzyme techniques used by different investigators. It appears that enzyme treatment may, on occasion, leave the S and s antigens still detectable. Some examples of anti-S, however, may show reactions resembling those of anti-U when tested against enzyme-treated cells [16]. Fy^a and Fy^b, like M and N, are also inactivated by enzyme treatment, as is the sex-linked blood group factor Xg^a.

READING OF AGGLUTINATION

Proper reading of agglutination tests is critical, particularly when positive reactions are weak. Vigorous agitation or shaking must be avoided. Agglutination may be dispersed by shaking, thereby converting a weak positive test to a negative one. The tube must be *gently* rolled between the fingers until the cell button has been completely resuspended, while constantly observing the resuspension. In positive reactions, agglutinates break away from the cell button, whereas in negative tests, free cells are seen trailing smoothly away from the cell button.

An optical aid will make reading the tests easier. Magnifying mirrors or hand lenses are most often used. With slides a microscope may be used with a low-power objective and either $10 \times$ or $5 \times$ eyepieces. Microscopic reading must be quick, as drying on the slide may be falsely interpreted as a positive test result. This problem can be minimized by the use of coverslips. Some serums may cause red cells to stick together nonspecifically. Overinterpretation of microscopic findings, especially in these cases, may cause tests to be falsely interpreted as positive.

At times, especially when the test results are doubtful, there is a temptation to recentrifuge and read the test again, or to have another observer read the test. This operation may be effective, but it is usually better to assume that the first reading is the only reliable one. Recentrifuging with the object of reading again is a bad practice, particularly in antiglobulin procedures. When there is doubt about a test result, it is always best to repeat the entire test. *Second readings are notoriously unreliable.*

In reading test results, the presence of agglutination should be recorded using a system of grading that recognizes differences in the strength of the reaction. Many laboratories have developed their own system of recording agglutination. A suitable scheme is given on page 207.

AUTOMATED TEST SYSTEMS

For over twenty years, the mass processing of donor blood has been aided by automated equipment capable of carrying out ABO and Rh tests (and, in some cases, other required testing for donors). The design of the earliest automated blood grouping equipment was aimed at the needs of large blood centers, providing the ability to process numerous samples daily under the supervision of a single operator. Serum and cells from anticoagulated blood specimens were mixed with reagent antiserums and red cells through a system of plastic tubing and glass coils in a series of parallel channels, each leading eventually to an outlet from which agglutinated or unagglutinated red cells were discharged onto a roll of absorbent paper. By examining the pattern of agglutinated and unagglutinated cells appearing in each row on the paper, the operator was able to interpret the ABO and Rh group of each specimen, and to identify each test result with the specimen to which it belonged from the positioning of the specimens in the sampling area of the instrument. In a similar fashion, the instrument also carried out a serologic test for syphilis, using a cardiolipin antigen containing carbon particles to enable flocculation of the antigen (in a positive test) to be recognized in the mixture expelled on the absorbent paper.

Automated equipment applying this principle is still in use in some blood centers, but instruments having increasingly sophisticated capabilities have been introduced in more recent years, along with others designed to meet the lighter workload of smaller centers, accordingly priced more modestly.

The newer instruments provide for the more reliable identification of specimens through the electronic reading of barcode labels, and the ability to transmit data to a computer is provided as a feature of even the least expensive of them. The numerous automated blood grouping instruments currently available (in 1987) apply varied methods in sampling, carrying out and interpreting blood grouping results. Their features are summarized in Table 4–3.

Table 4-3. Automated Blood Grouping Instruments Currently in Use in the United States

Manufacturer (alphabetical order)	Instrument*	Intended Use	Reaction Principle	Required Sample	Sample ID	Sample Dispensing Method	Reaction Vessel	Reaction Mixing Method	Reading Method
Cetus Corporation, Emeryville, CA	ProGroup™ System	ABO and Rh** grouping on donors	Agglutination	EDTA <72 hours old	Barcode reader	Automated	U-bottom wells	Agitation	Photometric/visual
Dynatech Laboratories, Inc., Chantilly, VA	MicroBank™ 220 System	ABO and Rh** grouping on donors	Agglutination	EDTA <72 hours old	Position only	Automated	U-bottom wells	Agitation	Photometric/visual
Gamma Biologicals, Inc., Houston, TX	Gamma STS-M™	ABO and Rh** grouping on donors	Streaming patterns	EDTA <48 hours old or donor anticoagulant up to exp. date	Barcode reader	Automated	Tear-shaped	Agitation	Photometric
Kontron Instruments, Inc., Everett, MA	MicroGroupamatic	ABO and Rh** grouping	Agglutination	EDTA <72 hours old	Barcode reader	Manual	U-bottom microplate	Agitation	Photometric/visual
	Groupamatic G360-C™, G2000™, MiniGroupamatic (MG-50™)	ABO and Rh grouping, including detection of D^u	Agglutination	EDTA <72 hours old	Barcode reader	Automated	U-bottom wells	Agitation	Photometric/visual
Olympus Corporation of America, Lake Success, NY	Olympus PK7100™	ABO and Rh grouping, including detection of D^u	Agglutination	EDTA <72 hours old	Barcode reader	Automated	Stepped microplate wells (amphitheater effect)	Air jet	Photometric
Technicon Instrument Corporation, Tarrytown, NY	Technicon AutoGrouper™ 16C	ABO and Rh** grouping on donors	Agglutination	EDTA <72 hours old	Barcode reader	Automated	Plastic tubing	Movement of continuous flow	Photometric
	Technicon AutoAnalyzer™ BG9 and BG15	ABO and Rh** grouping on donors	Agglutination on filter paper	EDTA <72 hours old	Position only	Automated	Plastic tubing	Movement of continuous flow	Visual only

*All instruments listed, except the Gamma STS-M, are approved for testing whole blood samples on donors only.
**Not approved by the Food and Drug Administration for detection of D^u.

Blood Grouping

A critical part of blood processing is the determination of the ABO blood group and the Rh(D) type of each donor unit, since the results of these tests will be recorded on the label and will be used in selecting the blood for a recipient. Such testing must be carried out with antiserums that meet FDA requirements. It is unnecessary to consider blood groups other than ABO and D in the process of selection, except in the case of patients who have already produced one or more antibodies in response to pregnancy or to an earlier transfusion. Hence, red cell typing beyond that mentioned is not carried out as a matter of routine on all donors, but may be done to meet the needs of a particular recipient, or to compile a list of donors known to be negative for other antigens. Such negative phenotypes may be useful for patients with blood group antibodies.

Blood group testing may be carried out manually or by an automated test procedure, depending on the resources of the donor center and its needs. It would be hard to cope with grouping several hundred donors each day without the aid of automation; and difficult to justify the cost of automated equipment where the number of donors is considerably less. Yet all blood drawing centers, large and small, must complete the processing of donors as soon after drawing as possible. To this end, microplate techniques have been adopted in smaller blood banks as a means of improving the efficiency with which blood grouping tests are completed.

Conventional tube test methods are preferred in many laboratories, and a diminishing number still use slides. Slide tests are convenient because they can be interpreted almost immediately without using a centrifuge. On the other hand, there are several disadvantages. For example, exposure to the air on a slide causes drying of the reaction mixture, leading to pseudoagglutination and the possibility of false-positive test results. This limits the ability to extend incubation as a means to allow weaker reactions to develop, and makes a slide test procedure particularly unsuitable for the ABO reverse (serum) grouping test. Drying is especially likely to occur in Rh tests carried out on slides, since these must be incubated with the aid of a heated Rh view box, which accelerates the evaporation of fluid from the test mixture.

ABO BLOOD GROUPING

ABO grouping tests are always carried out using both serum and red cells from the test specimen. Because anti-A and anti-B occur naturally in the serum whenever the corresponding antigen is absent from the red cells, the ABO blood group of a sample can, in theory, be determined either by testing the cells with anti-A and anti-B (*forward grouping*) or by testing the serum with group A and group B cells (*reverse grouping*). In practice, variable strength in the natural agglutinins, as well as the possible presence of other agglutinins in the serum, make the reverse grouping test less consistently dependable than for-

Table 4–4. The Most Commonly Observed Reaction Patterns
in ABO Blood Grouping Tests (Forward and Reverse)

Forward (Cell) Grouping		Reverse (Serum) Grouping		Blood Group
Anti-A	Anti-B	A_1 Cells	B Cells	
+	0	0	+	A
0	+	+	0	B
+	+	0	0	AB
0	0	+	+	O

ward grouping. Taken together, however, the results of cell and serum grouping tests complement each other and provide a means of recognizing false or misleading results.

The common patterns of reaction observed in ABO grouping are listed in Table 4–4.

Cell (Forward) Grouping

The red cells of donors must be tested at each donation with anti-A and anti-B serums. A test with anti-A,B (group O) serum is also commonly done as a means of recognizing weak subgroups of the ABO system. The anti-A and anti-B in group O serums agglutinate cells belonging to certain subgroups more strongly than the antibodies in A and B serums; some subgroups, indeed, are recognized *only* by a positive reaction with anti-A,B serum. The A_x subgroup is the one most commonly considered to justify testing with anti-A,B serum, but A_x is exceedingly rare and of debatable significance. Agglutination of A_x cells by anti-A,B is comparatively feeble, and usually develops only after a period of incubation at room temperature, so A_x is frequently missed, even by anti-A,B testing. There is one report of a case in which a hemolytic transfusion reaction occurred when a unit of A_x blood was given to a group O recipient [17]. The lack of similar reports may indicate that this was an exceptional event, despite the difficulty that exists in consistently recognizing the A_x phenotype. It is hard to rationalize testing *all* donor bloods routinely with anti-A,B serum. On the other hand, we believe the use of anti-A,B to confirm donor bloods that appear to be group O is justified, because units labeled as group O may be transfused in emergencies without crossmatching.

Serum (Reverse) Grouping

Testing the serum of all donors against A and B cells enables the expected antibodies of the ABO system to be detected, and provides confirmation of reactions obtained in forward grouping. The group A cells must be of the A_1 subgroup. Red cells of the A_2 phenotype may be used as an optional *extra* test, if desired, but not as a substitute for A_1. We do not recommend the inclusion of a test with A_2 or with O cells as part of reverse grouping, because this creates as many problems as it solves.

Commercial reverse grouping cells are always Rh-negative, supposedly to avoid any complication that might be caused by the presence of a saline-reactive Rh antibody in the serum being tested. This is an unnecessary precaution. In fact, Rh-positive cells are perfectly satisfactory for reverse grouping.

THE INVESTIGATION OF DISCREPANT REACTIONS

The purpose of carrying out both cell and serum grouping tests in the determination of ABO groups is to strengthen the reliability of the final test result by taking advantage of Landsteiner's Law. If serum grouping confirms the results obtained in cell grouping, the likelihood of error is considerably reduced. If the results of cell and serum grouping are discrepant, there may be an erroneous reaction in some part of the test, and the possibility exists that the ABO group of the blood could be interpreted incorrectly. Any such discrepancy must be investigated and resolved before a conclusion is reached as to the ABO group of the blood being tested, and before the donor unit is labeled.

Since discrepant reactions may be caused by technical errors in carrying out the test, the specimen should simply be retested before embarking on a complex investigation that may not be required. Retesting should be carried out with conscious attention to the errors of technique most likely to occur in ABO grouping. Both serum and cells must be tested, and this time the cells may be washed in several changes of isotonic saline before being suspended in saline for testing. This, in itself, will eliminate some of the more obvious causes of discrepant results, and may enable the problem to be resolved without additional testing.

The most common technical errors in forward and reverse ABO grouping tests are listed in Table 4–5.

If the results of retesting the cells and serum are not discrepant, the ABO group may be interpreted; no further investigation is necessary. If the discrepant reactions persist, however, they are most likely to be attributable to some unusual characteristic of the test sample, affecting either the red cells or the serum and giving rise to aberrant reactions in the forward or reverse grouping test, or in both. Further investigation of the problem must be approached objectively, without drawing a premature conclusion as to whether the unexpected reactions are those observed in the cell or the serum grouping test. While it is true that the cell grouping results are most often correct, this is not invariably the case. It may be necessary to test the cells with additional antiserums (most often anti-A_1 and anti-H) to determine their subgroup status. In addition, the serum may have to be tested against A_2 and selected group O cells, as well as A_1 and B cells in the reverse grouping test. In such a case, an autologous control test is a useful means to enable a cold autoagglutinin to be

Table 4–5. The Most Common Technical Errors in Forward and Reverse ABO Grouping

Source of Technical Error*	Observed Result
Incorrect matching of reverse grouping results from one test sample with forward grouping results from another	Uninterpretable test results
Incorrect recording of one or more test reactions	Uninterpretable test results
Failure to add serum from the test sample to one or more of the tubes in the reverse grouping test	False negative
Failure to add antiserum to one or more tubes in the forward grouping test (unlikely, as antiserums are colored to prevent this error)	False negative
Failure to recognize hemolysis as being equivalent to a positive test	False negative
Improper ratio of serum to cells	False positive or false negative
Improper warming of the test mixture	False negative
Over- or undercentrifugation, leading to either a cell button that is hard to resuspend, or one too easily dispersed	False positive or false negative
Bacterial or serologic contamination of antiserums or reverse grouping cells	False positive or false negative

*The first two sources of error listed occur frequently. The others are less common.

recognized. The identification of a cold-reactive alloagglutinin may be aided by extending the incubation time to 30 minutes or longer, and perhaps by reducing the incubation temperature to 4°C, as a means of enhancing its reactivity.

The most common sources of discrepant ABO grouping results are listed in Table 4–6, in each case, with brief details of the features that will enable them to be recognized.

Further Testing to Resolve Discrepancies

COLD AUTOAGGLUTININ IN THE TEST SERUM. When discrepant ABO grouping is caused by a cold autoagglutinin in the serum of the test sample, thorough washing of the red cells in warm saline should permit the correct results to be obtained in forward grouping. The specificity of the autoagglutinin will most often be anti-I, which can readily be absorbed using group O red cells to leave a serum that should give the expected reactions with A and B red cells, according to the ABO group of the test sample.

FACTORS CAUSING ROULEAUX IN THE TEST SERUM. This is not a common problem in testing blood from healthy donors. When rouleaux are observed, however,

Table 4–6. The Most Commonly Encountered Causes of Discrepant ABO Grouping Tests and Their Effects on Test Results

Source of Discrepant Test Results	Effect on Red Cells in Forward Grouping Test	Effect on Serum in Reverse Grouping Test
Cold autoagglutinin in the test serum	False positive if cells are tested unwashed or suspended in their own serum or plasma	False positive
Protein imbalance* or intravenous use of substance causing rouleaux formation	False positive if cells are tested unwashed or suspended in their own serum or plasma	False positive
Antibody in test serum to dye in antiserum (e.g., tartrazine)	False positive if cells are tested unwashed or suspended in their own serum or plasma	None
Antibody in test serum directed at an ingredient in suspending medium used for reverse grouping cells (e.g., Neomycin chloramphenicol, EDTA)	None	False positive
Alloantibody in test serum that is active as an agglutinin in a saline test system at room temperature	None	False positive with any reverse grouping cells positive for the relevant antigen
Weak or absent expected agglutinin(s) in test serum, caused by immunodeficiency* or age (newborn or elderly)	None	False negative with either or both reverse grouping cells
Weakly expressed antigen on test cells (as in subgroups)	False negative	Misleading positive reaction if an unexpected alloantibody is present (e.g., anti-H, anti-A_1)

*These causes of discrepant reactions are unlikely to be encountered when testing normal healthy donors.

washing the test red cells should enable correct results to be obtained in the forward grouping test. The presence of rouleaux may still make it difficult to interpret the reverse grouping test straightforwardly, but by replacing the supernatant serum with saline after centrifugation, it may be possible to disperse rouleaux and obtain correct reverse grouping results. An alternative course of action is to test doubling dilutions of the test serum with group O cells to determine the lowest dilution at which rouleaux formation is no longer occurring. If the expected antibodies are of normal potency, it may be possible to obtain correct reverse grouping results by testing the serum against reverse grouping cells at the determined dilution.

ANTIBODY IN THE TEST SERUM DIRECTED AT A COLORING AGENT. Two yellow dyes (tartrazine and acriflavine), both used as coloring agents in anti-B serums, have been implicated in reports of false-positive reactions that do not occur when the test cells are washed before testing. The reverse grouping test gives the correct reactions.

ANTIBODY IN TEST SERUM DIRECTED AT AN INGREDIENT IN THE CELL-SUSPENDING MEDIUM. Antibodies to the antibiotics commonly used as preservatives in commercial Reagent Red Blood Cell suspending mediums, or to EDTA (sometimes included in the formulation to prevent hemolysis in the reverse grouping test) may cause false-positive reactions in the reverse grouping test only. Forward grouping will give correct results (unless the test cells are suspended in a medium containing the offending substance). Correct reverse grouping is obtainable by the simple expedient of washing the A and B cells and resuspending them in isotonic saline for testing.

AGGLUTINATING ALLOANTIBODY IN THE TEST SERUM. Unexpected alloantibodies such as anti-P_1, anti-Le^a and anti-Le^b, and anti-M are relatively common, and may occasionally be strong enough to interfere with the reverse grouping test. In such cases, the forward grouping results are correct, but the reverse grouping results may not correspond if one or both cells possess the antigen at which the antibody is directed. The discrepancy is easily resolved by testing the serum against a panel of group O cells at room temperature to identify the antibody responsible. Valid reverse grouping results can then be obtained by using reverse grouping cells that lack the relevant antigen.

WEAK OR ABSENT EXPECTED AGGLUTININ(S) IN TEST SERUM. In such conditions as agammaglobulinemia, or hypogammaglobulinemia, the expected agglutinins of the ABO system may be absent or depleted.

If the expected antibodies are merely reduced in potency, it may be possible to demonstrate their presence by extending incubation of the reverse grouping test to 30 minutes or longer, or by lowering the temperature of incubation to

4°C. This may create a further problem by enhancing the reactivity of some unexpected alloantibody besides, but a useful control would be to test a set of group O screening cells in parallel with the group A and group B cells, and to regard the reverse grouping test as valid only if the group O cells are negative. An autologous control test will recognize activity due to an autoagglutinin that may be brought to light by incubation at low temperature. If anti-A or anti-B cannot be demonstrated, it will be necessary to interpret the ABO group from the forward grouping test alone.

SUBGROUPS, WITH OR WITHOUT UNEXPECTED ALLOANTIBODIES. Subgroups of both A and B may be associated with weak expression of the antigen, and sometimes with the presence of an unexpected antibody that may be the cause of the discrepant reaction by which the anomaly is recognized. Bloods of the A_2 subgroup, for example, may have anti-A_1 in the serum in approximately 2 percent of cases; in A_2B, the incidence of anti-A_1 is as high as 26 percent. Serums from people of the A_1 and A_1B subgroups may contain anti-H. The antibodies mentioned are seldom as potent as the expected antibodies of the system, but when detectable in tests carried out at room temperature, they may confuse the interpretation of the test. Subgroups of B are less common than subgroups of A, but present similar features (see p. 91).

Aids to the resolution of problems associated with subgroups may include testing the cells with anti-A_1 (and possibly also with anti-H), as well as identifying the unexpected antibody as anti-A_1. In the case of very weak expression of A, as in the subgroup A_x, agglutination of the red cells may occur only with anti-A,B serums, and even that is likely to be weak and to require a period of incubation to develop.

RH TYPING

Testing for the D Antigen

The D antigen is known to be strongly immunogenic; therefore, it is important to protect D-negative recipients from making anti-D by giving them only D-negative blood. Accordingly, routine blood processing includes testing for D with an antiserum that is capable of detecting D by direct agglutination, and can also react by the antiglobulin test with the weaker forms of D known collectively as D^u. Since the vast majority of people who are D-negative do *not* have anti-D in their serum, there is no confirmatory serum test, as in ABO grouping, and the accuracy of the result depends on the care with which the test with one antiserum is carried out. Although potentiated high-protein antiserums have the disadvantage of being pronc to causc spontaneous agglutination of red cells coated with immunoglobulin, they are the most suitable reagents to use for Rh typing of donor blood. Such antiserums show strong reactivity by whatever test procedure they are used, and in tube or microplate tests commonly agglutinate D-positive red cells directly on centrifugation without incubation. The presence of immunoglobulin on the red cells seldom causes error among healthy blood donors. When it does, the only consequence is that a D-negative donor unit is labeled as D-positive, which errs on the side of safety. Accordingly, although a control test to detect spontaneous agglutination is mandatory when testing recipients, it is commonly and appropriately omitted when testing donors.

THE D^u TEST. If a donor's red cells fail to agglutinate directly when tested for the D antigen, a test for weaker forms of D is required before concluding that the blood is D-negative and labeling the donor unit accordingly. The test for D^u involves incubating a suspension of the donor's red cells with a suitable anti-D serum for a specified period (usually 15 minutes) at 37°C, then washing the cells preparatory to carrying out an antiglobulin test. This may be done with either a polyspecific anti-human globulin or anti-IgG. If the test gives a negative result, the donor is D-negative, and the unit may accordingly be labeled Rh-negative. If agglutination occurs at the antiglobulin phase of the test, a *direct antiglobulin test* (DAT) is carried out. If the DAT is negative, the D^u test is confirmed to be positive, and the blood is labeled Rh-positive. If the DAT is positive, the cells were coated with IgG in vivo, and the test for D^u cannot be interpreted. This is of no importance, however, because such a unit would not be released for transfusion.

Testing for Other Rh Antigens

RH-NEGATIVE. A practice that has now been discontinued in the United States is that of testing all D-negative donor blood for the presence of the C and E antigens. The purpose of such testing was to recognize donor units having C or E in the absence of D, with the object of labeling them Rh-positive. This policy was founded on the principle that D-negative recipients, most of whom lack C and E, as well as D, must be protected from receiving C-positive or E-positive blood. The C and E antigens, however, are substantially less immunogenic than D. There is no evidence that they are any more likely to bring about an immune response in D-negative recipients than in D-positives, to whom C-positive and/ or E-positive blood is given without a second thought. Therefore, the practice of treating these donors as Rh-positive is without merit.

RH-POSITIVE. The frequency with which antibodies to the Rh antigens other than D are produced after transfusion does not justify *routinely* typing donors and recipients for these antigens. E and c are the Rh antigens after D that most often cause an immune response, but even to take these into account in the routine selection of donor blood is unnecessary.

Typing for Antigens of Other Blood Group Systems

After D, the antigen most likely to produce an immune response in a susceptible recipient is probably K, of the Kell blood group system. That is not to say, however, that recipients and donors should be routinely tested for K, and that donor blood should be selected accordingly.

Selective Additional Antigen Typing

In presenting arguments against the practice of testing donors *routinely* for antigens other than A,B and D, it is not our intention to condemn the practice of testing donors for other antigens as a means of preparing a list of people who are known to be negative for certain antigens. Recipients who have produced a clinically significant antibody have to be given blood lacking the corresponding antigen; and if they have made *more than one* antibody, the choice may be very limited unless there is a list of available donors who have been tested and are known to be negative for the relevant antigens. In deciding which donors to test, it is sensible to choose those of group O, whose red cells can be given to recipients of any ABO group, and to give preference to people having a consistent record of attendance as a donor. This ensures that the labor and the antiserums involved are put to the best possible use. If extensive additional testing is contemplated, it is an economy to carry out Rh phenotyping first, as a means of restricting further typings to donors already established to be c-negative or e-negative, or to those known to be dce. If the cells of selected donors are to be tested for K, Fy^a and Fy^b, Jk^a and Jk^b, etc., it is most advantageous if these are all DCe, DcE, or dce, since the typed blood will then be equally useful for recipients who have made multiple antibodies that include an Rh specificity.

Antigens of High Frequency

If a recipient produces an antibody to a high-frequency antigen, no effort should be spared to obtain one or more blood donations to be used in the preparation of an antiserum. Once such a serum becomes available in quantity, there is a strong obligation on any blood center having the necessary resources to undertake systematic screening for donors whose cells lack the antigen in question. Alternatively, the serum should be passed on to a blood center that *does* have the necessary resources, rather than being stored away in the freezer as a valuable but neglected resource. The availability of donor blood for immunized patients through a rare-donor registry is wholly dependent on using such serums to screen for donors who can be available when needed.

Quality Control of Blood Typing Procedures

It is a sound practice that all antiserums be tested on each day of use against red cells of appropriate phenotypes, in each case to demonstrate both a positive and a negative reaction. A cell suspension possessing weak expression of the relevant antigen is preferable as the positive control to one having strong expression. In blood group systems other than ABO, this normally implies heterozygous expression, although if cells known to have even weaker expression of the antigen are available, they would be more suitable.

In the case of ABO grouping, the tests largely control themselves, in that the results of forward and reverse grouping complement each other and provide a means to recognize unexpected or aberrant results. Elaborate testing to verify the potency and specificity of the reagents is not indicated, but may be required by some accreditation agencies.

Quality control testing is obviously of greatest importance in smaller laboratories, where a vial of antiserum may last for several days and the widest range of possible phenotypes may not be encountered frequently. In large and small laboratories alike, it is important for the quality control testing to be carried out by the test methods used in the regular routine. It is also essential that the results of all quality control testing not only be systematically recorded in a laboratory workbook but be scrutinized regularly by someone in authority, so that appropriate corrective measures can be taken if any reagent is performing unsatisfactorily. Daily quality control testing is not undertaken solely to satisfy inspectors from the various regulatory agencies that drop in from time to time. The true purpose is to facilitate early recognition of reagent problems that may give rise to erroneous results. That purpose is not fulfilled if the results are merely recorded slavishly in a book that nobody ever reviews, and if the significance of those results is only vaguely understood.

Detection of Blood Group Antibodies (Antibody Screening)

The screening of donor serums is required at each donation on all donors with a history of exposure (such as pregnancy or blood transfusion) that could have resulted in their making a blood group antibody. Many laboratories find it more convenient to test serums from all donors for antibodies, as this is less trouble than selecting on the basis of history. This practice also ensures that an unreliable history does not cause a significant antibody to go unrecognized.

Unlike the situation in screening recipients (see p. 181), it is permissible to use a pool of screening cells representing the required antigens, because sensitivity is less important when screening donors. Testing is carried out by incubating each donor serum with the indicator cells at 37°C, then examining for hemolysis and agglutination before proceeding to the antiglobulin test.

The reasons for blood collection facilities to test for antibodies in donors are as follows:

1. A proper antibody screening test will detect donor antibodies that might impair the survival of the recipient's own red cells, or those of another donor when transfused to the same recipient.
2. Whether or not the antibody detected by screening is potentially harmful to

a recipient's red cells, its presence identifies a donor whose red cells lack the corresponding antigen. This information contributes toward maintaining a list of donors whose blood is suitable for selection in emergencies for patients who have made antibodies.
3. Again, whether or not the antibody is significant, the donor's plasma may provide a useful and recurring source of raw material for a reagent that can be used in further antigen typings, assuming it is of acceptable potency. This is of particular value when the specificity is one that is not available commercially, or is rare. Such a resource should be shared liberally with any blood center having the capability and willingness to join in the search.
4. Donors may later be patients. Prior knowledge that the serum has been found to contain a blood group antibody may save time if a transfusion is indicated.
5. The discovery of a "new" antibody, and a study of the antigen it detects may be of scientific interest.

When an antibody detection test has been done, the container label should state the result, whether positive or negative. If positive, the specificity of the antibody should be stated, whether determined by the blood drawing center itself or by a consulting laboratory.

USE OF DONOR BLOOD CONTAINING UNEXPECTED ANTIBODIES

When unexpected antibodies are detected in the serum of a donor, it is advisable to remove the plasma and use the unit as red blood cells, preferably washed. In blood banks equipped to freeze and reconstitute red cells, the red blood cells from units that contain unexpected antibodies may be frozen. These may be useful because of their negative phenotype, and will contain almost no trace of the original plasma. This is also true of washed red blood cells.

Tests for Transmissible Disease

At the present time, testing for transmissible disease on donors may include serologic tests for syphilis, for hepatitis B surface antigen (HBsAg), for antibody to human immunodeficiency virus (anti-HIV), for antibody to hepatitis B core antigen (anti-HBc), and for alanine aminotransferase (ALT), an enzyme released when liver cells are destroyed, as would be occurring in chronic hepatitis. Although the presence of anti-HBc and an elevated level of ALT are not directly associated with non-A,non-B hepatitis, there is a statistical relationship that is considered to justify the adoption of the two tests as a means of reducing the incidence of transfusion-associated hepatitis, pending recognition of the causative agent(s) of non-A,non-B hepatitis and the development of a suitable specific screening test [18–20]. The term *surrogate testing* is applied to describe indirect measures of this kind. Table 4–7 summarizes the tests currently used to screen for donors that may be carriers of disease.

Table 4-7. Tests Used to Screen Donor Blood for Transmissible Disease

Test for	Required By	Recommended By
Syphilis	FDA	
HBsAg	FDA and AABB	
Anti-HIV	AABB	FDA
Anti-HBc	AABB	
ALT	AABB	
Anti-CMV		AABB*

*In special situations.

The tests used to screen donor bloods for infectious agents, or for antibodies to them, are not sensitive enough to detect the infective or carrier state in all cases. In the case of the hepatitis B surface antigen, for example, Alter and his associates found that as few as 10^6 particles per milliliter could infect chimpanzees [21]. It would be surprising if the tests currently used have the required sensitivity to detect so few particles; hence, it is to be expected that some potentially infective donors go unrecognized. Tests for other infective agents also have their limitations, and those that detect only antibody to a virus have limitations of another kind. The presence of antibody merely indicates past exposure to the virus. It does not always signify that the blood is infectious now.

It is important always to handle human blood and any components and products derived from it as though they could be infectious. Scrupulous attention to cleanliness and sanitary conditions is necessary in all laboratories where human blood is handled. Blood from donors found to give a confirmed positive test result for infectious agents must be autoclaved or incinerated before being disposed of (see Addenda).

SEROLOGIC TESTS FOR SYPHILIS

The causative organism of syphilis, *Treponema pallidum,* may be in the blood of apparently healthy donors, even when their serum is nonreactive by any of the serologic tests for syphilis. The organism is delicate, however, and does not survive refrigerated storage for more than 96 hours; hence, transmission of the infection from donor to recipient is limited to transfusions of fresh blood or components. This is a very rare complication of transfusions (see Chap. 7).

The methods most commonly used to test for syphilis are the Venereal Disease Reference Laboratory (VDRL) and the rapid plasma reagin (RPR) tests. Both use cardiolipin antigen, which is prepared by alcohol extraction of normal beef heart. The fact that the antigen is not prepared from material containing the causative organism means that neither test is truly specific, but these and tests like them have proved sensitive and reliable over the years for the detection of treponemal infection.

Of the two test procedures, the RPR test is the easier to carry out and interpret. Unlike VDRL antigen, which has to be prepared by adding a measured volume of saline buffered at a pH that is critical to the accurate performance of the test, the RPR antigen is already made up and usually contains charcoal particles to facilitate recognition of the flocculation that occurs in a positive test. Serums known to be reactive, weakly reactive, and negative should be tested in parallel with each batch of tests, both by way of quality control and to provide known reactions with which to compare unknowns.

TESTS FOR HEPATITIS B SURFACE ANTIGEN

With the accumulation of overwhelming evidence associating a positive test for HBsAg with the transmission of posttransfusion hepatitis came the adoption of the test as a requirement on all blood donations. When such routine testing first began, in 1972, the test was carried out by counterelectrophoresis, a more sensitive adaptation of the simple gel diffusion procedure by which HBsAg was initially recognized.

The test methods mentioned are now history, having soon been replaced by more consistently sensitive procedures, as measured by their ability to recognize all the samples containing HBsAg that comprise the FDA reference panel. The more sensitive tests mentioned are referred to as *third-generation tests*. Several were developed, and screening by one or another of them became mandatory in 1975. The first third-generation test to be introduced was the radioimmunoassay (RIA); but currently, increasing numbers of tests are carried out by the enzyme-linked immunosorbent assay (ELISA).

Radioimmunoassay

RIA tests for HBsAg are founded on the sandwich method of Ling and Overby, a solid-phase procedure that may vary according to the surface used as the carrier to which anti-HBs is bound [22]. One popular method uses plastic beads, whereas others use columns, tubes, or microplates in various configurations.

In the plastic bead method, each serum to be tested is incubated with a coated bead, during which time HBsAg, if present in the serum, becomes bound to the antibody coating the bead. The beads are then washed to remove unattached protein and fluid, and ^{125}I-labeled anti-HBs is added. In a positive test, the radioactive antibody attaches to the antigen bound during incubation and may be detected by means of a gamma radiation counter. In a negative test, where no antigen is bound during incubation, no radioactive antibody is taken up.

The method is very sensitive and quite specific, but suffers from the disadvantage that it involves the handling and disposal of radioactive materials. Proper precautions must be taken in handling all radioactive solutions and radioactively contaminated solid materials. Beads, plates, or tubes must be autoclaved and then disposed of as required by the Nuclear Regulatory Commission, either by storage in appropriate containers until the radioactivity has decayed sufficiently (about 6 months for ^{125}I) or by removal by a licensed disposal company.

Enzyme-Linked Immunosorbent Assay

The ELISA is essentially similar to the RIA, except that the anti-HBs added after incubation is labeled with an enzyme, instead of ^{125}I. As in the RIA, this attaches to any HBs that becomes bound during incubation in a positive test, and remains bound during washing. A substrate is then added, which is oxidized in the presence of the enzyme, resulting in a color change if the test result is positive. The density of color is measured in a spectrophotometer, and the result is interpreted by comparing the absorbance of each unknown with that shown by several (usually three) negative control serums.

This test procedure, like the RIA, has excellent sensitivity and specificity. Both can be read objectively; automated equipment is available that can read the tests and print out the results. A method using a plastic bead coated with anti-HBsAg is illustrated in Fig. 4–3.

Test for Antibody to Hepatitis B Core Antigen

The most commonly used test for anti-HBc is an ELISA based on competitive inhibition of the reaction between hepatitis B core antigen and an antibody to it (anti-HBc). An inert plastic carrier (wells in a tray, test tubes, plastic beads, etc.) is coated with hepatitis B core antigen prepared from infected tissues or, more commonly, by recombinant DNA technology. This antigen-coated carrier is incubated with a mixture of the serum (or plasma) to be tested and a reagent consisting of anti-HBc that has been conjugated with horseradish peroxidase. Antibodies, both from the reagent and from the patient's serum, bind to the antigen-coated carrier. The unbound material is washed away, a reagent that develops color in the presence of horseradish peroxidase is added, and the amount of color read in a spectrophotometer. If the patient's serum contains *no* anti-HBc, all the HBc sites on the carrier bind peroxidase-labeled reagent anti-HBc, resulting in the development of an intense color. Anti-HBc, if present in the test serum, competes for antigen with the labeled anti-HBc, so that less labeled anti-HBc is bound, and correspondingly less color is developed. Thus in a competitive inhibition test, more color is a *negative* test and less color indicates a *positive* test. Most samples are clearly negative or positive, although in some cases, there is difficulty evaluating results near the cutoff value that separates negative from positive.

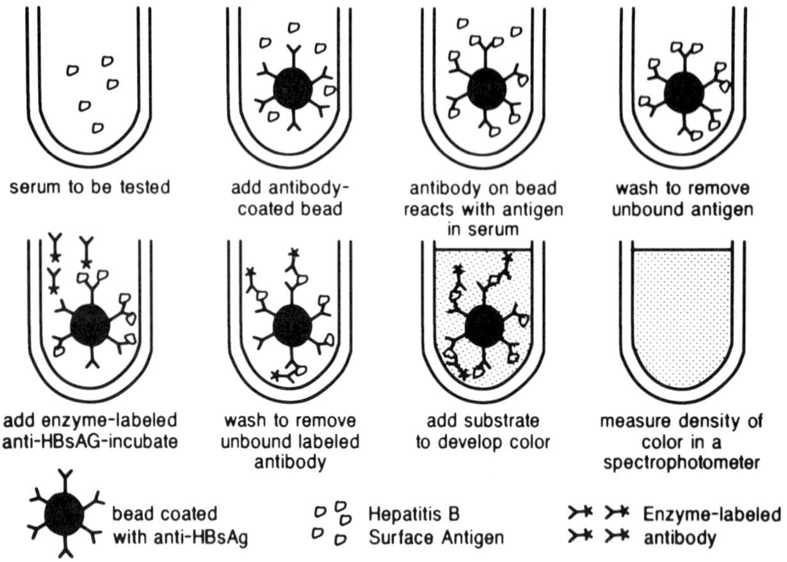

Figure 4-3
Enzyme-linked immunosorbent assay (ELISA) procedure using a bead coated with anti-HBsAg. If hepatitis B surface antigen is present in the test serum, it becomes bound to the bead during incubation, and then takes up enzyme-labeled anti-HBsAg in the next phase of the test. Unbound anti-HBsAg is then washed away and a substrate is added that causes color to develop in the presence of the enzyme label. The color is then measured spectrophotometrically. Absence of color indicates a negative test because no HBsAg was present to bind the labeled antibody.

TEST FOR ANTIBODY TO HUMAN IMMUNODEFICIENCY VIRUS

The principle of the test for anti-HIV is basically similar to that of the ELISA test for HBsAg, except that the protein bound in solid phase is *antigen,* rather than antibody, in this case derived from multiple antigens of the virus, disrupted and purified. Anti-HIV, if present in a serum being tested, binds to one or more antigens during the incubation phase, and remains bound during washing to remove free protein. Enzyme-labeled anti-human globulin is then added, which attaches itself to any human globulin present on the test surface, and the enzyme label is detected by the color change that takes place through oxidation when the substrate is added.

Any serum that yields an initially reactive result must be retested to establish whether it is repeatably reactive. Blood drawn from repeatably reactive donors must not be used for transfusion. It, and any associated samples, test materials, etc., must be discarded after first being autoclaved to destroy any infectious agents that may be present.

A reactive test for anti-HIV is not diagnostic of AIDS, nor does a negative test exclude infection with HIV. Serums that show repeatably reactive tests may be subjected to additional testing, such as for antibodies to specific virus proteins by the Western Blot technique. Due to the sensitivity of the test procedure, a proportion of reactive serums will be found *not* to contain antibody to HIV. The rate of false reactivity is dependent on the sensitivity of the test kit being used for screening, but is also influenced by the prevalence of anti-HIV in the population from which the test samples are drawn.

TESTING FOR ALANINE AMINOTRANSFERASE

A test now being carried out as one of two surrogate tests intended to reduce the incidence of transfusion-associated hepatitis, in particular non-A,non-B hepatitis, is quantitation of ALT. This enzyme is released when hepatic tissue is damaged; hence, a level of ALT that is higher than normal may be indicative of a chronic infection of the liver, and in turn, may suggest a carrier state of hepatitis. The test is a straightforward chemical determination that is easily automated. Although studies have shown a clear relationship between elevated levels of ALT in the donor and hepatitis in the recipient there is no specific level of donor ALT that separates high-risk from low-risk donors. For this reason it has been difficult to select a value for ALT above which donors are considered unacceptable, and cutoff values separating acceptable from unacceptable donor units may vary from blood bank to blood bank or from region to region.

TESTING FOR ANTIBODY TO CYTOMEGALOVIRUS

Although ELISA test kits are available to test for anti-CMV, the test is most often carried out by a latex agglutination procedure. The screening procedure for anti-CMV is not mandatory, and is normally applied selectively to a sufficient proportion of donors bled to yield a supply of known seronegative units from which to draw when needed.

The incidence of anti-CMV among healthy donors varies depending on age, geographic location, and socioeconomic status. For example, in one metropolitan area, CMV antibodies were found in 25 percent of donors under the age of 36. As donor age increased, the percentage of anti-CMV positive persons increased to a high of 70 percent. In most donor populations, the incidence of anti-CMV-positive donors is about 30 to 40 percent. Donor units found to be reactive are suitable for transfusion, but should not be selected for recipients considered to be at risk if they contract the infection (see Chap. 7).

Recording of Laboratory Results

Test results must be recorded accurately and systematically, using a form that permits the entry of symbols denoting actual observation as the tests are carried out and read. It is important to make a clear distinction between *observations* and *interpretations,* using symbols to recognize differing degrees of agglutination, if present, or to denote its absence. Each observation must be recorded *directly* into the laboratory work record, whether or not it coincides with the expected test result. No test results should be written on scraps of paper with the intention of transferring them into the official record later, perhaps when some unexpected result has been resolved. Although this practice generates *tidier* records, it can lead to serious transcription errors.

The work record should allow space to enter the identity of the personnel who carried out, read, and interpreted the tests. Space should be provided to enter the identity of all reagents used, with lot numbers, in case some unexpected reaction necessitates tracing the source, and possibly investigating further any bloods tested with the same reagent(s). The workbook is also the most suitable place to enter the results of quality control testing.

Symbols used to denote serologic observations vary widely, based on the past experience of each person. There is no right or wrong way to do it, but the adoption of a standardized system within each laboratory is important as a means to ensure that the terminology in use is interpreted in the same way by everybody. The symbol " − " is not a satisfactory way to indicate a negative test result, as it is too easily altered to " + " by a single vertical stroke, and can be mistakenly understood to mean "not done." The notation "0" is preferred; or the abbreviation "neg" is acceptable. "H" is commonly used to denote the presence of hemolysis, and a slash, "/" or, perhaps preferably, the notation "ND" is used to indicate a test not done. The symbol " ± " (plus-minus) is confusing and should never be used.

Testing for Sterility

The fact that most blood transfusion supplies are now disposable largely absolves blood banks and transfusion centers from the responsibility to test for sterility, since everything is supplied both sterile and pyrogen-free by the manufacturer. So long as blood is collected, and components prepared, in a closed system, sterility testing is not required. Only if a container is entered, or if contamination of a blood or component is suspected, is it necessary to undertake sterility testing. Visible signs of bacterial growth in a unit of blood might be a purplish discoloration at the interface between the red cells and the plasma, frank hemolysis, or the formation of clots in the plasma layer after a few days of storage. Certain gram-negative organisms (such as *Pseudomonas*) may grow at refrigerator temperatures, and produce powerful endotoxins that are extremely dangerous if transfused (see Chap. 7).

Whenever a culture is positive, the organisms must be identified. If other units of blood drawn at the same time are still available, it may be advisable to culture some of them as well. To permit a check on individual techniques, a record should be kept of the results of all cultures, together with the name of the phlebotomist. Contamination of a unit of blood may indicate poor phlebotomy technique or (less likely) nonsterile supplies.

RETENTION OF RECORDS

Laboratory work records may be required for reference at some later time, and should be filed in such a way that particular records can be located. Such records should be retained for at least 5 years, or for however long a period the original findings may be required.

Labeling of Donor Blood

The attachment of the final label to a donor unit is an indication that the unit is ready for issue. *This must therefore not be done until all required laboratory testing has been completed and interpreted.* Labels must adhere securely to the container, in such a way that their removal would be obvious. There are specific labeling requirements issued by various accrediting agencies. The act of affixing the label should be the responsibility of a senior member of the blood bank staff, who should be assisted by a second person to compare it with the laboratory work record and verify the accuracy of the information on the label.

Retention of Test Samples

Donor tube segments from all donor units should be retained until the expiration date of the unit. This will occupy very little space in the refrigerator and, since the contents of a segment derive from those of the donor unit itself, the cells should remain in satisfactory condition. Antigen integrity will be preserved, and the red cells will be available for any rechecking that may be required.

References

1. Reckel RP, Harris J. The unique characteristics of covalently polymerized bovine serum albumin solutions when used as antibody detection media. *Transfusion* 1978; 18:397–406.
2. Stroup M, MacIlroy M. Evaluation of the albumin antiglobulin technic in antibody detection. *Transfusion* 1965; 5:184–91.
3. Jørgensen J, Nielsen M, Nielsen CB, Nørmark J. The influence of ionic strength, albumin and incubation time of the sensitivity of the indirect antiglobulin test. *Vox Sang* 1979; 36:186–91.
4. French EE. Anti-globulin cross-matching test. Its usefulness for urgent blood-transfusions. *Lancet* 1958; 1:664–7.
5. Moore SB, Taswell HF, Pineda AA, Sonnenberg CL. Delayed hemolytic transfusion reactions. Evidence of the need for an improved pretransfusion compatibility test. *Am J Clin Path* 1980; 74:94–7.
6. Beattie KM, Zuelzer WW. The frequency and properties of pH-dependent anti-M. *Transfusion* 1965; 5:322–6.
7. Atchley WA, Bhagavan NV, Masouredis SP. Effect of ionic strength on the reaction between anti-D and D-positive red cells. *J Immunol* 1964; 93:701–12.
8. Elliot M, Bossom W, Dupuy ME, Masouredis SP. Effect of ionic strength on the behavior of red cell isoantibodies. *Vox Sang* 1964; 9:392–414.
9. Hughes-Jones NC, Polley MJ, Telford R, et al. Optimal conditions for detecting blood group antibodies by the antiglobulin test. *Vox Sang* 1964; 9:385–95.

10. Löw B, Messeter L. Antiglobulin test in low ionic strength salt solution for rapid antibody screening and crossmatching. *Vox Sang* 1974; 26:53–61.
11. Rosenfield RE, Shaikh SH, Innella F, et al. Augmentation of hemagglutination by low ionic conditions. *Transfusion* 1979; 19:499–510.
12. Lalezari P, Jiang AF. The manual Polybrene test: A simple and rapid procedure for detection of red cell antibodies. *Transfusion* 1980; 20:206–11.
13. Ferrer Z, Wright J, Moore BPL, Freedman J. Comparison of a modified manual hexadimethrine bromide (polybrene) and a low-ionic-strength solution antibody detection test. *Transfusion* 1985; 25:145–8.
14. Malde R, Kelsall G, Knight RC. The manual low-ionic strength polybrene technique for detection of red cell antibodies. *Med Lab Sci* 1986; 43:360–3.
15. Swanson J, Polesky HF, Tippett P, Sanger R. A "new" blood group antigen, Do[a]. *Nature* 1965; 206:313.
16. Case J. The behavior of anti-S antibodies with ficin treated human red cells. In: Abstracts of Volunteer Papers; 30th Annual Meeting of the American Association of Blood Banks, Atlanta GA. Abstract No. 71, Nov. 11–16, 1977.
17. Schmidt PJ, Nancarrow JF, Morrison EG, Chase G. A hemolytic reaction due to the transfusion of A_x blood. *J Lab Clin Med* 1958; 54:38–41.
18. Aach RD, Szmuness W, Mosely JW, et al. Serum alanine aminotransferase of donors in relation to the risk of non-A,non-B hepatitis in recipients: the transfusion-transmitted virus study. *N Engl J Med* 1981; 304:989–94.
19. Trépo C, Vitvitski L, Hantz O. Non-A,non-B hepatitis virus: identification of a core antigen-antibody system that cross reacts with hepatitis core antigen and antibody. *J Med Virol* 1981; 8:31–47.
20. Vyas GN, Perkins HA. Non-B post-transfusion hepatitis associated with hepatitis B core antibodies in donor blood. *N Engl J Med* 1983; 306:749–50.
21. Alter HJ, Tabor E, Meryman H, et al. Transmission of hepatitis B virus infection by transfusion of frozen-deglycerolized red blood cells. *N Engl J Med* 1979; 301:393–5.
22. Ling CM, Overby LR. Prevalence of hepatitis B virus antigen as revealed by direct radioimmunoassay with ^{125}I antibody. *J Immunol* 1972; 109:834–41.

5. Pretransfusion Testing

Pretransfusion testing includes procedures to determine the group and Rh(D) type of the recipient, a test on the recipient's serum to ascertain whether or not unexpected antibodies are present, and some kind of test to ensure that there is not potentially significant incompatibility between the recipient's serum and the cells of donors whose blood has been selected for transfusion. The latter is the *crossmatch,* an outmoded term that persists but reflects older procedures. More detailed testing may be indicated in selected cases, including typing for additional antigens and procedures for the identification of blood group antibodies.

The precise format of pretransfusion testing has varied somewhat over the years, as has the manner in which the individual tests have been carried out. Such changes presumably reflect constant professional reevaluation of the factors considered deserving of priority in the cause of transfusion safety, and the implementation of reforms, whether to improve safety directly or to eliminate costly and unnecessary measures. The past few years have witnessed a radical departure from standards once considered essential, but before embarking on a discussion of that issue, we should examine the various elements that comprise pretransfusion testing, and examine the reasons they may be considered necessary.

The Recipient's Blood Sample

The selection of blood for transfusion begins with laboratory tests carried out on a blood sample drawn from the patient. If the patient has received blood or a component containing red cells within the preceding three months, or has been pregnant within the same period, or if the history is uncertain or unobtainable, pretransfusion testing must be done on a sample drawn within two days of the scheduled transfusion. This is to ensure the best possible chance of detecting any antibodies that may be developing as a result of the earlier event. Naturally, a recipient who is receiving multiple transfusions over a period of time must have fresh blood samples drawn every two days, and all required testing must be carried out on each sample, however frequently the recipient's blood may have been tested in the past.

Procedures essential to the safety of blood transfusion include correct identification of the patient when the sample is drawn, and of the sample itself through all subsequent manipulations, as well as care and accuracy in carrying out the required tests.

Laboratory testing before transfusion must be done by personnel with proper training who are thoroughly familiar with the sources of error and who can recognize the significance of unexpected reactions. Proper quality control procedures, designed to facilitate the recognition of substandard performance on the part of personnel or reagents, are also essential. It is a matter of record, however, that most serious transfusion reactions result from nontechnical errors in the identification of patients, samples, or donor blood [1]. Thus, it is also essential that only persons trained to appreciate the importance of proper identification should be permitted to collect blood samples for compatibility testing.

COLLECTION OF THE SAMPLE

Venipuncture Site
Blood specimens are usually drawn from one of the large veins in the antecubital fossa, but it may sometimes be necessary to use the smaller veins on the back of the hand or in the wrist. This makes the operation more painful for the patient. Veins in the jugular or femoral area may be used as a last resort, but in such cases, the venipuncture needs to be done by a specially trained person. Special care is needed when drawing blood from a patient receiving intravenous medication, as contamination of the blood specimen with intravenous fluids may cause difficulty in the interpretation of laboratory tests. Withdrawal of the blood specimen from the self-sealing rubber adapters provided in many administration sets is almost certain to result in such contamination. If possible, the blood sample should be drawn from the other arm. If the use of the same arm is unavoidable, a vein other than the one receiving the infusion should be chosen. In cases where a large part of the body is bandaged or otherwise inaccessible, or where venipuncture is difficult for some other reason, nonvenous blood may have to be used.

Nonvenous Collection of Blood
When it is necessary to draw blood from a small infant, the specimen may be collected by sticking the heel, big toe, or ear with a sharp instrument, such as a disposable lancet. The heel is the best site for the incision, and if a small amount of petroleum jelly is rubbed over the skin before the puncture, the drops of blood are easier to collect into capillary tubes, of which several should be collected to ensure enough blood for testing. When it is necessary to collect nonvenous blood in adults, a finger or an earlobe is usually chosen for the incision.

The Sample
Blood for pretransfusion testing is most often collected into a clean, dry tube without an anticoagulant, because certain disadvantages attend the use of plasma in antibody detection tests, including the crossmatch. If the participation of complement is considered necessary to the detection of blood group antibodies, serum separated from a clotted sample is required, since anticoagulants are anticomplementary. Plasma may be used otherwise, although this has

other disadvantages. One is that fibrin may form in the mixture of plasma and cell suspension during incubation. This enmeshes red cells and presents an appearance that can be mistaken for agglutination, or may entrap serum in the clot that may remain through the washing phases of the test and neutralize the antiglobulin reagent.

The volume of blood drawn should be enough for all pretransfusion testing, with a sufficient excess of serum to allow for any posttransfusion testing that may be needed. A 5 to 7 ml sample is normally sufficient. If extensive pretransfusion testing is anticipated, however, as in a recipient believed from earlier testing to have made an alloantibody, or when crossmatching many donor units, a larger volume of blood will have to be drawn. An anticoagulated sample may be drawn in addition, if required.

IDENTIFICATION OF THE PATIENT AND THE SAMPLE

At the Bedside

Proper identification of the patient, as well as the blood sample, is crucial. Each tube must be clearly and legibly labeled in an indelible manner. Wax pencil on glass is unacceptable. Paper labels must be firmly glued to the tubes, and not attached by rubber bands or stuck on with small pieces of adhesive tape. The label must be large enough to accommodate the required information, yet not be so large as to prevent inspection of the contents of the tube. The required information includes the patient's full name (first and last), an identification number or code, the date on which the specimen was drawn, and some identification of the person drawing the sample.

Before drawing the blood, the phlebotomist must confirm that the person from whom blood is going to be drawn is the person whose name appears on the requisition. The patient, if conscious, should be asked to state his or her name and, if possible, to spell it out as a means of verifying the information on the requisition. It is not appropriate to ask "Are you so-and-so?" because a person who is hard of hearing, or who does not comprehend the question, may answer misleadingly in the affirmative. In most hospitals, all patients wear an identifying wristband. This should always be checked as a matter of routine, but not considered to be the most infallible means of correctly identifying the person wearing it. Identification cards on the bed or on the wall are unreliable, because the patient may have been moved from another bed and his card left behind. If the patient is unconscious, or otherwise incapable of answering questions, some responsible person must confirm the patient's identity.

The blood sample must be placed in an unlabeled tube, which is then immediately labeled, before leaving the bedside. *Prelabeling of tubes is dangerous,* because if several prelabeled tubes are on the tray, the risk of placing the sample into the wrong one is very real. Several ingenious systems have been

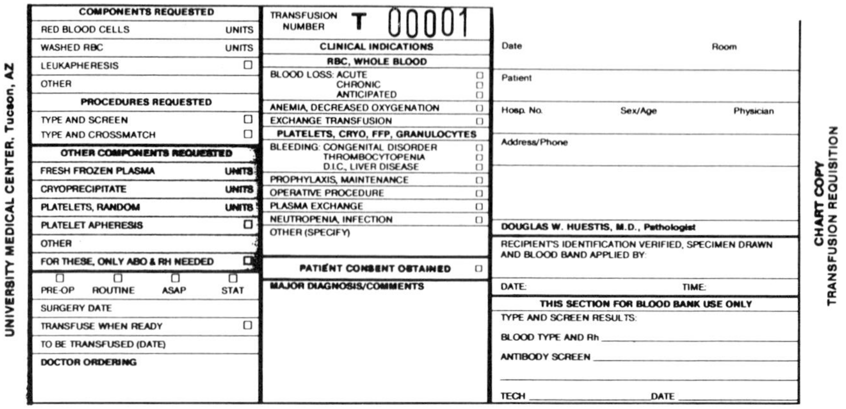
UNIVERSITY MEDICAL CENTER, Tucson, AZ

COMPONENTS REQUESTED
RED BLOOD CELLS UNITS
WASHED RBC UNITS
LEUKAPHERESIS □
OTHER
PROCEDURES REQUESTED
TYPE AND SCREEN □
TYPE AND CROSSMATCH □
OTHER COMPONENTS REQUESTED
FRESH FROZEN PLASMA UNITS
CRYOPRECIPITATE UNITS
PLATELETS, RANDOM UNITS
PLATELET APHERESIS □
OTHER
FOR THESE, ONLY ABO & RH NEEDED □
□ PRE-OP □ ROUTINE □ ASAP □ STAT
SURGERY DATE
TRANSFUSE WHEN READY □
TO BE TRANSFUSED (DATE)
DOCTOR ORDERING

TRANSFUSION NUMBER T 00001
CLINICAL INDICATIONS
RBC, WHOLE BLOOD
BLOOD LOSS: ACUTE □
CHRONIC □
ANTICIPATED □
ANEMIA, DECREASED OXYGENATION □
EXCHANGE TRANSFUSION □
PLATELETS, CRYO, FFP, GRANULOCYTES
BLEEDING: CONGENITAL DISORDER □
THROMBOCYTOPENIA □
D.I.C., LIVER DISEASE □
PROPHYLAXIS, MAINTENANCE □
OPERATIVE PROCEDURE □
PLASMA EXCHANGE □
NEUTROPENIA, INFECTION □
OTHER (SPECIFY)
PATIENT CONSENT OBTAINED □
MAJOR DIAGNOSIS/COMMENTS

Date Room
Patient
Hosp. No. Sex/Age Physician
Address/Phone
DOUGLAS W. HUESTIS, M.D., Pathologist
RECIPIENT'S IDENTIFICATION VERIFIED, SPECIMEN DRAWN AND BLOOD BAND APPLIED BY:
DATE: TIME:
THIS SECTION FOR BLOOD BANK USE ONLY
TYPE AND SCREEN RESULTS:
BLOOD TYPE AND Rh
ANTIBODY SCREEN
TECH DATE

CHART COPY
TRANSFUSION REQUISITION

Figure 5–1
A transfusion requisition with detachable labels on the back, as a means of ensuring proper identification of the patient, test samples, and donor units. Please note that this requisition also documents the clinical indications for transfusion and the fact that consent has been obtained.

devised to aid in the identification of patients and blood samples, not only at the collection stage but through all subsequent procedures in the laboratory and, ideally, extending to the blood selected for transfusion. As an example, the requisition form may come with a page of adhesive-backed tabs attached to it, each printed with the same unique identifying number (Fig. 5–1). The first of these is attached to the patient's body (usually the wrist) when the blood sample is drawn, while the second goes on the tube containing the blood sample. Further numbered tabs remain attached to the requisition to be used in the laboratory to identify the tube into which the patient's serum is placed after being separated from the original sample, as well as the laboratory workbook entry, the test tube rack used for crossmatching, and any donor units subsequently released as being compatible for that patient.

Systems like the one described are of particular value when blood samples are collected by personnel other than those of the laboratory, as is commonly the case in large hospitals. Such systems are also useful in a situation where several persons of uncertain identity require transfusion, as may occur in a busy emergency room, or where a patient is unconscious and cannot be questioned as to identity. The ultimate purpose of the system is to enable the numbered tab attached to the recipient to be checked against those on the blood sample, the requisition form, the laboratory test report, and selected donor units, to verify that all the steps of the procedure were carried out on blood drawn from the proper patient.

On Arrival in the Laboratory

Once the blood sample is delivered to the laboratory, the information on the label is checked carefully against that on the accompanying requisition. This procedure is as critical as the identification of the patient before venipuncture. The importance of a fully and accurately labeled sample cannot be overemphasized. Clearly, the ideal situation is that in which the person identifying the patient has drawn the sample and attached the identifying label *at the patient's bedside*. As a matter of routine, nothing less is acceptable, yet there may be circumstances that would justify a relaxation of the normal rules. If an exception appears to serve the best interests of the patient, it may be appropriate to make one, subject to the preparation of signed records explaining the circumstances and justifying the decision. A sample bearing no label at all must be rejected.

A thought worth remembering is that the times when departures from established routine are most likely to occur are often the very ones in which *additional care* is needed. In the case of multiple casualties from a single accident, for instance, apparently insignificant deviations from the normal routine may be especially dangerous. Such an accident may involve a family, so that more than one victim could have the same last name, or even same first and last names.

In normal circumstances, a delay of at least 10 minutes between drawing the sample and separating the serum is sufficient to allow adequate clotting. If serum is separated sooner, threads of fibrin may form in the test mixture on incubation at 37°C, which interferes with interpretation of the results. In patients with coagulation disorders, it may take longer for coagulation to proceed to completion. In an emergency in such cases, thrombin may be added to accelerate the process and allow the serum to be separated. A convenient method of adding sufficient thrombin to promote clotting is to place two applicator sticks into a vial of dried thrombin so that a small amount of thrombin becomes attached to their tips. This is then transferred to the blood sample, which can normally be expected to clot completely within a few minutes.

A similar problem may arise with blood samples from heparinized patients. In this case, the addition of protamine sulfate to the sample may be necessary to neutralize the heparin and allow clotting to take place. One drop of a 1 percent (10 mg/ml) solution of protamine sulfate should be sufficient to achieve the desired effect. It is important not to add too much protamine, however, as an excess may itself inhibit coagulation. Moreover, protamine in the serum may cause rouleaux that will interfere with the interpretation of serologic tests. Curiously, cells possessing the N antigen, namely, those of the MN and N phenotypes, aggregate more readily in protamine than those of the M phenotype; hence, a serum containing protamine sulfate may be mistakenly assumed to contain anti-N. The phenomenon presumably results from some difference in the strength of the negative charge borne on the N sialoglycoprotein in comparison with that on the M sialoglycoprotein, since the protamine molecule carries a strong positive charge.

On the Administration of the Transfusion

In labeling the donor unit, the laboratory must take care that the information coincides precisely with that on the sample used for pretransfusion compatibility testing. In turn, at the patient's bedside, the person who administers the transfusion must again check the label on the donor unit to see that it corresponds in every particular to the identity of the proposed recipient.

Testing the Recipient's Blood Sample

ABO GROUPING

ABO grouping on recipients is carried out in essentially the same manner as on donors, with the cells being tested with anti-A and anti-B, and the serum being tested against A_1 and B red cells. It is wasteful in this context to test the cells with anti-A,B serum as well as anti-A and anti-B. Although proficiency testing surveys occasionally give the opposite impression, there is no need to distinguish between group O and such weak subgroups as A_x among recipients of blood transfusion. Since the proper donor blood to choose for transfusion in such cases is without question group O, it would be better if recipients belonging to such subgroups were typed as O in the first place. The potential for antibody activity in the plasma of group O donors to destroy the red cells of a group A_x recipient is purely a theoretical one, and no such case has ever been reported in the literature.

DISCREPANT AND UNUSUAL REACTIONS

The investigation of discrepant ABO reactions is treated in detail in Chapter 4. The causes listed there are as equally likely to arise in testing recipients as in testing donors. Some additional causes, however, are unlikely to arise in testing blood from donors. These are appropriately examined in detail here. For example, in disease there is an increased likelihood of a protein imbalance or some kind of hemagglutinin in the serum, and certain forms of medication can cause aberrant serologic reactions. Also, the expected antibodies of the ABO system may be absent in the newborn, or sometimes become diminished in potency in the elderly or as the result of immunosuppressive therapy. They may therefore not be detected in the reverse (serum grouping) test.

In testing recipients, the following causes of discrepant ABO reactions must be considered *in addition* to those already listed in Chapter 4 as being common to both donors and recipients.

Polyagglutinability (Including Acquired B)

Polyagglutinability caused by the exposure of hidden receptors on the cell surface by a bacterial enzyme (such as in T-, Th-, and Tk-activation) is seldom recognized in the ABO grouping test. The natural agglutinins directed at these receptors are destroyed during the manufacture of commercial antiserums. This occurs more by accident than by design, usually as a side effect of the solvent treatment used by manufacturers to remove lipoproteins from the raw material. Accordingly, unless systematically screened for with a lectin made from *Arachis hypogaea* (peanut) lectin, these kinds of polyagglutinability are most often detected when the cells are tested with a noncommercial antiserum for some reason, or with a fresh normal serum.

By contrast, Tn polyagglutinability is of nonmicrobial origin. It will almost invariably present appearances superficially suggesting a subgroup of A since weak agglutination may be expected to occur with anti-A serums because of a similarity between the Tn and A antigens. In these cases, however, anti-A,B serum will *not* show stronger reactivity, and testing with the *Dolichos biflorus* anti-A_1 lectin will provide a clue to the correct explanation by unexpectedly showing relatively strong agglutination.

Acquired B is a form of polyagglutinability that occurs only in group A bloods, since one explanation for the acquired antigen is that it originates through the conversion of A receptors by a bacterial enzyme (see p. 91). The forward grouping result, therefore, will suggest group AB (although the B antigen is usually weaker than normal), but the reverse grouping test will show the presence of anti-B, thereby calling attention to the anomaly.

Recent Blood Transfusion or Bone Marrow Transplant

The most likely explanation of mixed-field agglutination in a forward grouping test on a patient is a recent blood transfusion. The administration of group O red blood cells to a group A or group B recipient would have this effect, which would gradually diminish over the life span of the transfused cells. An alternative explanation to be considered is an ABO incompatible bone marrow transplant.

A less common cause of a mixed-field reaction not due to a subgroup is a condition known as *chimerism,* wherein two distinct cell populations are produced by the bone marrow. This phenomenon may also be encountered in donors, and can be caused either by an exchange of erythropoietic tissue between twin fetuses in utero, or by fertilization of the ovum by two sperm.

As with donor blood, discrepancies must be resolved before a conclusion is reached as to the ABO group of the blood, and such resolution should be reached before transfusion. That is not to say that any patient should be allowed to bleed to death while the laboratory personnel try to unravel a problem. Group O red blood cells are almost always safe in such cases. Like most other rules, this one should be applied with discretion and common sense, always with the welfare of the patient uppermost in mind.

RH TYPING

Since the administration of D-positive blood to D-negative patients is likely to produce an immune response in a high proportion of cases [2], the red cells of all recipients are tested for D in order to enable D-negative blood to be selected in appropriate cases. Except in special circumstances, testing for D^u, for other antigens of the Rh system, or for those of other blood group systems is unnecessary. Such special circumstances may exist, for example, in a patient whose serum contains an unexpected antibody, where the red cells would need to be tested for other antigens as part of the investigation to establish the identity of the antibody.

Controlling the Test for D

In testing for the D antigen in recipients, an appropriate control test to detect spontaneous agglutination must be used as a routine, to prevent false interpretation of D-negative cells as D-positive. If the red cells are being tested unwashed or suspended in their own serum, spontaneous agglutination may be caused by cold autoagglutinins in the recipient's serum and lead to false-positive test results, or rouleaux caused by a protein imbalance in the patient's serum may be mistaken for agglutination. These sources of possible misinterpretation occur regardless of the protein concentration of the anti-D serum. Spontaneous agglutination caused by a coating of immunoglobulin on the test cells, on the other hand, is most likely to occur when the antiserum is a high-protein one, and is not greatly lessened by washing the cells before testing.

In appropriate circumstances, a simultaneous ABO grouping test may be a sufficient control of the test for D. Such would ordinarily be the case when the test for D is done with a low-protein antiserum, based on the premise that a low-protein anti-D serum is no more capable of promoting spontaneous agglutination than the reagents used for ABO grouping. By that reasoning, a negative test result with either anti-A or anti-B, or with both, is sufficient to validate a positive test result with the anti-D serum. In the case of a group AB test sample that gives a positive reaction with anti-D, some additional control is required, but a simple control test with the patient's own serum would usually be sufficient in a test system using a protein concentration similar to that of normal human serum.

The foregoing argument applies not only to antiserums made from traditional saline-reactive (IgM) antibodies, but also to those made from chemically modified IgG [3], providing these are formulated in a diluent that contains approximately the same total protein concentration as human serum and lacks macromolecular additives. The mere fact that an antiserum is represented as being "saline reactive," or is stated to have been manufactured by the reduction and alkylation of IgG, does not necessarily mean that it has been formulated in a low-protein diluent. Some chemically modified IgG reagents are made up in a diluent that contains macromolecular compounds or an elevated level of protein to improve the avidity of agglutination. In either case, the control precautions needed for high-protein reagents are applicable, since these measures increase the likelihood that the reagent will cause spontaneous agglutination. The manufacturer's directions should state what routine control tests are required when using all antiserums, and these must be strictly followed.

When using high-protein Rh antiserums, a parallel control test is *always* required when typing potential recipients. These reagents have developed from the discovery, in the mid-1940s, that the incorporation of albumin into the test mixture enables "incomplete" Rh antibodies to agglutinate antigen-positive red cells [4, 5]. An application of this principle enabled Rh typing reagents to be made from serums containing these otherwise nonagglutinating, but abundantly available, antibodies [6]. The earliest Rh reagents so made were prepared by a procedure involving simple dilution, with human or bovine albumin, of the human serum known to contain Rh antibodies. Antiserums so prepared proved to be acceptably sensitive test reagents for D, providing the total protein concentration was above 20 percent and the test cells were suspended in their own serum or plasma to avoid introducing saline into the test system.

A simple parallel control test with bovine albumin was initially considered to be a sufficient means of identifying spontaneous agglutination. Soon, however, manufacturers began enhancing the performance of their anti-D reagents by incorporating macromolecular additives into them. Understandably, just as the speed and strength of specific agglutination were enhanced by the additives, so also were the speed and strength of spontaneous agglutination caused by autoagglutinins or by an immunoglobulin coating on the cells. In a study involving Rh phenotyping serums, White, Issitt, and McGuire found that red cells could be sufficiently coated with immunoglobulin to agglutinate spontaneously in the test environment containing the additives present in Rh reagents, yet might show no agglutination in control tests with bovine albumin that did not contain such additives [7]. Other manifestations of spontaneous agglutination caused by additives present in Rh antiserums, but usually absent from bovine albumin, soon came to light [8, 9].

These observations led manufacturers to begin offering Rh control reagents formulated to contain their own preferred additives at concentrations to match their anti-D serum. Such reagents enable the Rh control test to provide a reliable means of recognizing potentially false-positive reactions caused by spontaneous agglutination, but only when the control reagent corresponding to the anti-D in use is chosen for the test. The control reagent of another manufacturer may not be wholly suitable.

OTHER TYPING

When testing for additional antigens is indicated, appropriate controls are required. For example, Rh antiserums other than anti-D, if formulated in a high-protein diluent, are just as likely to promote the spontaneous agglutination of immunoglobulin-coated cells as an anti-D reagent of similar composition. The same control precautions as those described for anti-D are therefore needed. Understandably, red cells having a positive direct antiglobulin test due to an anti-IgG coating cannot be reliably tested for antigen status using the indirect antiglobulin test procedure, which would ordinarily be the only method of testing for antigens belonging to the Kell, Duffy, or Kidd systems. In such cases, it may be possible to elute the antibody causing the positive direct antiglobulin test without damaging the cell membrane, as a means of enabling the cells to be tested with appropriate antiserums. A method by which this may be attempted using chloroquine diphosphate is described on page 203. The procedure is not invariably successful, and it may prove to be impossible to determine the antigen status of red cells having a positive direct antiglobulin test.

Detection of Unexpected Antibodies

Tests for the detection of unexpected antibodies include the *major crossmatch,* a procedure that involves the direct testing of a recipient's serum against red cells taken from donor units selected for transfusion. This is the most straightforward method of testing for incompatibility, but provides information applying only to the selected donor units and may not assure the absence of significant unexpected antibodies from the serum.

The *minor crossmatch* is the procedure in which the plasma of each donor is tested for reactivity against the red cells of the recipient. This is seldom done nowadays mainly because it has become part of the routine to screen serums from all donors for unexpected antibodies, or at least from those who have a history of pregnancy or of being transfused themselves. Since fewer transfusions nowadays are of whole blood, there is less likelihood of a recipient's own red cells being destroyed by an antibody present in the plasma of a donor. The minor crossmatch has always suffered from the defect that it does not safeguard against *interdonor incompatibility,* where a donor unit containing a potent antibody is administered to the recipient ahead of one of which the red cells possess the corresponding antigen, potentially a more significant source of hemolysis than a minor incompatibility. Anti-K has twice been reported to cause a severe reaction by this means, but the circumstances are rare [10, 11].

Antibody screening involves the systematic testing of serum from potential recipients for unexpected blood group antibodies by testing against red cells selected for the combination of antigens they possess. In the earliest application of the principle, in the mid-1940s, screening tests were designed solely to detect anti-Rh in pregnant women. At that time, the routine was simply to test the recipient's serum, by the relatively primitive test procedures then commonly used, against a suspension of D-positive red cells chosen without regard for other antigens. In truth, few other blood group antigens had been recognized at that time, as any blood group antibodies depending on the indirect antiglobulin test for their detection had to await the adoption of that test after its introduction in 1945 [12]. Rh antigens other than D were as yet poorly characterized.

Gradually, as unexpected antibodies began to be detected with greater frequency and in greater variety with the exposure of more people to foreign blood group antigens through transfusion, the advantages of systematic antibody screening on all bloods submitted to the laboratory for blood grouping became apparent. By screening against red cell suspensions prepared from the blood of donors with blood group antigens corresponding to the antibodies most commonly found, preexisting immunization could be recognized in advance of a major crossmatch, thereby permitting the antibody to be identified, and enabling donor blood negative for the appropriate antigen to be obtained.

The commercial availability of appropriately selected reagent red cell suspensions was a major factor enabling the antibody screening procedure to be adopted as a routine, beginning in the late 1950s. Routine screening for unexpected antibodies is still not universally practiced outside the United States, but is gaining currency throughout the world wherever commercial reagents are available, or where regional blood transfusion centers undertake the responsibility of distributing appropriately chosen sets of screening cells to institutions within the regions they serve.

Methods Used in Antibody Detection

Traditionally, the test procedures used in detecting unexpected blood group antibodies have been those capable of recognizing all antibodies considered to be clinically significant in blood transfusion. No single test procedure is ideal for the detection of all blood group antibodies. Most "immune" blood group antibodies, being usually IgG, react best at 37°C and most often require the indirect antiglobulin test for detection. Accordingly, this test is the most important aspect of any antibody detection procedure. On relatively rare occasions, the recognition of an antibody by the antiglobulin technique depends on the binding of complement to the cells, a condition requiring the serum being tested to be fresh enough to contain active complement. It also requires the use of a polyspecific antiglobulin reagent, rather than the anti-IgG that is perfectly suitable in virtually all other cases.

The ability to agglutinate antigen-positive red cells directly in a saline or low-protein test medium is a property confined mainly to antibodies of the IgM class of immunoglobulin, which also tend to show better reactivity at cold temperatures than at 37°C.

Some immune antibodies, especially those of the Rh blood group system, agglutinate antigen-positive cells directly, but only in a high-protein test system, or in saline, if the cell membrane is modified by a proteolytic enzyme. Enzyme treatment enhances the sensitivity of detection procedures for Rh antibodies, those of the Kidd and Lewis blood group systems, and also certain cold-reactive specificities such as anti-P_1 and anti-I. A few blood group antigens, particularly those of the Duffy and MNSs systems, as well as anti-Xg^a, are inactivated by treatment with proteases. This makes an enzyme test procedure useless for the detection of the corresponding antibodies, but of some value in helping to separate the components of antibody mixtures as a means of identifying them.

Testing at Room Temperature and Below
Since some blood group antibodies react preferentially in the cold, it was for many years considered necessary to include as part of the antibody detection routine a test in which the serum was incubated with the indicator cells at room temperature. Depending on the time of year and the laboratory temperature, many unexpected antibodies that were of no clinical significance were detected, which means that time had to be taken to identify them, thereby delaying transfusion in some cases. Most common among the antibodies detected were cold autoagglutinins, often those of anti-I, anti-H, or anti-HI specificity, as well as examples of anti-P_1, and of Lewis specificities that were not detectable at 37°C. On the rare occasions that these antibodies are clinically significant, it is likely they will be reactive in the 37°C or antiglobulin phases of the antibody detection test, or show hemolysis. Accordingly, routine testing for unexpected antibodies at room temperature is no longer a required feature of antibody screening.

These remarks do not apply to the reverse (serum) grouping phase of the ABO test, whose purpose is to test for the *expected* antibodies of the system. If a discrepancy is observed between the results obtained in the serum and cell grouping tests, the required resolution of the matter may properly include testing against group O red cell suspensions at room temperature as a means to identify a cold-reacting agglutinin that is causing an unexpected reaction with either or both of the reverse grouping cells. Similarly, the investigation of an unexpected antibody initially found after incubation at 37°C, whether it was observed to be reactive as a direct agglutinin or only at the antiglobulin phase, may need to include testing at room temperature as an aid to the resolution of the problem.

Tests Using Bovine Albumin
The advantages and disadvantages of bovine albumin as a potentiator are discussed in Chapter 4. It is still commonly used, most often as an additive in the form of a 22 percent solution, which fails to achieve the desired effect of potentiating direct agglutination by IgG antibodies.

Low–Ionic Strength Test Systems

Antibody detection tests carried out in a low–ionic strength environment as a means of reducing incubation time without sacrificing sensitivity are gradually replacing methods in which bovine albumin is used. The required test milieu can be achieved either by using one of many available commercial additives, some of which contain macromolecular substances to potentiate direct agglutination by Rh antibodies, or by suspending the test red cells in a special low–ionic strength suspending medium.

Polybrene and Protamine Methods

Some antibodies that would ordinarily be detectable only by the indirect antiglobulin test can be made to show direct agglutination of antigen-positive cells by using positively charged molecules like those of Polybrene (hexadimethrine bromide) or protamine sulfate to cause red cells to aggregate. Minimal incubation is required to sensitize the cells, but the method requires special skill to achieve its full potential, and has the limitation that it may not detect anti-K reliably. The procedure is discussed in greater detail on p. 145.

Enzyme Test Procedures

Proteolytic enzymes remove sialic acid from the red cell surface, thereby reducing the negative surface charge and making the cells agglutinable, when suspended in a saline medium, by some IgG antibodies. Applications and limitations of enzyme tests are discussed on p. 146.

REAGENT RED BLOOD CELLS FOR ANTIBODY SCREENING

The group O red cells chosen for routine antibody screening should possess, between them, as many of the common blood group antigens as possible. This necessitates using at least two individual cell suspensions, as the needed combination of antigens would be cumulatively uncommon, even if the FDA did not consider it necessary for both Le^a and Le^b to be represented, a feature not attainable with the red cells of a single donor. The pooled cells of two donors, though acceptable for screening donor serums, are not sensitive enough for the screening recipients.

Such antigens as C^w, Lu^a, Kp^a, V, and Js^a are most often absent from red cells used for antibody screening, mostly because it would be impossible for manufacturers to meet the demand for screening cells if these relatively uncommon antigens had to be represented along with all the others. The inability of screening tests to detect antibodies directed at these antigens does not appear to be causing a significant incidence of hemolytic transfusion reactions.

Although homozygous expression of certain selected antigens would help to improve the sensitivity of the test procedure for the detection of weak antibodies showing dosage, this is not required, and indeed, would not be feasible on a regular basis with only two cell suspensions. The Rh antigens are commonly represented in double dose on commercial screening cell sets, however, and homozygous expression of other significant antigens may occur as a matter of chance on individual pairs of cells. The consistent representation of other significant antigens in double dose would require the extension of testing to include at least three red cell suspensions.

CHOICE OF TECHNIQUES

The methods used in antibody screening are largely a matter of personal preference. A test involving room temperature incubation is no longer required, but is sometimes included for completeness, or where there is a reason to do so. A separate test mixture for each cell suspension is required in this case. An immediate-spin test is not useful. In fact, centrifugation and examination of the test mixture before incubation may enable nonsignificant cold agglutinins to cause complement to be bound to the cells, and remain bound, which later complicates the interpretation of the antiglobulin phase of the test.

It is not essential to examine the test mixture for agglutination after incubation at 37°C, although many workers do so before proceeding to the antiglobulin phase. The test mixture does have to be centrifuged at this point, however, because it is essential to check for hemolysis after incubation, and it is no hardship to examine at the same time for agglutination. *Examination for hemolysis must not be omitted,* because a few clinically significant antibodies may cause distinct hemolysis due to their ability to bind complement. The most commonly quoted examples are anti-Le^a, anti-Jk^a, and anti-Vel.

An antiglobulin test is mandatory, as is the need to carry out an antiglobulin control test on all test mixtures interpreted as negative. The required control test involves the addition of red cells coated with IgG to all tubes showing a negative result in the antiglobulin test, to confirm that active antiglobulin is still present. The control test supposedly demonstrates the efficacy with which the test cells were washed free of unbound protein, but is often carried out with control cells so strongly coated with IgG that they could be agglutinated by partially neutralized anti-human globulin. This defeats the purpose of the control test, and engenders a false sense of confidence in the efficacy of the antiglobulin test procedure. We recommend the use of *lightly coated* control cells, which do provide a valid control for residual antiglobulin activity.

AUTOLOGOUS CONTROL

The purpose of an autologous control test in blood group serology is to facilitate discrimination between autoantibodies and alloantibodies. It is therefore unnecessary to run one with most antibody screening tests, as almost all serums are expected to show a negative reaction with either or both screening cells. In the event that a positive reaction is observed with one or more of the cells, identification of the antibody will necessitate testing the serum with further typed cell suspensions. In almost all cases, this is the earliest point at which an autologous control test can be rationally justified. The one significant exception could be in the case of a patient who has recently been transfused and is in the process of mounting an immune response. In this situation, the only detectable antibody may be attached to any antigen-positive donor cells still surviving. This is unlikely to be recognized except by means of a mixed-field positive indirect antiglobulin test with the recipient's own posttransfusion red cells. In such a case, however, it may take exceptional visual acuity on the part of the technologist, even if an autologous control test *is* included as part of the routine.

Identification of Antibodies

When unexpected antibodies are detected in the course of screening or crossmatching, the next step is to determine their specificity by testing against a battery of separate group O red cell suspensions chosen for their combinations of phenotypes in the common blood group systems. Such a battery of cells is called a red cell *panel*. The antigen combinations of the individual cells are chosen to facilitate the recognition of the commonly encountered antibodies in the presence of each other. There is usually a preponderance of D-negative cells, for example, since anti-D is still the most commonly encountered immune antibody.

Any given cell panel may not provide the ability to identify all antibody mixtures, as it is not practicable to provide a wide range of antigen combinations with so limited a number of cell suspensions. It may not be consistently feasible, for example, for anti-K to be identified in the presence of anti-e, nor both anti-Jk^a and anti-Fy^a in the presence of anti-c.

In deciding which test procedures to use in identifying an unexpected antibody, it seems reasonable to give priority to those by which reactivity was first observed. But test methods by which no reactivity was observed initially should not automatically be left out. For instance, even though a test incubated at room temperature is no longer necessary as part of screening for antibodies, it is still a useful adjunct to antibody identification. Incubation at 4°C may be helpful if there is reason to suspect that a cold agglutinin may be responsible for weaker and less readily reproducible reactions occurring at higher temperatures.

In all cases, an autologous control is required for each procedure, to recognize reactions due to an autoantibody. The mere fact that a recipient's serum is found to agglutinate the autologous red cells does not preclude the possibility of an alloantibody as well as an autoantibody. In such a case, it may be necessary to absorb the serum with the recipient's red cells, to ascertain that an alloantibody is not being concealed by the autoantibody. In a recently transfused patient, the results of autoabsorption need to be interpreted cautiously, as surviving donor cells could cause an alloantibody to be removed.

On most occasions, antibodies tend to show the reaction characteristics for which they are best known, based on experience with past examples. Thus, the behavior of an antibody in different test procedures may provide a valuable clue that will aid in its identification. Table 5–1 shows the usual reaction characteristics of some of the more commonly encountered blood group antibodies. Bear in mind the possibility of exceptions to the rules. For instance, anti-Xg^a is almost always reactive by the indirect antiglobulin test, but examples have been reported that showed direct agglutination of Xg(a+) red cells in a saline test medium.

STRAIGHTFORWARD ANTIBODY IDENTIFICATION

In many cases, the identification of an antibody is a straightforward matter of comparing the positive and negative reactions shown when the serum is tested against the cell panel. As an aid to the comparison, it is useful to strike out the antigens *present* on any cell suspensions of the panel that *do not* show reactions with the recipient's serum, on the premise that if an antibody is *nonreactive* with a cell suspension possessing certain antigens, that antibody cannot be directed at those antigens. This is not unfailingly true, but when it is so, the antibody is directed at an antigen among those *not* struck out. If there are enough cell suspensions showing negative results, we may find only one such antigen. Table 5–2 exemplifies the straightforward identification of a single antibody in a serum.

More often, several antigens will remain not struck out. In this case, we have a list of antigens against which the antibody *might* be directed, or an indication of what specificities *have not been excluded* as components of a possible mixture of antibodies. We now need to examine the antigen combinations of cell suspensions that did react to see if there is a clear-cut match, and whether additional selected panel cells must be tested to ascertain that multiple antibodies are not present.

VARIABLE REACTIVITY AND DOSAGE

In the first example, the pattern of antibody reactivity would have enabled E-negative blood to be selected for crossmatching with probably compatible results. Sometimes the identification of an antibody is less straightforward. If, for example, a cell suspension on the panel does possess the antigen at which the antibody is directed, yet for some reason gives a negative reaction, the procedure of striking out the antigens of cells giving a negative test result will be misleading. Technical error in carrying out the tests, or mistyping of the cells themselves, may not be the only cause of this. For example, a weak antibody that reacts detectably only with red cells possessing the strongest expression of the antigen may not react with cells showing heterozygous expression. This situation is depicted in Table 5–3.

Here, the pattern of test results observed does not correspond with any of the antigens for which the panel cells have been tested, which raises the possi-

Table 5–1. Serologic and Clinical Behavior of Blood Group Antibodies

Antibody	In Vitro Hemolysis	Saline 4°C	Saline 22°C	Albumin 37°C	Albumin AGT	Enzyme 37°C	Enzyme AGT	Associated with HDN	Associated with HTR
Anti-M	0	Most	Some	Few	Few	0	0	Few	Few
Anti-N	0	Most	Few	Occ.	Occ.	0	0	Rare	
Anti-S	0	Few	Some	Some	Most	See text		Yes	Yes
Anti-s	0	0	Few	Few	Most	See text		Yes	Yes
Anti-U	0	0	Occ.	Some	Most	Most	Most	Yes	Yes
Anti-P_1	Occ.	Most	Some	Occ.	Rare	Some	Few	No	Rare
Anti-P	Some	Most	Some	Some	Some	Some	Some	No	
Anti-PP_1P^k	Some	Most	Some	Some	Some	Some	Some	Rare	
Anti-Lu^a	0	Some	Most	Few	Few	Few	Few	No	
Anti-Lu^b	0	Few	Few	Few	Most	Few	Few	Mild	Yes
Anti-K	0		Few	Some	Most	Some	Most	Yes	Yes
Anti-k	0		Few	Few	Most	Some	Most	Yes	Yes
Anti-Kp^a	0		Some	Some	Most	Some	Some	Yes	
Anti-Kp^b	0		Few	Few	Most	Some	Some	Yes	Yes
Anti-Js^a	0		Few	Few	Most	Few	Few	Yes	
Anti-Js^b	0		0	0	Most	Few	Few	Yes	
Anti-Le^a	Some	Most	Most	Some	Many	Most	Most	No	Few
Anti-Le^b	Occ.	Most	Most	Few	Some	Some	Some	No	No
Anti-Fy^a	0		Rare	Rare	Most	0	0	Yes	Yes
Anti-Fy^b	0		Rare	Rare	Most	0	0	Yes	Yes
Anti-Jk^a	Some		Few	Few	Most	Some	Most	Yes	Yes
Anti-Jk^b	Few		Few	Few	Most	Some	Most	Yes	Yes
Anti-Xg^a	0		Few	Few	Most	0	0	No report	
Anti-Di^a	0			Some	Some	Most	Some	Some	Yes	Yes
Anti-Di^b	0				Most	Some	Some	Yes	Yes
Anti-Yt^a	0		0	0	Most	0	Some	No	
Anti-Yt^b	0				All			No report	
Anti-Do^a	0		0	0	Some	Some	Most		Yes
Anti-Do^b	0				All		All	No report	
Anti-Co^a	0		0	0	Some	Some	Most	Yes	
Anti-Co^b	0		0	0	Some	Some	Most	No report	
Anti-Sc1	0				All			No report	
Anti-Sc2	0		Some	Some	Most	Most	Most	No report	

The reactivity shown is based on the tube methods in common use. If tests are carried out by more sensitive test procedures, direct agglutination (prior to the antiglobulin phase) may be observed more often with some antibodies. Blank spaces indicate a lack of sufficient data to make generalizations.

AGT = Antiglobulin test; HDN = Hemolytic disease of the newborn; HTR = Hemolytic transfusion reaction.

Table 5–2. The Identification of a Single Antibody in a Serum

Panel Cells	D	C	E	c	e	Cw	M	N	S	s	P1	Leª	Leᵇ	Luª	Luᵇ	K	k	Kpª	Jsª	Fyª	Fyᵇ	Jkª	Jkᵇ	SRT	37°C	AGT	F37	FAG
1	0	+	0	+	+	0	+	0	+	+	+	0	+	0	+	0	+	0	0	+	0	+	0	0	0	0	0	0
2	+	+	0	+	+	0	0	+	0	+	+	+	0	0	+	0	+	0	0	+	0	+	+	0	0	0	0	0
3	+	+	0	0	+	0	0	+	+	0	+	+	0	0	+	+	+	0	0	0	+	+	+	0	0	0	0	0
4	+	0	+	+	+	0	0	+	0	+	0	0	+	0	+	0	+	+	0	+	+	+	0	0	0	2+	3+	1+
5	0	0	+	+	+	0	+	0	+	0	0	+	0	0	+	0	+	0	0	0	+	+	+	0	0	1+	3+	0
6	0	0	0	+	+	0	0	+	0	+	+	0	+	0	+	0	+	0	0	+	0	0	+	0	0	0	0	0
7	0	0	0	+	+	0	+	0	0	+	0	0	+	+	0	+	0	0	+	+	+	0	+	0	0	0	0	0
8	0	0	0	+	+	+	0	+	+	0	+	+	0	0	+	0	+	0	0	+	+	+	+	0	0	0	0	0
9	0	0	0	+	+	0	+	+	0	+	+	0	+	0	+	0	+	0	0	+	+	+	0	0	0	0	0	0
10	0	0	0	+	+	0	0	+	+	+	+	+	0	0	+	0	+	0	0	+	0	+	+	0	0	0	0	0
Auto																												
Screening Cells																												
I	+	+	0	+	+	0	0	+	0	+	+	0	+	0	+	0	+	0	0	+	0	+	0	0	0	0	0	0
II	+	0	+	+	+	0	+	0	+	0	+	+	0	0	+	0	+	0	0	0	+	+	+	0	0	2+	3+	1+

Only cells 4 and 5 of the panel and cell II of the screening cell pair have shown positive reactions; hence, the antibody is not directed at any antigen present on cells 1, 2, 3, 6, 7, 8, 9, or 10 of the panel, nor on cell I of the screening cell pair. If those antigens are struck out in the column headings on the antigen sheet, the only antigens remaining *not* struck out are E and Kpª. Thus the antibodies not excluded are anti-E and anti-Kpª. All three of the reactive cell suspensions are E+. We may therefore be reasonably confident that this serum contains anti-E. We have no evidence that anti-Kpª *is* present, as the only Kp(a+) cell suspension here is also E+, so anti-Kpª is not excluded. An E-negative Kp(a+) cell suspension would be required to prove the point, which is not at all important.

SRT = Saline room temperature; AGT = Antiglobulin test; F37 = Ficin-treated cells at 37°C; FAG = Antiglobulin test on ficin-treated cells.

Table 5-3. Identification of a Serum Containing a More Complicated Antibody

Panel Cells	D	C	E	c	e	C^w	M	N	S	s	P_1	Le^a	Le^b	Lu^a	Lu^b	K	k	Kp^a	Js^a	Fy^a	Fy^b	Jk^a	Jk^b	SRT	37°C	AGT	F37	FAG
1	0	+	0	+	+	0	+	0	+	+	+	0	+	0	+	0	+	0	0	+	0	+	0	0	0	1+	0	0
2	+	+	0	+	+	+	0	+	0	+	+	+	0	0	+	0	+	0	0	0	+	+	+	0	0	0	0	0
3	+	+	0	0	+	0	+	+	+	+	0	0	0	0	+	+	+	0	0	+	0	+	+	0	0	1+	0	0
4	+	0	+	+	0	0	0	+	0	+	0	0	+	0	+	0	+	+	0	0	+	+	0	0	0	0	0	0
5	0	0	+	+	+	0	0	+	0	+	0	0	0	0	+	0	+	0	0	0	+	+	+	0	0	0	0	0
6	0	0	0	+	+	0	+	+	+	0	+	+	0	0	+	0	+	0	0	0	+	0	+	0	0	0	0	0
7	0	0	0	+	+	0	+	+	+	+	+	0	0	+	+	+	0	0	0	+	0	0	0	0	0	0	0	0
8	0	0	0	+	+	0	0	+	0	+	+	0	0	0	+	0	+	0	+	+	+	+	+	0	0	0	0	0
9	0	0	0	+	+	0	+	0	+	+	0	+	+	0	+	0	+	0	0	+	0	+	+	0	0	0	0	0
10	0	0	0	+	+	0	0	+	+	+	+	+	0	0	+	0	+	0	0	+	+	+	0	0	0	0	0	0
Auto																								0	0	0	0	0
Screening Cells																												
I	+	+	0	0	+	0	+	0	+	+	+	0	+	0	+	+	+	0	0	+	0	+	0	0	0	1+	0	0
II	+	0	+	+	0	0	+	+	0	+	+	+	0	0	+	0	+	0	0	0	+	0	+	0	0	0	0	0

Here we have struck out all the antigens in the panel. Close examination, however, reveals that the reactive cells are all Fy(a+b−), suggesting the possibility that we are dealing with a weak example of anti-Fy^a that is only reacting convincingly with cells having homozygous expression of the Fy^a antigen. This antibody is showing reactions only at the antiglubulin phase, and there is no reactivity at any phase with ficin-treated cells. This behavior is what would be expected of anti-Fy^a, but there is one Fy(a+b−) cell suspension that is not reactive. That cell suspension is Js(a+), a phenotype that occurs predominantly in blacks. More than two-thirds of blacks belong to the phenotype Fy(a−b−), so the gene Fy is more common than either Fy^a or Fy^b in blacks, and in this population group, the genotype of a person of the phenotype Fy(a+b−) is much more likely to be Fy^aFy than Fy^aFy^a.

SRT = Saline room temperature; AGT = Antiglobulin test; F37 = Ficin-treated cells at 37°C; FAG = Antiglobulin test on ficin-treated cells.

bility that one or more of the reactions may not be correct. The negative results with the cells numbered 8, 9, and 10 on the panel, and with the second screening cell suspension, are leading away from the proper identification of this antibody.

MULTIPLE SPECIFICITY

When a serum contains more than one antibody, the method of systematically dismissing antibodies directed at all antigens known to be present on cell suspensions showing a negative test result is particularly useful, as illustrated in Table 5-4. The same results also demonstrate the importance of recognizing and recording any variation in the strength of agglutination with different cells. Such evidence, combined with recognition of the fact that reactivity is occurring at different phases of the test, may indicate that more than one antibody is present.

Antibody mixtures are common. Once a patient produces one immune blood group antibody, other specificities may also appear. In theory, the patient may have antibodies to any other antigen for which his or her cells are negative and to which he or she has been exposed. But it should not be routine to select donor blood on the basis of what antibodies a patient *might* produce. Such lengths are not justified as a matter of routine, even in recipients expected to need multiple transfusions in the future, although opinion is divided about whether it may be appropriate to apply the principle on a limited basis.

ANTIBODIES TO HIGH-FREQUENCY ANTIGENS

Panel testing occasionally gives uniformly strong reactivity against all the cells. In the absence of reactivity with the patient's own cells, this could indicate an unexpected antibody directed at an antigen of high frequency, although multiple antibodies of more or less equal potency and reactivity may still be the explanation. Identifying the antibody or antibodies, and locating suitable donor blood in such cases, is difficult. Accordingly, it is important to recognize at an early stage when outside help, such as a reference laboratory or a rare-donor registry, is needed.

ANTIBODIES TO LOW-FREQUENCY ANTIGENS

The opposite situation occurs when a serum previously found to contain an antibody shows no reactivity with any of the cells in the panel. This may be due to an antibody directed at an antigen on the cells tested originally but not represented on the panel. Absence of such an antigen in the panel does not imply that the antibody is of no clinical significance. Indeed, it *could* be significant, for example, if it has reactivity at 37°C, either as a direct agglutinin or by the antiglobulin test, and it is prudent to assume that it could cause red cell destruction. The antigen is likely to be one having a low frequency, which means that the selection of blood for transfusion will present little difficulty.

Table 5-4. Identification of a Serum Containing Two Antibodies

Panel Cells	D	C	E	c	e	C^w	M	N	S	s	P_1	Le^a	Le^b	Lu^a	Lu^b	K	k	Kp^a	Js^a	Fy^a	Fy^b	Jk^a	Jk^b	SRT	37°C	AGT	F37	FAG
1	0	+	0	+	+	0	+	0	+	+	+	0	+	0	+	0	+	0	0	+	0	+	0	2+	0	0	0	0
2	+	+	0	0	+	+	0	+	0	+	+	+	0	0	+	0	+	0	0	0	+	+	+	0	0	0	0	0
3	+	+	0	0	+	0	+	+	+	+	+	+	0	0	+	+	+	+	0	0	+	+	+	0	0	3+	1+	2+
4	+	0	+	+	0	0	0	+	0	+	0	0	+	0	+	0	+	0	0	0	0	+	0	2+	0	0	0	0
5	0	0	0	+	+	0	0	+	+	0	0	0	+	0	+	0	+	0	0	0	+	+	+	2+	0	0	0	0
6	0	0	0	+	+	0	+	0	+	+	+	0	0	0	+	+	0	0	0	0	+	+	0	0	0	0	0	0
7	0	0	+	+	+	0	0	+	0	+	0	+	0	+	+	0	+	0	+	+	0	0	+	2+	0	4+	2+	3+
8	0	0	0	+	+	0	+	+	+	0	+	0	0	0	+	0	+	0	0	+	0	+	+	0	0	0	0	0
9	0	0	0	+	+	0	0	+	+	+	0	0	0	0	+	0	+	+	0	+	+	+	+	2+	0	0	0	0
10	0	0	0	+	+	0	+	0	+	+	+	+	0	0	+	0	+	0	0	+	+	+	0	0	0	0	0	0
Auto																								0	0	0	0	0
Screening Cells																												
I	+	+	0	0	+	0	+	0	+	+	+	0	+	0	+	+	+	0	0	+	0	+	0	2+	0	3+	1+	2+
II	+	0	+	0	+	0	0	+	0	+	+	0	0	0	+	0	+	0	0	+	+	0	+	0	0	0	0	0

One antibody is a direct agglutinin that reacts best in the cold, as indicated by the reactivity observed with cells 1, 4, 5, 7, and 9. Cell 3 is showing its strongest reactivity at the antiglobulin phase, with some agglutination of ficin-treated cells after 37°C incubation and at the antiglobulin phase. Cell 7 (and also cell I of the screening cell set) look as if they may possess both antigens. The antigens not struck out in the column headings are Le^b, Lu^a, K, and Kp^a. Further study confirms the presence of anti-Le^a and anti-K, with anti-Lu^a and anti-Kp^a remaining unexcluded. There is a hint that anti-Kp^a is probably *not* present because the only Kp(a+) cell here is also Le(b+), and is showing only the reactivity shown by other Le(b+) cells that are Kp(a−).

SRT = Saline room temperature; AGT = Antiglobulin test; F37 = Ficin-treated cells at 37°C; FAG = Antiglobulin test on ficin-treated cells.

Even if the antibody were anti-Co^b or anti-Yt^b, both directed at antigens having a frequency between 5 and 10 percent that are not required to be present on cells used for detection and identification of antibodies, the blood of more than 90 percent of randomly selected donors would be compatible. If the antigen is one having a *very* low incidence, such as Wr^a (Wright) or Vw (Verweyst), it would be an extraordinary coincidence if an antigen-positive donor unit were among those selected for transfusion. Antibodies to low-frequency antigens occur commonly, often without a demonstrable immune stimulus; yet, even so, they sometimes behave like immune antibodies in belonging to the IgG class of human immunoglobulin. Multiple specificity is quite common, especially in serums from persons suffering from autoimmune hemolytic anemia or among those with any kind of autoimmune disease.

ANTIBODIES TO BG ANTIGENS

A problem similar to that created by a low-frequency antigen in a red cell suspension used for screening or crossmatching is that caused by the so-called Bg antigens. The antigens collectively called "Bg" are manifestations of HLA antigens, occurring at variable strength on the red cells.

A curious feature of the Bg antigens is that they are variable in the strength of their expression, not only between different persons, but at different times in the same person. To make things more complex, Bg antibodies are commonly of multiple specificity, often showing inconclusive and inconstantly reproducible reactions by the indirect antiglobulin test (see p. 115). Because of these features, a reaction initially observed in a screening test may not necessarily be reproducible at the same strength on all occasions.

The various forms of anti-Bg occur so commonly in serums from patients who have recently received a transfusion, or been pregnant, that the use of a red cell suspension having strong expression of a Bg antigen can be a recurring source of aggravation during the shelf-life of the particular set of screening cells. Its presence leads, all too frequently, to the testing of a reactive serum against a panel of cells, with the only conclusion being that the observed reactivity is attributable to an antibody that is not clinically significant. The waste in terms of labor, reagents, and other disposables may be considerable, not to mention the delay this causes in providing blood for transfusion. Because it is better *not* to detect anti-Bg during antibody screening, manufacturers now try to avoid issuing screening cells that possess a strong Bg antigen. This objective may not be achieved consistently, as it is difficult to be certain that a particular suspension of screening cells will not detect Bg antibodies with unacceptable frequency, however thoroughly it is tested with examples of anti-Bg.

HIGH-TITER LOW-AVIDITY ANTIBODIES

Of somewhat similar reactivity to the various forms of anti-Bg are the specificities that have been collectively called *high-titer low-avidity* (HTLA) antibodies.

The name is descriptive, and should possibly be allowed to fall into disuse. It derives from the fact that, although the serum may exhibit reactivity to a high dilution, the actual strength of reactivity at any dilution is poor, unlike most other blood group antibodies, which show progressively weaker reactivity with dilution. HTLA antibodies are often as ephemeral as those directed at Bg, but cause more difficulty because their corresponding antigens are of much higher frequency; hence, it is harder to find crossmatch-compatible blood. Several antibodies fall under this heading, and to deal with their identification would not be profitable. The HTLA antibodies most often encountered are those directed at the antigens Yk^a/Cs^a (York/Cost-Stirling) and Kn^a/McC^a (Knops/McCoy). The clinical significance of these antibodies has sometimes been the subject of lively debate, but there is little evidence that any of them has ever been involved in a hemolytic transfusion reaction. The important thing is to identify the antibody as showing the characteristic behavior of the group, by showing in a titration that it shows weak reactivity over a wide range of dilutions (i.e., to at least 1 in 64). It is not appropriate to dismiss as being of no significance an antibody reacting weakly with all red cells except the patient's own without first demonstrating that similar reactivity does indeed extend to high dilutions. The observed characteristics could just as easily reflect the first signs of a developing immune response to some high-frequency antigen, such as Vel, Kp^b, or Lan, that deserves to be taken more seriously. Once an HTLA antibody has been adequately characterized, blood may be issued despite the incompatible crossmatch, with the recipient under careful clinical observation.

The Chido and Rodgers Antigens

Two other antibodies that show relatively feeble reactions, often to high dilutions, are those directed at the Chido (Ch) and the Rodgers (Rg) antigens. These antigens actually reside on the C4d fragment of the C4 molecule of human complement [13, 14]. Because C4 is taken up by the red cells to some extent, anti-Ch and anti-Rg will react by the antiglobulin test with the red cells of Ch-positive and Rg-positive persons, but there is no report of them causing a hemolytic transfusion reaction. Reactivity of both antibodies can also be demonstrated by direct agglutination if the indicator red cells are deliberately coated with human C4.

Since C4 is present in abundance in the serum, the antibodies are inhibited by serums from people whose C4 possesses the appropriate antigens. The ability of serums of known Ch and/or Rg status to inhibit or not to inhibit reactions suspected to be caused by anti-Ch or anti-Rg is useful in the identification of both specificities. Inhibition by antigen-positive serum or plasma may be complete or only partial, which provides an indication of complex heterogeneity among the antigens represented on the C4 molecule [15]. The principle may also be applied to the determination of Ch or Rg antigen status of unknown bloods using known examples of the relevant antibody.

The Sd^a (Sid) Antigen

Sd^a occurs at variable strength on the red cells of more than 90 percent of the population. The corresponding antibody is comparatively common, but has been reported to be of no clinical significance, except for one case in which anti-Sd^a was implicated in a hemolytic transfusion reaction [16]. The antigen may have been expressed at greater than its usual strength in that case.

A curious feature of anti-Sd^a is that it can be inhibited by the urine of Sd(a+) persons, and by all guinea pig urine, because the Sd^a antigen appears to be associated with the normally present Tamm and Horsfall urinary glycoprotein [17]. Accordingly, one approach to the identification of anti-Sd^a is an agglutination inhibition test using urine from an Sd(a+) person. Because such factors as pH and salt concentration can cause urine to inhibit agglutination by other antibodies too, however, the urine sample must first be dialysed against phosphate-buffered saline and, if necessary, have its pH adjusted to neutral [18].

The serologic behavior of anti-Sd^a is unique, so that an inhibition test with urine is seldom needed. Anti-Sd^a produces mixed-field agglutination that is unusual in being composed of distinctive, small, spherical agglutinates against a background of unagglutinated cells. This characteristic reaction is most often seen when the antiglobulin phase of the antibody detection test is examined microscopically, but that is only because the agglutinates are difficult to see with the naked eye, and agglutinating tests in saline are seldom examined microscopically. In reality, anti-Sd^a is a direct agglutinin of saline-suspended Sd(a+) cells, which is detected at the antiglobulin phase only because the agglutinates it produces survive the washing phase. If anything, the washing improves the integrity of the agglutinates. They are just as readily recognized if saline instead of antiglobulin serum is added to the dry button of cells after washing. In fact, a useful method of recognizing agglutination due to anti-Sd^a is to set up the test with a 10 to 15 percent cell suspension instead of the more commonly used 3 to 5 percent suspension, incubate for 15 minutes at room temperature instead of 37°C before washing the cells, and add two drops of saline before examination. [J. Case, unpublished observation].

AUTOANTIBODIES

When a serum is tested against a panel and the autologous control test is positive, the serum probably contains an autoantibody. Interpretation may not be entirely straightforward, however, as the reactivity of the autoantibody may be concealing some clinically significant alloantibody. The direct antiglobulin test will be positive if the thermal range of the autoantibody enables it to attach to red cells at a temperature close to that of the human body. A positive direct antiglobulin test in a recently transfused recipient could indicate that a developing *allo*antibody is coating surviving donor cells.

In discussing the steps to be taken in resolving the problems that arise when the autologous control test is positive, it is convenient to adopt a systematic approach based on the observed reactivity, in particular, the phase of testing at which it is most prominent. Special techniques, such as autoabsorption, or elution and the subsequent testing of the eluate, will be determined by the characteristics of the particular autoantibody.

Cold Autoagglutinins

When autoantibody reactivity takes the form of direct agglutination in tests at room temperature or lower, the cause is most often anti-I, an autoantibody commonly present in healthy persons but ordinarily detectable only in tests at 4°C. Anti-I is the most common specificity associated with cold hemagglutinin disease, where its potency increases and its thermal range broadens until agglutination occurs in tests carried out at 37°C. Anti-I is seldom, if ever, truly reactive at 37°C, even though direct agglutination may be seen in tests incubated at that temperature. The reason is that the temperature of the test mixture falls rapidly below 37°C during centrifugation, not that the autoagglutinin is actually causing agglutination at the temperature of the human body.

Anti-I, which is almost always wholly IgM, binds complement to red cells; hence, may be detected by the antiglobulin test when the antiglobulin serum contains an anti-C3 component. An eluate from the red cells most often contains no antibody reactivity. A measure sometimes adopted to determine that an IgG alloantibody does not accompany a complement-binding cold autoagglutinin is to carry out the antiglobulin test with anti-IgG instead of a polyspecific reagent. In many cases, the ability of the autoagglutinin to bind complement to the cells can be defeated by prewarming the serum and cell suspension to 37°C before mixing them and by carrying out all subsequent manipulations, including centrifugation, at 37°C. Since the test mixture never falls to a temperature that is within the thermal range of the cold-acting autoantibody, complement is never bound by it.

A valuable aid to the identification of anti-I is the knowledge that the I antigen is expressed weakly on the red cells of newborn infants, and that anti-I therefore shows weaker reactions against cells from cord blood than against adult cells. Cord cells are not entirely devoid of I, however, and where the anti-I is of exceptional potency it may not be possible to recognize the discrepancy in reactivity without first diluting the serum.

Some examples of cold agglutinins appearing superficially to be anti-I may in reality be directed at an antigen that has been called HI (or IH) because it occurs only when both I and H are present on the cells. Unless it is particularly potent, this form of "anti-I" may not even be recognized as an autoagglutinin, because it usually occurs only in serums from A_1 or A_1B persons and reacts more feebly with red cells of those phenotypes than with the group O cells most often used for testing.

Warm Autoantibodies
Warm autoantibodies most often belong to the IgG class of immunoglobulin, and hence do not generally show direct agglutination except in a high-protein medium or by an enzyme technique. The autoantibody may show a specificity relating to the Rh system, most often because red cells lacking the e antigen give weaker reactions with the patient's serum (or with an eluate from the cells) than do cells of the more common Rh phenotypes. The autoantibody is thus directed at e, or at least part of it is so directed. This conclusion may not be precisely correct, but is valid enough in the context of transfusing "least incompatible" blood. More often, however, cDE cells are not perfectly compatible; although if there were an opportunity to test the serum with D-- or with Rh_{null} cells, either or both may be nonreactive. This appears to validate the relationship with Rh, but such a finding is of purely academic interest. Testing autoantibodies with cells of these rare phenotypes is neither required nor clinically useful. It is almost always impractical, besides.

As in the case of cold autoagglutinins, powerful warm autoantibodies may not show differing grades of reactivity when tested undiluted, yet when titrated against cells chosen for their phenotypes, may appear to show specificity within the Rh system. Warm-type autoantibodies with apparent specificity against one of the common blood group antigens not of the Rh system (e.g., Jk^a or Xg^a) have also been reported. In some cases, there may be little or no antibody in the patient's serum even though the direct antiglobulin test on the patient's red cells is distinctly positive. Here, the task of excluding accompanying alloantibodies presents few difficulties. Sometimes, the specificity of the antibody in the patient's serum does not coincide exactly with that of an eluate prepared from the cells. There are several explanations for this besides the presence of an alloantibody in the serum. It is not uncommon for the antibody in an eluate to be less potent than that in the serum, for example; and if the autoantibody should be one that shows variable strength of reactivity with red cells of different phenotypes, the native serum may appear to contain a specificity lacking from the eluate.

Antibody-Coated Donor Cells (Mixed-Field Antiglobulin Reaction)
When the red cells of a recently transfused recipient have a positive direct antiglobulin test, it is worth looking for the typical mixed-field reaction that may indicate the presence of immunoglobulin on only *some* of the red cells in the recipient's blood. In the case of an alloantibody developing from a recent transfusion, there may be no free antibody detectable in the serum because it has all been adsorbed to antigen-positive donor cells still circulating. And since the recipient's red cells are usually more numerous than the coated donor cells, the direct antiglobulin test is perceptibly positive on only the minority population, resulting in a reaction in which relatively small agglutinates are seen

against a distinct background of unagglutinated cells. This is a *mixed-field* reaction.

AGGLUTINATION CAUSED BY OTHER INFLUENCES

Drugs and Antibiotics

Treatment with certain drugs, especially alpha-methyldopa, may cause the red cells to take up immunoglobulin, with or without overt clinical manifestations of autoimmune hemolytic anemia. The serum and the eluate may contain an autoantibody having apparent specificity in the Rh system. Other drugs, such as phenacetin, quinidine, stibophen, dipyrone, and some of the sulfonamides, may cause a positive direct antiglobulin test (and sometimes severe hemolytic anemia) without a detectable antibody in the serum or in eluates.

Penicillin sometimes becomes attached to the red cells and stimulates the production of antibodies, particularly in subjects who are given large doses of the antibiotic intravenously. The antibodies so produced bind, in their turn, to the penicillin still attached to the red cells, causing a positive direct antiglobulin test and sometimes hemolysis. Anti-penicillin in the serum, and in an eluate from the cells, may be demonstrated by appropriate testing against red cells coated in vitro with penicillin.

Neomycin, chloramphenicol, and hydrocortisone, used as ingredients in the suspending mediums of commercial reagent red cells, have all been separately reported as causing test results simulating blood group antibodies when the cells were tested with serums containing antibodies to the substance in question [19–21].

Anticoagulants, Saline, and Bovine Albumin

Nonspecific reactivity has been reported with red cells from blood samples in EDTA, and with cells recently washed in saline [22–24]. Of various other common laboratory solutions reported to have caused misleading reactivity in hemagglutination tests, bovine albumin may be one of the most significant. The phenomenon of albumin autoagglutination was first reported in 1956, when three serum samples were found to agglutinate all red cell suspensions tested, including the patients' own, whenever bovine albumin was present in the test mixture. The indirect antiglobulin test on saline suspensions was consistently negative [25]. Sodium caprylate, a short-chain fatty acid added to stabilize some bovine albumin solutions during manufacture, was found to be responsible for the reactivity. A later study showed that a complex formed between the albumin molecule and sodium caprylate acted in combination with an antibody to caprylate in the reactive serums [26, 27]. Caprylate is not invariably implicated in albumin autoagglutination; other (undetermined) factors have also been implicated [28].

Microbial Contamination

Certain bacteria and viruses produce enzymes that alter the red cell membrane in such a way that the cells are directly agglutinated by many normal human serums. This is called *polyagglutinability,* the most common form of which occurs when the enzyme neuraminidase activates hidden cell-surface receptors called *T-receptors,* thereby causing the cells to become agglutinable by the anti-T agglutinins in most normal adult human serums [29]. This effect can occur in red cells in vivo as a result of bacteremia, and in vitro, in blood samples stored without adequate aseptic precautions. It can also occur when fresh red cells are incubated with serums heavily contaminated with bacteria that produce enzymes capable of T-transforming red cells, or of bringing about other forms of microbial polyagglutinability (such as Th- or Tk-transformation). Polyagglutinable red cells are likely to be agglutinated with most *fresh* human serums, but not with commercial reagent antiserums (see p. 175). It may not be possible to store blood and serum samples in a sterile condition, but samples should always be kept in the refrigerator when not in use, to minimize bacterial growth. Any sample that has become obviously contaminated should not be used.

PSEUDOAGGLUTINATION

Rouleaux

The formation of red cells into aggregates resembling piles of coins is called *rouleaux,* and is most often caused by an excess of certain proteins in the serum, particularly globulins. Rouleaux formation, if unusually pronounced, may interfere with blood typing because of difficulty in distinguishing it from true agglutination. A useful way to make the distinction between rouleaux and true agglutination is to examine the test mixture microscopically under a coverslip, using pressure applied to the coverslip with a pencil tip to put the aggregates into motion. Unlike most true agglutinates, rouleaux have a shining appearance because they refract light. This feature usually makes it easy to recognize rouleaux. As with autoagglutination, however, a possibility exists that true agglutination caused by an alloantibody is being concealed by the aggregation. A drop of physiologic saline added gently to the reaction mixture is sometimes successful in dispersing rouleaux while not affecting true agglutination. Alternatively, a technique called *saline replacement* is sometimes used: the reaction mixture is centrifuged and the supernatant serum aspirated and carefully replaced with physiologic saline before the cell button is resuspended and examined in the usual way. This procedure, by reducing the protein content of the test mixture, usually enables the cell button to be resuspended without rouleaux.

The formation of rouleaux occurs less often in a test mixture that includes bovine albumin than in one having a lower protein concentration. It appears that the presence of a protein having a lower molecular weight than that of the globulin causing the rouleaux tends to even out the imbalance. Rouleaux formation normally affects only the examination of the test for direct agglutination. Rouleaux are hardly ever seen in an antiglobulin test, as the abnormal serum proteins are removed during the washing phase. In myeloma, however, additional washing may be needed to remove the excess of globulin present.

Colloidal Silica

When saline or other electrolytic solutions are autoclaved in glass bottles, colloidal silica may be released into the solution and subsequently adsorbed to red cells that may be suspended or washed in it. Red cells so coated may show spontaneous agglutination [30].

Other Forms of Pseudoagglutination

When the test sample is imperfectly clotted, as sometimes occurs in coagulation disorders, or when the patient is anticoagulated with heparin, fibrin strands may develop during incubation. If the test red cells become enmeshed, this leads to clumping that resembles true agglutination. A similar appearance can result from an excess of polymorphonuclear leukocytes in the red cell suspension; these, too, may form clumps that involve red cells. Contamination of the serum or cell suspension with particles of dirt or calcium stearates (which sometimes precipitate during frozen storage of serum), or with chemical crystals or foreign bodies on the glassware, may produce similar misleading effects.

Crossmatching

The earliest reported application of crossmatching was to detect ABO incompatibility [31]. In the ensuing years, with the discovery of many other antigens, came the realization that no single test procedure could detect all blood group antibodies. This led to the perception of a need to detect all agglutinating, coating, and hemolyzing antibodies, and to the development and adoption of methods that, between them, would attempt to achieve the desired objective. Test methods in crossmatching are essentially the same as those used in antibody screening. The only difference is that in crossmatching, the test is carried out against red cells from donor units intended for transfusion, whereas in screening, the test is carried out against group O reagent cells selected to react with the most commonly encountered unexpected antibodies. Plainly, antibody screening is more comprehensive in its coverage, since the indicator cells carry most of the important blood group antigens, whereas donor cells are selected only for ABO and D types and possess other antigens only by chance. But these same donor cells may possess one of the less-common antigens (such as C^w and Kp^a), or even an antigen of very low incidence that is usually absent from screening cells. Thus, a crossmatch, which uses the actual red cells to be transfused, may detect a clinically significant antibody that would not be recognized by a routine screening test.

In practice, the antiglobulin phase of the major crossmatch only rarely detects a clinically significant antibody that was not recognized during screening. Hence, if a recipient has no history indicating past blood group immunization, and the serum has given a negative result on being appropriately screened for unexpected antibodies by test procedures that included an antiglobulin phase, an antiglobulin crossmatch is no longer mandatory. A test *is* still required, however, to exclude ABO incompatibility before transfusion, in case a chosen donor unit should have been incorrectly labeled as to ABO.

The favored means of excluding ABO incompatibility in many institutions is an immediate-spin test using the recipient's serum and a suspension of donor cells; but the sensitivity of this procedure has been called into question, particularly when it is done with group B serums and cells of the A_2B subgroup. In one study, 204 of 531 immediate-spin tests failed to detect the incompatibility between these two groups [32]. A second study found that when 84 unselected group B serums were examined, their reactivity with A_2B cells in a LISS test was recognized only 37 percent of the time by immediate-spin. Incubation of the test for 5 minutes at room temperature enabled 69 percent of the incompatibilities to be detected, but incubation for 15 minutes at 37°C reduced the figure to 42 percent. Even at the antiglobulin phase, the incompatibility between group B serums and A_2B cells was missed 27 percent of the time with anti-IgG and 5 percent of the time with polyspecific anti-human globulin. Agglutination at the antiglobulin phase was recognized only by microscopic examination in a significant proportion of the cases [33].

To view these observations in proper perspective, it must be a rare event indeed for a group A_2B donor unit inadvertently labeled as B to escape detection before being selected to be crossmatched for a group B recipient. And if it *were* to get that far, there is clearly no guarantee that even an indirect antiglobulin test would detect the incompatibility. All things considered, we believe that an immediate-spin test is sufficient to meet the requirement to exclude ABO incompatibility before transfusion.

THE IMMUNIZED RECIPIENT

A full crossmatch, including an antiglobulin phase, is essential for recipients whose serum contains an unexpected antibody, or has been reported to contain one in the past. Once an antibody has been recognized, transfusion should ideally be postponed until the antibody specificity has been determined and appropriate donor units have been selected by typing with appropriate antiserum(s) and crossmatching with the recipient's serum. The application of this rule is, naturally, to be guided by common sense. No delay can be allowed that will compromise the recipient's chances of survival. The decision whether or not the risks of postponing transfusion outweigh those resulting from possibly significant serologic incompatibility should be made by the recipient's physician, in consultation with the physician in charge of the transfusion service. If a transfusion is urgently required, crossmatch-compatible blood may be released before the antibody has been identified. The crossmatch is the most important part of any subsequent testing, because it has the potential to recognize incompatibility even when the recipient has made an antibody that is difficult to identify, or more than one.

The main purpose of testing apparently compatible donor units with a reagent antiserum of appropriate specificity is to ensure recognition of the incompatibility when the patient's antibody is relatively weak. Sometimes, the patient's antibody may be *more potent* than the commercial antiserum, in which case testing compatible donor cells with the latter merely adds verification to the specificity of the antibody. In any case, once the antibody has been identified, it is needlessly extravagant to use a reagent antiserum to screen for potentially suitable donors. The patient's serum should be used in the first instance, reserving the more costly testing with a commercial antiserum for donor units selected as being nonreactive.

Autoimmunity

If a recipient's serum contains autoantibodies showing equal reactivity with all donor cells, there may be no choice but to give blood that is incompatible with the serum. Assuming that appropriate steps have been taken to exclude concomitant alloantibody, and that the "autoantibody" is not in reality an alloantibody developing in response to a recent transfusion, the administration of "incompatible" blood in this setting is seldom harmful. At least, the donor blood is usually no more incompatible than the recipient's own red cells. In these cases, the necessity of giving incompatible blood should be discussed with the recipient's physician. Cold autoagglutinins not active at 37°C are hardly ever clinically significant and, so far as recipients with warm autoantibodies are concerned, we see no purpose in postponing transfusion to select "least incompatible" blood.

THE URGENT TRANSFUSION

The clinical indications for a transfusion are occasionally so pressing that there is no time to test the recipient's blood at all. More often, there is time to draw a blood sample but not to complete the pretransfusion compatibility-testing routine. Such emergencies must be handled on an individual basis, as the measures to be taken will depend on the tests that can be completed in the time available. This is discussed in Chapter 6.

Special Techniques in Investigating Unexpected Antibodies

ABSORPTION, ELUTION, AND INHIBITION

Absorption of a serum is a procedure by which unwanted antibodies can be removed from a serum, or a mixture of antibodies separated. For example, the components of a serum containing two antibodies can be separated by adding washed, packed red cells possessing one of the corresponding antigens but lacking the other. One antibody is adsorbed to the red cells while the other remains in the serum. The adsorbed antibody can then be removed from the red cell surface by *elution,* thereby enabling each antibody to be identified. The description oversimplifies the procedure, which may not achieve the desired separation without repetition. Moreover, the potency of the eluted antibody is dependent on many variables, including the affinity of the antibody for its antigen and the method chosen to dissociate it once it has been adsorbed.

The terminology bears clarification. We say that a serum is *ab*sorbed with red cells that *ad*sorb the antibody to their surfaces, from which it may be recovered by eluting it into an appropriate *substrate*. The process of mixing the serum and washed, packed red cells for this purpose is referred to as *ab*sorption, and the serum that remains after you have separated the red cells is called *ab*sorbed serum. The antibody that was removed from the serum had been *ad*sorbed to the red cells.

Autoabsorption is a further application of the absorption principle, in which a serum is absorbed with its own red cells to remove an autoantibody, as a means to determine whether an alloantibody is also present. Absorption of unwanted ABO antibodies from a serum containing a potentially useful alloantibody may be used in the preparation of a reagent antiserum, to make it suitable to use for the typing of bloods of all ABO groups.

Absorption is always carried out under conditions that favor the antibody it is desired to *remove* from the serum. If, for example, the antibody to be removed reacts preferentially in the cold, the absorption would be done at 4°C. Similarly, if the activity is enhanced by treatment of the test cells with an enzyme, then enzyme-treated cells should be used. If the antibody to be left in the serum is directed at an antigen known to be *destroyed* by enzyme treatment, the cells do not have to be negative for the antigen concerned when they are treated with an enzyme before the absorption is carried out.

The red cells chosen for absorption are first thoroughly washed to remove antibodies contained in the plasma. After the last wash, they are centrifuged with sufficient force to permit removal of as much saline as possible, to minimize dilution of the serum during absorption. The ratio of washed, packed red cells to serum, and the duration of exposure to the cells, are chosen to minimize the need for repeated absorption. A volume of packed cells equal to the volume of serum being absorbed is most often suitable, and an incubation time of 30 minutes is usually adequate. Absorption is often more effective if done twice, each time using a half volume of packed cells for half the incubation time. Leaving the red cells in contact with the serum for prolonged periods (e.g., overnight) does not improve the efficacy of the procedure. If cells for absorption are in short supply and an eluate from them is not required, they can often be regenerated after use by rewashing them. This is particularly the case when the purpose is to remove cold autoagglutinins. Rewashing the cells with saline at 37°C dissociates adsorbed antibody and permits effective reuse.

After each absorption, test the absorbed serum with a suspension of the cells being used for the procedure, using a suitably sensitive technique to establish whether or not absorption has proceeded to completion. Some antibodies are more difficult to remove than others, depending, among other variables, on their potency and their affinity.

Elution is a procedure by which the antibody adsorbed to red cells during absorption is *dissociated* from the cells into a suitable substrate, in order to enable the antibody to be identified by testing the *eluate* against a cell panel. For example, if a serum is suspected to contain a mixture of anti-Fy^a and anti-c, absorption with c-negative $Fy(a+)$ cells should remove anti-Fy^a and leave anti-c to be identified in the serum. Absorption with cells that are c-positive and $Fy(a-)$ should remove anti-c and leave behind anti-Fy^a. Eluates prepared from the cells used for absorption in each case should confirm the identity of the adsorbed antibody as anti-Fy^a and anti-c, respectively.

There are many elution procedures, all having varying degrees of effectiveness. The general approach is always fundamentally the same. The red cells are first thoroughly washed to remove any unattached antibody, centrifuged to pack them tightly, and then exposed to conditions that will cause the bound antibody to dissociate into the substrate. A small sample of saline from the last wash is always saved to test as a control, in parallel with the eluate. Negative reactions in the control test demonstrate that any antibody reactivity in the eluate has been truly dissociated from the cells and was not merely left behind as the result of inadequate washing.

An alternative purpose for an elution procedure is to help identify an antigen that is, for example, so feebly expressed that it gives a significantly weaker reaction than expected with the corresponding typing serum. In such a case, an eluate is made from the red cells after they have been incubated with the particular antiserum. If this shows reactivity that corresponds to the specificity of the antiserum, it may be concluded that the antigen in question is present on the test cells, although at an atypical level of expression. The *last-wash control* is especially important in this context, as failure to wash away all unbound antibody would lead to a false-positive test result.

The potency of an eluate may be influenced by the volume of fluid (substrate) added to the packed cells after they have been washed free of unattached immunoglobulin. The usual practice is to elute the antibody into a volume of substrate equal to the volume of coated packed cells. With some elution methods this ratio is critical to the successful recovery of as much antibody as possible. With other methods, however, the eluted antibody may be concentrated by being taken up into a lesser volume of substrate. This is useful when the antibody adsorbed to the cells is weak.

The simplest elution procedure is the *heat method,* originally described by

Landsteiner and Miller in 1925, in which the washed packed cells are suspended in saline and placed in a waterbath at 56°C [34]. This method was initially designed for eluting antibodies of the ABO system, and is still one of the best for that purpose, but it is less effective at recovering immune antibodies.

By contrast, Weiner's *cold ethanol precipitation method* is relatively ineffective with anti-A and anti-B, but is particularly successful for recovering Rh antibodies. This method uses cold ethanol to precipitate the immunoglobulin released when coated red cells are lysed by freezing and thawing [35].

A method developed by Kochwa and Rosenfield uses digitonin to lyse the washed, coated red cells, followed by dissociation of the antibody into an acid solution [36]. The original method necessitated high-speed centrifugation and dialysis, but a modification enables the procedure to be more readily applied in a routine laboratory [37]. This method is effective for the recovery of most antibodies, but necessitates additional preparation, as the stroma have to be washed free of digitonin before attempting to recover the antibody. If this step is omitted, the test cells are likely to be lysed by residual digitonin when the eluate is subsequently tested. A further modification eliminates the digitonin step and simply uses glycine-HCl solution to dissociate the antibody directly from the intact washed red cells [38]. The foregoing acid-elution methods depend on a measured volume of substrate to achieve the low pH required for elution and therefore provide little opportunity to concentrate the dissociated antibody. This is because any deviation from the required 1:1 ratio of substrate to cells alters the pH of the mixture. In particular, decreasing the volume of substrate increases the proportion of red cells and results in a pH above the 3.0 level at which dissociation of antibody occurs most efficiently.

Other successful methods of elution have been reported. Each has its adherents, although no single technique is the most effective for eluting *all* blood group antibodies. In choosing an elution method it makes good sense to avoid any procedure that carries a significant risk to the health and welfare of the technologist, such as one that uses a known carcinogenic solvent (dichloromethane, chloroform, or xylol), or a dangerously flammable one (ether).

Inhibition of antibody reactivity may be used in place of absorption as an aid to the separation of antibody mixtures whenever the relevant antigen is available in soluble form. The principle is similar, in many ways, to absorption, except that the unwanted antibody is not removed but is bound to the soluble antigen in a complex that remains in the serum. Soluble A and B substances are to be found, respectively, in porcine and equine gastric mucin, as well as in saliva and other human body fluids from secretors of appropriate ABO groups. Synthetic A and B substances are also available commercially.

Also present in human body fluids are Lewis substances, Le^a most abundantly in nonsecretors possessing the *Le* gene, and Le^b, like A, B, or H, only in secretors. Anti-P_1 is also readily inhibitable by soluble P_1 substance present at high concentration in the eggs of the turtle dove [39] or pigeons. Soluble P_1 substance may also be obtained from hydatid cyst fluid, either from humans or from sheep [40].

TREATMENT OF RED CELLS TO REMOVE IMMUNOGLOBULIN

Chloroquine Treatment

In the course of making eluates for testing, the red cells from which the antibody is dissociated are either destroyed or their antigens are damaged. A method involving treatment of the cells with chloroquine diphosphate, however, may dissociate enough antibody from coated cells to enable them to give a negative direct antiglobulin test, in turn permitting them to be tested for their antigen status by antiserums that cannot be used with coated cells [41]. The method was derived from an earlier application designed for preparing eluates from the red cells in autoimmune hemolytic anemia [42]. The required reagent is a solution containing 20 percent chloroquine diphosphate, adjusted to a pH of 5.1 with $1N$ NaOH. This solution is stable if stored refrigerated.

Incubation of red cells with chloroquine for longer than 2 hours, or raising the incubation temperature to 37°C, may cause lysis and loss of red cell antigens. The technique is not always effective; and there have been reports that tests with saline-reactive Rh antiserums (whether manufactured from IgM or from reduced and alkylated IgG) may show false-negative test results after chloroquine treatment of the test cells [43, 44]. Testing with such reagents can normally be undertaken without treating the cells to remove coating immunoglobulin, however. It is usually only to enable the cells to be tested by the indirect antiglobulin procedure that it is necessary to remove the coating protein. The original authors found no impairment of antigen reactivity when reagent-grade antiserums were used following the treatment, but the reports of impaired Rh antigen reactivity as measured by saline-reactive antiserums may indicate that chloroquine treatment causes some damage to the surface antigens. This conclusion is supported by a report that "home-made" antiserums that are of less-than-optimal potency may be less reliable than commercial-grade reagents, even though they yield acceptable reactions with untreated red cell suspensions [45].

"ZZAP" Treatment

"ZZAP," a reagent containing a mixture of cysteine-activated papain and dithiothreitol, may be used to remove immunoglobulin from red cells [46]. This treatment, too, is not invariably successful, and has certain disadvantages, not the least being that it subjects the red cells to enzyme treatment, thereby making them unsuitable for testing for antigens that are destroyed by proteases. Unlike the usual enzyme treatment procedures, the "ZZAP" reagent also destroys all antigens of the Kell system except Kx, thereby precluding subsequent testing for them. Red cells treated in this way show strongly enhanced reactivity with antiserums corresponding to their Rh antigens, but this is because they have become enzyme-treated during the process. This may be a source of false-positive test results with commercial antiserums, as manufacturers seldom extend their specificity testing to include an enzyme test procedure. The technique is most useful when applied to the preparation of cells for autoabsorption to remove an unwanted autoantibody, because not only is the coating protein removed, but the cells are also treated with an enzyme during the same operation, enhancing their ability to adsorb most autoantibodies.

Treatment of Red Cells to Remove Kell System Antigens

Antigens of the Kell blood group system (except for Kx) are inactivated by 2-aminoethylisothiouronium bromide (AET) [47]. The required reagent is a 6 percent solution of AET in distilled water, adjusted to a pH of 8.0 with 5 N NaOH and used in the proportions of 4 ml to 1 ml of washed, packed red cells. The reagent, which must be prepared immediately before use, is allowed to remain in contact with the cells for 20 minutes at 37°C, after which it is washed away and the red cells are resuspended as desired. The ability of AET to destroy the reactivity of a cell suspension with an antibody does not invariably place that antibody in the Kell system. Antigens not belonging to the Kell system, such as LW^a, have been observed to show a loss of reactivity subsequent to AET treatment [J.J Moulds, personal communication].

TITRATION

When it is necessary to determine the potency of a blood group antibody, the method most commonly used in routine serology is *titration*. A series of doubling dilutions of the serum is prepared in a suitable diluent, and a measured volume of each dilution is tested against selected red cell suspensions. The *endpoint* of the titration is the highest dilution (meaning the weakest concentration of serum) that still shows distinct macroscopic agglutination, usually defined as a 1 + reaction or stronger, and the *titer* of the antibody is the reciprocal of that dilution.

In carrying out a titration, the range of dilutions prepared should be sufficient to extend one or more dilutions beyond the expected endpoint. It is usual, as a routine, to make a series of 10 doubling dilutions in the first instance, ranging from 1 in 1 (meaning the undiluted serum) through 1 in 512 at the tenth tube. An eleventh tube contains only the diluent fluid, to demonstrate that the diluent itself is not causing agglutination. If an antibody is expected to have a titer less than 128 or so, it is not necessary to carry the dilutions to 10 tubes.

In determining the endpoint of a titration, the additional dilution caused by the volume of cell suspension added to each tube is not taken into account. Thus, if an antibody were observed to show 1 + or stronger agglutination up to the fourth tube (namely, that containing the 1 in 8 dilution), with possibly a weak reaction at 1 in 16 and nothing beyond, then the titer of the serum is expressed as 8, not as 1 in 8 or 1/8, and most especially not as 1:8. The use of a colon between two digits implies a ratio, not a dilution, and its use to describe dilutions is a misleading practice that gives rise to error. The ratio 1:2 means one part of something to two parts of something else; in other words (in the context of a serum dilution) one part of serum to two parts of diluent, meaning a dilution of *1 in 3*, not 1 in 2.

In reading the results of a titration, it is always best to start with the blank tube (i.e., with a negative result) and to proceed backward from the weakest to the strongest dilution of the serum, as this facilitates the objective recognition of the endpoint.

Applications of Titration

Not every unexpected antibody detected in routine screening and crossmatching needs to be titrated, but there are situations in which titrations yield useful information.

   1. *To determine the response to antigenic stimulation.* In pregnancy, particularly, it may be useful to know whether the patient's antibody is increasing in potency, as this could indicate continuing exposure to the antigen, implying that the cells of the fetus are positive for it. An increase of two dilutions in the titer of an antibody may be interpreted as indicating a significant rise (see Chap. 9).

   The follow-up of a recipient who has apparently developed an immune antibody as a result of blood transfusion may call for the application of a similar comparison, to determine whether the immune response is primary or secondary. The rate at which the potency of an antibody increases in a secondary response is always faster than in a primary response (see Chap. 2).

   2. *As an aid in the identification of antibody mixtures.* The identification of antibody mixtures commonly calls for selective absorption of the serum, as a means of separating the individual specificities comprising the mixture. Titration with cells representative of different antigens may aid in the selection of suitable red cells for absorption, since it is always easier to remove the weakest antibody first from the serum.

   3. *To study the strength of antigen expression on red cells.* The method of titrating an antiserum against a cell suspension, in parallel with control cells known to be representative of homozygous and heterozygous expression of the corresponding antigen, is not a reliable method of establishing zygosity, even under optimal conditions. The reason is that the number of antigen sites produced by a given blood group gene varies to the extent that the minimum number in a homozygote may overlap the maximum possible number in a heterozygote. There are also influences of other alleles to be taken into account, particularly in the MNSs blood group system, in which titration as a

means of determining zygosity is applied with the most confidence. The traps that exist for the unwary should be of concern to those who attempt to attach genetic significance to apparent differences in antigen expression.

Methods of Titration

As a general rule, the prepared dilutions of the serum will be tested by whatever test procedure has shown the best reactions, and the diluent will be chosen appropriately. If the purpose of titration is to compare the titers of an antibody against several cell suspensions, a series of *master dilutions* should be prepared in sufficient volume to enable all the selected indicator cells to be tested. If the serum dilutions are each to be tested against only one cell suspension, 0.1 ml of each dilution is an adequate volume, and the dilutions may be made in the same tubes in which they are going to be incubated with the indicator cells. To achieve maximum accuracy, and prevent carryover of antibody, separate pipettes are used to prepare each dilution. If the titer of a serum exceeds 512, it is best to discontinue the series of doubling dilutions at that point, and begin again with an accurately prepared 1 in 1,000 dilution.

Scoring of Agglutination

Comparative titrations may show the same endpoints but have marked differences in the strength of agglutination at the different dilutions. Hence, to make a titration quantitatively more informative, it is useful to assign a numerical value to each grade of agglutination as a means of scoring the reactions at each dilution. The scores obtained from each series of dilutions against each indicator cell suspension are then added together and the resulting total is expressed as the titration score of the antibody against the cells in question. Several investigators have devised their own scoring systems and reported them in the literature. Any of these may be adopted, or a system suited to the special requirements of a particular laboratory may be developed. The only important thing is that a regular system should be adopted and followed consistently. The numerical values assigned by Marsh to the grades of agglutination are shown in Table 5–5. Finer gradations of reaction are allowed for by intermediate numerical values, thereby enabling results to be recorded using a continuous gradient from 0 to 12. This scoring system is simple and convenient [48].

As an example, Table 5–6 gives the results of comparative titrations of two serums against the same cells, together with titration scores assigned in accordance with the numerical scoring system of Marsh. These two serums show a difference in titer of only a single dilution, yet the titration score of serum 2 (titer 16) is more than one and a half times that of serum 1 (titer 8), indicating a substantially greater difference in potency than is suggested by the titration endpoints.

Table 5–5. A Numerical System of Scoring Hemagglutination Reactions, as Proposed by Marsh [48]

Score*	Symbol	Macroscopical Appearance	Microscopical Appearance
12	C	Complete agglutination; a single large agglutinate	No free cells detected
11			
10	+++	Strong reaction; 1 or 2 large agglutinates	A few detached masses of agglutinated cells
9			
8	++	Strong reaction; a number of large agglutinates	Large agglutinates in a sea of smaller clumps and unagglutinated cells
7			
6			
5	+	Many small agglutinates	Many agglutinates of up to 20 cells in a background of small clumps and free cells
4			
3	(+)	Weak granularity in the cell suspension	Scattered agglutinates of 6–8 cells, with mostly free cells
2	W	An even cell suspension	A few small clumps of 3 or 4 cells in a sea of free cells
1			
0	0	An even cell suspension	No agglutination detected

*Note that no description of macroscopic appearance is shown alongside some score values. These values are intended to be assigned to intermediate grades of agglutination, in order to provide a continuous gradient from 0 to 12.

Table 5–6. Two Serums with Similar Titers but Different Scores

	Reaction Strength										
	Serum Dilution										
Serum	Undil.	1/2	1/4	1/8	1/16	1/32	1/64	1/128	1/256	1/512	Score
Serum 1	+++	++	+	(+)	W	0	0	0	0	0	28
Serum 2	C	C	+++	++	+	W	0	0	0	0	49

There is only one dilution in the difference between titration endpoints; yet when numerical values are assigned to the graded agglutination reactions, as in Table 5–5, there is a significant difference in antibody potency.

Record Keeping

It is important to keep accurate and detailed records of results obtained in all pretransfusion testing. Such records need to be kept for at least the length of time required by applicable laws, and must be readily accessible for reference as required.

PATIENT RECORDS

Records of test results on all recipients should be maintained in the laboratory, even though all blood typing and antibody screening tests must be repeated each time a new specimen is received in the laboratory. The length of time for which records must be kept may be influenced by local requirements.

The ability to refer to earlier test results is especially useful in the case of people whose serum has been found to contain an unexpected antibody, but is also of some value when earlier findings were negative. Once an unexpected antibody has been identified, and a policy established for transfusion to the patient, that policy must be followed, *even if the antibody concerned should become undetectable by some later date*. Certain clinically significant antibodies (notably those of the Kidd blood group system) may disappear once the red cells carrying the stimulating antigen are no longer present, but reexposure can bring about a strong and rapid secondary immune response, which may lead to a delayed hemolytic transfusion reaction [49].

DONOR UNIT RECORDS

Records identifying all units of donor blood passing through the blood transfusion service must be maintained, including details as to source of each one, whether drawn by the transfusion service itself or acquired from an outside source. The source blood service keeps its own accurate donor records to facilitate tracing a donor if that should become necessary, but records of any retesting and additional processing are the responsibility of the institution in which such testing or processing is done. The record for each donor unit should include a note as to its disposition, whether it was released for transfusion to a patient, discarded, returned to its source, or shipped to another transfusion service. If the donor unit was transfused, the identity of the recipient and the date of release are needed. If a unit is separated into components, the record must include details about what components were prepared, by whom and when, as well as separate disposition information for each component.

References

1. Honig CL, Bove JR. Transfusion-associated fatalities: Review of Bureau of Biologics Reports 1976–1978. *Transfusion* 1980; 20:653–61.
2. Pollack W, Ascari WQ, Crispen JK, et al. Studies on Rh prophylaxis. II. Rh immune prophylaxis after transfusion with Rh-positive blood. *Transfusion* 1971; 11:340–4.

3. Romans DG, Tilley CA, Crookston MC, et al. Conversion of incomplete antibodies to direct agglutinins by mild reduction. Evidence for segmental flexibility within the Fc fragment of immunoglobulin G. *Proc Nat Acad Sci USA* 1977; 74:2531–5.
4. Diamond LK, Abelson N. The demonstration of Rh agglutinins—an accurate and reliable slide test. *J Lab Clin Med* 1945; 30:204–12.
5. Diamond LK, Denton RL. Rh agglutination in various media with particular reference to the value of albumin. *J Lab Clin Med* 1945; 30:821–30.
6. Cameron JW, Diamond LK. Chemical, clinical and immunological studies on the products of human plasma fractionation. XXIX. Serum albumin as a diluent for Rh typing reagents. *J Clin Invest* 1945; 24:793–801.
7. White WD, Issitt CH, McGuire D. Evaluation of the use of albumin controls in Rh phenotyping. *Transfusion* 1974; 14:67–71.
8. Reid ME, Ellisor SS, Frank BA. Another potential source of error in Rh-Hr typing. *Transfusion* 1975; 15:485–8.
9. Case J. Albumin autoagglutinating phenomenon as a factor contributing to false positive reactions when typing with rapid slide reagents. *Vox Sang* 1976; 30:441–4.
10. Zettner A, Bove JR. Hemolytic transfusion reaction due to interdonor incompatibility. *Transfusion* 1963; 3:48–51.
11. Franciosi RA, Awer E, Santana M. Interdonor incompatibility resulting in anuria. *Transfusion* 1967; 7:297–303.
12. Coombs RRA, Mourant AE, Race RR. A new test for the detection of weak and incomplete Rh agglutinins. *Br J Exp Pathol* 1945; 26:255–66.
13. O'Neill GJ, Yang SY, Tegoli J, et al. Chido and Rodgers blood groups are distinct antigen components of human C4. *Nature* 1978; 273:668–70.
14. Tilley CA, Romans DC, Crookston MC. Localisation of Chido and Rodgers determinants to the C4d fragment of human C4. *Nature* 1978; 276:713–5.
15. Giles CM. "Partial inhibition" of anti-Rg and anti-Ch reagents. II. Demonstration of separable antibodies for different determinants. *Vox Sang* 1985; 48:167–73.
16. Peetermans ME, Cole-Dergent J. Haemolytic transfusion reaction due to anti-Sd^a. *Vox Sang* 1970; 18:67–70.
17. Soh CPC, Morgan WTJ, Watkins WM, Donald ASR. The relationship between the N-acetylgalactosamine content and the blood group Sd^a activity of Tamm and Horsfall urinary glycoprotein. *Biochem Biophys Res Comm* 1980; 93:1132–9.
18. Judd WJ. Urines for inhibition. *Transfusion* 1983; 23:404–5 (letter to the editor).
19. Hysell JK, Gray JM, Hysell JW, Beck ML. Neomycin-dependent antibody interference with routine ABO grouping and antibody screening. *Transfusion* 1975; 15:16–22.
20. Beattie KM, Ferguson SJ, Burnie KL, et al. Chloramphenicol antibody causing interference in antibody detection and identification tests. *Transfusion* 1976; 16:174–7.
21. Mann JM. Hydrocortisone-associated hemagglutination property of human sera. *Transfusion* 1973; 13:346 (abstract).
22. Gillund TD, Howard PL, Isham B. A serum agglutinating human red cells exposed to EDTA. *Vox Sang* 1972; 23:369–70.
23. Henry R, Freihaut BH, Pierce SR, et al. A second example of an agglutinin for red cells exposed to EDTA. *Transfusion* 1973; 13:345 (abstract).
24. Allan CJ, Lawrence RD, Shih SC, et al. Agglutination of erythrocytes freshly washed with saline solution. *Transfusion* 1972; 12:306–11.
25. Weiner W, Tovey GH, Gillespie EM, et al. Albumin autoagglutinating property in three sera: a pitfall for the unwary. *Vox Sang* 1956; 1:279–88.

26. Spence L, Jones D, Moore BPL. Effect of fatty acid salts on reactivity of albumin preparations with sera containing albumin autoagglutinating factor. *Transfusion* 1971; 11:193–5.
27. Golde DW, McGinniss MH, Holland PV. Mechanism of the albumin autoagglutination phenomenon. *Vox Sang* 1969; 16:465–9.
28. Golde DW, Greipp PR, McGinniss MH. Spectrum of albumin autoagglutination. *Transfusion* 1973; 13:1–5.
29. Beck ML. The technical problem of T-activation. *Transfusion* 1978; 8:109–10.
30. Stratton F, Renton PH. Effects of crystalloid solutions prepared in glass bottles on human red cells. *Nature* 1955; 175:722.
31. Hektoen L. Iso-agglutination of human corpuscles. *J Infect Dis* 1907; 4:297–303.
32. Berry-Dortch S, Woodside CH, Boral LI. Limitations of the immediate-spin crossmatch when used for detecting ABO incompatibility. *Transfusion* 1985; 25:176–8.
33. Steane EA, Steane SM, Montgomery SR, Pearson JR. A proposal for compatibility testing incorporating the manual hexadimethrine bromide (Polybrene) test. *Transfusion* 1985; 25:540–4.
34. Landsteiner K, Miller CP. Serological studies on the blood of primates. II. The blood groups of anthropoid apes. *J Exp Med* 1925; 42:853–62.
35. Weiner W. Eluting red-cell antibodies: a method and its application. *Br J Haematol* 1957; 3:276–83.
36. Kochwa S, Rosenfield RE. Immunochemical studies of the Rh system. I. Isolation and characterization of antibodies. *J Immunol* 1964; 92:682–92.
37. Jenkins DE Jr, Moore WH. A rapid method for the preparation of high potency auto and alloantibody eluates. *Transfusion* 1977; 17:110–4.
38. Rekvig OP, Hannestad K. Acid elution of blood group antibodies from intact erythrocytes. *Vox Sang* 1977; 33:280–5.
39. François-Gerard CH, Brocteur J. Description of a P_1-like antigen present in turtle dove eggs. XV International Congress of Blood Transfusion, Paris, 1978. (Abstract).
40. Cameron GL, Staveley JM. Blood group P substance in hydatid cyst fluids. *Nature* 1957; 179:147–8.
41. Edwards JM, Moulds JJ, Judd WJ. Chloroquine dissociation of antigen-antibody complexes: a new technic for typing red blood cells with a positive direct antiglobulin test. *Transfusion* 1982; 22:59–61.
42. Mantel W, Holtz G. Characterisation of autoantibodies to erythrocytes in autoimmune haemolytic anaemia by chloroquine. *Vox Sang* 1976; 30:453–63.
43. Sassetti R, Nicholls D. Decreased antigen reactivity caused by chloroquine. *Transfusion* 1982; 22:537–8 (letter to the editor).
44. Mallory D, Reid M. Misleading effects of chloroquine. *Transfusion* 1984; 24:412 (letter to the editor).
45. McShane K, Cornwall S. Chloroquine reduces antigen strength. *Transfusion* 1985; 25:83 (letter to the editor).
46. Branch DR, Petz LD. A new reagent (ZZAP) having multiple applications in immunohematology. *Am J Clin Pathol* 1982; 78:161–7.
47. Advani H, Zamor J, Judd WJ, et al. Inactivation of Kell blood group antigens by 2-aminoethylisouronium bromide. *Br J Haematol* 1982; 51:107–15.
48. Marsh WL. Scoring of hemagglutination reactions. *Transfusion* 1972; 12:352–3.
49. Kurtides ES, Salkin MS, Widen AL. Hemolytic reaction due to anti-Jk[b]. *JAMA* 1966; 197:816–7.

6. Red Blood Cell Transfusion

Transfusions of whole blood, red blood cells, or various red cell–containing components are indicated only when the patient's circulating hemoglobin level is low enough to compromise oxygen delivery to tissues. Although there may be additional benefits to transfusion, for example, an increase in the circulating blood volume, the only valid indication for red blood cell transfusion in any form is anemia of sufficient severity to compromise oxygen delivery to the tissues.

Blood Volume

All methods of measuring blood volume nowadays are indirect, and depend on the dilution of a known quantity of some labeling material in the patient's plasma or red cell volume. All methods in clinical use measure either plasma or red cell volume and calculate the total blood volume from it. Red cell volume measurements are particularly useful in the evaluation of patients with polycythemia, where it is important to know whether the polycythemia is from an increased red cell volume (primary polycythemia) or a decreased plasma volume (secondary polycythemia). Unfortunately, measurements of red cell or plasma volume are often inaccurate or hard to do when they are needed most, for example, in shock or acute severe bleeding. Despite this limitation, the test, carefully done and properly evaluated, can provide valuable clinical information. Standard techniques for the measurement of red cell and plasma volume have been prepared by the International Committee for Standardization in Hematology [1]. The publication describes, in detail, the proper approach to these determinations, and should be read by anyone with a serious interest in this subject.

PLASMA VOLUME

Human radioiodinated serum albumin (RISA) quickly dilutes into all areas of the body where serum albumin is found and is the substance most commonly used to measure plasma volume. In healthy persons, and in many patients as well, albumin is predominantly in the vascular compartment, and the dilution of RISA is an accurate measure of circulating plasma volume. Unfortunately, there are situations, particularly in shock, in which albumin easily and rapidly diffuses from the vascular system. The measured plasma volume is then overestimated, and the error introduced into the blood volume determination can be significant. If this limitation is kept in mind, RISA can give a clinically useful determination of plasma volume.

RED CELL VOLUME

After injection, a small volume of radiolabeled red cells will equilibrate quickly with the circulating erythrocytes. In this way, red cell volume can be measured

Table 6–1. Representative Values for Red Cell, Plasma, and Blood Volumes in Normal Subjects*

	Red Cell Volume	Plasma Volume	Blood Volume
Men	30 (25–35)	40 (34–46)	70 (59–81)
Women	25 (20–30)	40 (35–43)	65 (55–73)

*These are mean values in milliliters per kilogram of body weight, with 95% confidence limits.

and plasma or blood volume calculated. Radioactive chromium (^{51}Cr), usually used for this purpose, is safe and convenient. Technetium-labeled red blood cells can also be used to measure red cell volume and, because of technetium's short half-life (6 hours), can be used when repeated blood volume determinations are indicated [2]. When compared to ^{51}Cr, the total radiation dose received by the patient is less, and the surface counting to localize sites of red cell destruction is more effective.

Cells to be labeled with ^{51}Cr or ^{99m}Tc are mixed with a small tracer dose and incubated for a short time at room temperature or 37°C. These tagged cells are injected and, after a variable time, samples for radioactive counting are drawn. The measured red cell volume is accurate in most cases and can be used to calculate the blood and plasma volumes. This method, like all methods for red cell or plasma volume measurement, depends on adequate and complete mixing of the injected sample in the patient. Whenever this is not accomplished, the answer, no matter how it has been determined, will be inaccurate. Because mixing is usually complete within 10 minutes, it is customary to obtain samples for radioisotope counting about 10 minutes after injection of the isotope [3].

NORMAL VALUES

One set of normal volume values is given in Table 6–1. "Normal" values vary from laboratory to laboratory, depending on many factors, including the method used to measure the volume. The plasma volume is more variable than the red cell volume; hence, blood volume values based on the measurement of red cell volume are generally more accurate.

There is no entirely reliable method to predict what the normal value in any individual should be, since the blood volume varies with age, weight, body surface area, and body composition. Most reports are given in milliliters per kilogram of body weight, although a correlation between blood volume and lean body mass or body surface area is usually more valid.

A useful estimate of blood volume can be obtained by multiplying the body weight in grams by 7 percent. For example:

70-kg man = 70,000 gm × 7% = 4,900 ml (see Table 6–1).

Rationale for Red Cell Replacement

Blood transfusion is indicated "(1) to improve the stability of the circulatory system when the blood volume has been reduced in such a way as to imperil the patient and (2) to improve the oxygen-carrying capacity of the blood to prevent acute hypoxia or invalidism" [4]. Transfusion is not a tonic, nor is it a safe or efficient way to replace serum protein. Transfusion is almost never indicated to elevate a patient's hemoglobin or hematocrit value to some arbitrary level. An operation is not, in itself, an indication for transfusion, nor is asymptomatic anemia. There is no evidence that wound healing is improved when a postoperative patient has a normal hemoglobin value, and no basis for the often-repeated statement that postoperative patients "do better" when given a transfusion. Patients with chronic illness, such as cancer, leukemia, arthritis, or uremia, may be anemic, but transfusion will lead only to a temporary correction of the anemia, without general improvement of the patients' condition. The widespread practice of using blood transfusion as a tonic, to "get the hemoglobin up to normal," or to "make the patient feel better" are unjustified. Blood loss, hemolysis, or bone marrow failure with anemia are indications for transfusion only when the anemia is so severe that it represents a real risk to the patient. The goal of transfusion must be to treat the patient, not the abnormal laboratory data on the chart.

Recently there have been attempts to define specific indications for red cell products and to identify the reasons why clinicians order blood. Friedman has studied both the patterns of blood use in the United States [5] and the clinical and laboratory findings that induce physicians to order red cell or whole blood transfusions [6]. He terms the latter the *transfusion trigger* and has shown—not unexpectedly—that the hematocrit value is among the most important. Of interest is the finding that surgeons tend to use the same hematocrit trigger value in women and in men despite the well-known fact that normal values for women are lower.

Tissue oxygen need, rather than the hemoglobin or hematocrit value, should determine whether or not a patient should be transfused. Many variables, including (1) oxygen uptake, (2) blood flow, (3) hemoglobin mass, (4) hemoglobin-oxygen affinity, and (5) tissue demands, interact to determine whether oxygen transport and delivery are adequate and whether increasing the hemoglobin mass by transfusion is indicated. Another important variable is whether the patient is stable or unstable. One physiologic approach to determining the need for transfusion might be to evaluate several parameters of oxygen transport and delivery and use these as the transfusion trigger. For example, measurement of the mixed venous oxygen content ($P\bar{v}O_2$); the extraction ratio, i.e., the ratio of oxygen consumed to oxygen delivered; and the oxygen consumption (VO_2) can be useful in determining the need for transfusion [7, 8]. Although these measurements are not difficult to make, they are almost never used in deciding when to transfuse. Increasing concern about the risks of transfusion makes it mandatory to be more scientific when deciding which patients should be transfused.

Hemodilution techniques, particularly during open-heart surgery, have demonstrated the ability of many patients to tolerate low hemoglobin levels without difficulty. Not only is the severe anemia well tolerated, but it may even be advantageous because of improved flow characteristics of the diluted blood [9]. In critically ill postoperative patients, the optimal hematocrit value seems to be between 30 and 33 percent [10, 11]. At these levels, oxygen availability is optimal and neither oxygen delivery nor survival is improved by transfusing patients to attain higher values. But this may not be the case in patients with coronary insufficiency [12], in whom there is some evidence that hemodilution below 30 percent may contribute to cardiovascular strain, and jeopardize cerebral and myocardial oxygen supplies [13].

Taken together, many studies show that there is no critical hemoglobin or hematocrit value below which all patients should be transfused and above which transfusion is not indicated. Each decision must be individualized after careful consideration of many variables, only one of which is the hemoglobin or hematocrit value. We believe, however, that it will be difficult to find clinically valid indications for red cell transfusion in persons who have hematocrit values above 33 percent, and equally difficult to label a transfusion as not indicated, particularly in surgical patients, when the hematocrit value is below 30 percent. Transfusions are of no value for wound healing [14] or nutrition, although in some patients, they may be indicated for their beneficial effect on oxygen transport. (See Addenda.)

Although whole blood is acceptable and may have some advantages in the treatment of acute massive blood loss, it is of no value in the treatment of patients who need only red blood cell replacement [15–17]. For them, red blood cells are the component of choice, and in most hospitals, they should make up 75 to 85 percent of all red cell–containing transfusions [18].

Special Transfusion Problems

MASSIVE TRANSFUSION

Many factors affect the amount of hemorrhage that will cause shock, but rapid loss of 15 to 20 percent of the blood volume leads to symptoms in most persons [19] (Table 6–2). Almost all patients with hemorrhagic shock have lost at least 35 to 40 percent of their blood volume, and the average adult in severe hemorrhagic shock has probably lost about 2 liters of blood. In many cases, not all of the hemorrhage is visible, since serious blood loss accompanies fractures and internal injuries. For example, 1.5 to 2 liters is lost with a fractured pelvis, and about 1.5 liters with a fractured femur. These losses must be considered in addition to obvious bleeding from lacerations or gastrointestinal hemorrhage.

Table 6–2. Signs and Symptoms Seen in Experimental Situations after Measured Blood Loss

Blood Volume Lost (%)	Signs and Symptoms
5–15	None
15–20	Tachycardia, fall in systolic blood pressure
20–35	Borderline shock
35–40	Shock
40	50 percent mortality (dogs)

One of the earliest responses to hemorrhage is an attempt to restore the circulating blood volume to normal by shifting fluid from extravascular to intravascular spaces. Although this fluid does not have the oxygen-carrying capacity of whole blood, it does serve the all-important function of stabilizing the circulation. It will dilute the circulating red blood cells and, in so doing, cause the characteristic fall in the hemoglobin, hematocrit, and red cell count. Dilution begins almost as soon as the hemorrhage starts, and continues for as long as 72 hours after all bleeding has stopped, during which time the hemoglobin and hematocrit values are less reliable. These tests usually do not accurately reflect the *total* amount of bleeding for 3 days. In the first few hours, the hemoglobin and hematocrit values may be misleadingly high, despite obvious and significant bleeding.

Fluid volume replacement is the cornerstone of treatment in acute hemorrhagic shock. Volume replacement is more important than blood replacement, and the choice of fluid is less important than its rapid and appropriate administration. Early replacement with adequate volumes of crystalloid solutions is the resuscitative measure of choice [20]. Most trauma specialists advocate the rapid infusion of large volumes of lactated Ringer's solution for the initial management of hemorrhagic shock. Colloid solutions such as dextran, albumin, hydroxyethyl starch (hetastarch), or plasma protein fraction may be useful in later management, but have no obvious advantage in early resuscitation. In addition, they are expensive and can be associated with serious and even fatal anaphylactoid reactions [21]. Plasma of any kind, including fresh frozen plasma (FFP), is not indicated as a volume expander in the management of blood loss [22]. While is has been popular for some surgeons to use fresh frozen plasma in such cases, there is ample evidence that such a practice is not beneficial and may be dangerous [23–25].

Crystalloid solutions are important in early resuscitation after blood loss, but patients with serious injuries or bleeding, and many patients who undergo major surgery, will require large amounts of blood replacement. Transfusion that approaches or exceeds a total blood volume replacement in 24 hours is considered massive.

Use of Platelets

Much of our knowledge about massive transfusion has been gained from studies on wounded soldiers, a selected population of young men in good health at the time of injury. Their responses may, therefore, be different from those of the chronically ill or elderly, in whom mortality rates as high as 72 percent have been recorded after massive transfusion [26]. In both groups, an abnormal bleeding tendency is often seen after transfusion of 15 to 20 units of stored blood. In wounded soldiers, this is seen as a "mild tendency to ooze from cut surfaces," [27] but in civilians of varying ages and with associated diseases "generalized hemorrhage" was seen far more often [28]. Many of the latter ultimately died. The mechanism of the hemorrhagic tendency in either group is unknown, although abnormalities of prothrombin and partial thromboplastin time, and a low platelet count are almost always seen. Of these, the platelet count is the most frequently abnormal [23, 24, 29]. For this reason, the administration of platelets to such patients may be indicated [23, 24, 29]. It has not been possible to show a difference in platelet counts of patients who had abnormal bleeding and those who did not [30], but some authors state unequivocally that in patients who have abnormal bleeding, the bleeding is controlled shortly after platelet transfusions are given [24]. In addition, they advise that "Platelet concentrates are usually indicated if a patient receives over 20 units of blood in a 12 hour period" [24]. Similar findings have been reported in children who showed the expected correlation between blood volumes transfused and the reduction in platelet count along with the cessation of abnormal bleeding after platelets were given [29]. These papers are well known to surgeons and provide the documentation for the widespread requests for platelets in massive transfusion. Although the cited literature has not been confirmed, it corresponds to our observations and provides justification for the use of platelets in massive transfusion. Fresh (less than 24 hours old) blood, once considered appropriate as a source of platelets, is no longer advised, necessary, or available.

Use of Fresh Frozen Plasma

Although most patients who undergo massive transfusion also have abnormalities in coagulation function tests, there is no evidence that they benefit from the administration of fresh frozen plasma. The plasma is almost always used in doses that are too small to replace adequately the coagulation factors lost by dilution or consumed by clot formation, and clinical studies have shown that the administration of fresh frozen plasma has no beneficial effect [23]. A National Institutes of Health Consensus Development Conference on Fresh Frozen Plasma concluded that in massive transfusion, "the empiric use of FFP to reverse hemostatic disorders should be confined to those patients in whom factor deficiencies are presumed to be the sole or principal derangement. There is no evidence that the *prophylactic* administration of FFP decreases transfusion requirements . . ." [22].

Citrate Toxicity
Citrate toxicity is a potentially serious problem in massive transfusion, since bank blood is collected and stored in an excess of citrate (see Chap. 7). As a result, each transfusion not only replaces the shed blood with blood free of ionized calcium, but is also an infusion of excess citrate with its ability to bind the patient's circulating calcium. Hypocalcemia, however, is infrequently seen, since the body is quickly able to mobilize additional calcium from bone. In addition, all cells of the body rapidly metabolize the infused citrate, converting it first to bicarbonate and ultimately to carbon dioxide and water. There is a depression of ionized calcium during massive transfusion, but this probably has little clinical importance. There are reports of acute myocardial failure secondary to the rapid transfusion of citrated blood, especially in patients with heart disease and in infants, and there have been recommendations for the routine administration of calcium prophylactically in massive-transfusion situations [31, 32]. We accept the generalization that a warm adult with a normally functioning liver can tolerate a unit of whole blood every 5 minutes without needing supplemental calcium [33]. If red blood cells are used instead of whole blood, the amount of citrate infused will be less, and accordingly, the risk of hypocalcemia will be reduced. If the critical rate is exceeded in rapid and massive transfusion, or in the presence of hypothermia or severe liver disease, calcium infusion may be indicated. If so, it must be given directly to the patient and not added to the blood or to the transfusion tubing, where it might cause clotting. Either calcium chloride or calcium gluconate solutions can be used. One accepted dose is 10 ml of 10 percent calcium gluconate or 2.5 ml of 10 percent calcium chloride for each liter of citrated blood [34].

Acid-Base Abnormalities
Patients who undergo massive transfusion often have electrolyte and acid-base abnormalities, but the role of transfusion itself in causing these is difficult to define. Metabolic acidosis, whether from the associated shock syndrome or the immediate acid load of citrated blood, is a common early finding that is improved rapidly in patients when abnormal blood pressure and tissue perfusion are corrected [35]. If hemorrhage is not controlled and acidosis persists, the usually fatal outcome is not affected by the administration of alkalinizing solutions.

After massive transfusion, a relatively late finding is metabolic alkalosis, usually associated with hypokalemia. While it is logical to expect that citrate and lactate, both acidic, would contribute to an acidosis, these are rapidly metabolized to bicarbonate, leading to a metabolic alkalosis. This is accompanied by an exchange of intracellular hydrogen for extracellular potassium in an attempt to neutralize the excess base. As a result, metabolic alkalosis and hypokalemia often coexist in massive-transfusion situations and are made worse by the administration of exogenous bicarbonate in a mistaken attempt to correct for the presumed acid load [36].

Blood Warming

Massive blood replacement with cold blood has been associated with a high incidence of cardiac arrhythmias, including cardiac arrest [37]. In one study, the incidence of cardiac arrest during massive transfusion was lowered from 58 to 7 percent by warming the cold bank blood to body temperature as it was being infused [37]. The proper way to warm a unit of blood is by a properly monitored heat exchanger that includes disposable plastic inserts for the blood itself. Several varieties are available commercially. Coils of plastic tubing in containers of warmed water are safe only if the water temperature is carefully and constantly monitored, and this is almost never possible in massive-transfusion situations. Warming the entire container of blood in a water bath is not recommended, because the large volume of blood and the small surface area of the blood container result in inadequate heat exchange. In addition, blood warmed in this way and not used will have to be discarded. Red blood cells may also be warmed by the addition of warm (37 to 70°C) saline immediately before transfusion. Microwave ovens might seem appropriate, but to date, no oven is available that is acceptable for this purpose. In early work, severe hemolytic reactions were seen with the microwave ovens in use [38].

Whole Blood versus Red Blood Cells

Patients who require massive transfusion may be treated effectively with either whole blood or red blood cells [18]. There is no doubt that some physicians who treat such patients prefer to give whole blood because it is easier to administer and because it replaces both blood volume and oxygen-carrying capacity at the same time. We believe that whole blood does have these advantages and that, when available, it can be used in massive transfusion. But it is almost never available because of the need to prepare other components from as many donations as possible. Red blood cells do not flow as easily as whole blood and usually need to be diluted with saline (but not other fluids, see p. 238) before use. This should be done at the time of transfusion using a "Y" set with normal saline hung from one side of the set. As each unit of red cells is started, it is briefly held below the saline container and enough saline run into the unit to dilute the red cells to the point where they will flow easily. After a brief mixing, the saline line is reclamped and the red blood cell unit hung and administered as rapidly as needed. This procedure, once learned, does not interfere significantly with the speed at which blood can be given. Although either whole blood or red cells can be used, whole blood administration is restricted to situations in

Table 6–3. Rules and Suggestions for Transfusions that Are Not Identical with the Recipient's Blood Group

Rules

Red cells must be compatible with the recipient's plasma.

If whole blood is used, its plasma must also be compatible with the recipient's red cells.

Suggestions

Avoid Rh-positive red cells in Rh-negative recipients, especially women of childbearing age. Use O, Rh-negative red cells rather than ABO specific whole blood that is Rh-positive. Use Rh-positive red cells or blood when no compatible Rh-negative is available. Rh-negative may be used at any time for Rh-positive recipients.

Once O cells have been given to a non-O recipient, there will be a time when it is unwise or unsafe to return to the patient's original blood group. Group O red cells contain anti-A and anti-B, and at some point, the recipient will have passively transfused anti-A or -B. In an adult, after 4 or 5 units of O cells have been transfused, additional transfusions should be of group O. If a new sample shows no circulating anti-A or -B, it is safe to return to blood or cells of the patient's original type.

Consider the blood bank inventory when deciding which group to use. For example, in an AB recipient, it might be unwise to switch to B when the AB is exhausted, because supplies of group B are usually lower than those of group A. On the other hand, if there are large supplies of group B, its use might be preferred.

Check with the surgeons or anesthesiologists. Such consultations are essential in planning for anticipated needs.

---

which both red cells *and plasma* are compatible with the recipient. For example, when group O is selected for non-O patients, or those whose group is unknown, the transfusion must be with red cells and not whole blood.

Transfusions of Different ABO Groups

When faced with massive-transfusion situations, it is often indicated and sometimes necessary to select blood of an ABO or Rh type different from that of the recipient. Two simple rules and four suggestions (Table 6–3) govern the selection of what group of blood to use.

Group O whole blood is no longer considered the "universal donor," and its use in this way has been eliminated. Group O red blood cells, on the other hand, are safe to use in recipients of all ABO groups and can be given in cases when it is impossible to determine the patient's ABO group. At times, it will be necessary to decide whether to issue uncrossmatched O red cells or to use blood or cells of the recipient's group. O red cells should always be selected when the group is unknown or when there is any doubt about the recipient's group. In particular, previous records are unreliable and group-specific cells should *never* be given on the basis of information on driver's licenses, donation cards, or hospital medical records. If a particular patient is well known to the blood bank and has been grouped on this admission or on many occasions, if the blood bank records are unambiguous, and if the *patient identification is unquestionable,* it will probably be safe to issue group-specific uncrossmatched blood in an emergency without a new sample. In most cases, however, O red cells, Rh-negative if possible, are safer.

When a properly identified patient sample is available, one must decide whether to do a rapid ABO grouping and issue group-specific components or to issue group O red blood cells. Advantages of using group-specific transfusions are the ability to manage the patient with whole blood and the ability to use group A or B (or, at times, AB) components, which are often in better supply than those of group O. The disadvantage, of course, is the possibility of a typing error under the pressure of urgent demands for blood. The decision is best left to each blood bank director, but in situations where there is a rotating staff who rarely face such pressures, the selection of the group O red blood cell option seems safer.

Transfusions of Rh-Positive Blood into Rh-Negative Recipients
In massive-transfusion situations, Rh-negative recipients may have to be considered for Rh-positive transfusions because of limited supplies of Rh-negative blood. *Unimmunized* recipients can be given Rh-positive blood or red cells safely, although about 80 percent of them will produce Rh antibodies as a result. In cases where it has been determined that the recipient is unimmunized and it is anticipated that extensive blood use will be required, nothing is gained by using all of the blood bank's limited supply of Rh-negative units before switching to Rh-positive. If Rh-positive blood will need to be used eventually, it is appropriate to make that decision early so as not to deplete the inventory of Rh-negative blood, which may be better used for other patients. *This should be done only after it is established that the recipient has not been previously immunized to Rh.* In all other cases, transfusion with Rh-negative blood or cells is mandatory as long as supplies hold out.

If antibody detection cannot be done and *if blood replacement is essential,* Rh-positive should be used, although there is an increased risk.

After the acute transfusion episode is over, it is important to consider whether an Rh-negative recipient who received Rh-positive blood should be treated with Rh immune globulin (see Chap. 8). Each case must be considered individually. When large volumes of Rh-positive blood have been given, the amount of Rh immune globulin required is often more than the patient can tolerate intramuscularly, and the treatment is often unsuccessful. If only one or two units of Rh-positive cells or blood have been given to an adult, Rh immune globulin may be indicated. This is particularly true for women of the childbearing age or younger.

Microaggregate Filters
Because so much of the early work advocating microaggregate filtration was done on surgical patients who had received massive transfusion, there is a continuing interest in microaggregate filtration during massive transfusion.

A large body of data shows no convincing evidence for the use of microaggregate filters in massive transfusion and suggests that the acute respiratory distress syndrome seen in such patients is related to the type and magnitude of the injuries, not the presence of microaggregates in the transfused blood (see p. 239) [39, 40].

BURNS
The modern management of burns often involves early excision and grafting, a procedure associated with major blood loss. In such cases, the treatment of burns represents a special kind of massive transfusion. While early management is with crystalloid, rather than blood or colloid, the need for colloid replacement begins about 8 to 12 hours after the burn [41]. Early excision and grafting, the current procedure of choice, may occur as soon as 3 days after the burn and often causes major blood loss. We plan for red blood cell replacement in amounts equaling one to two units for each percent body surface area of burn tissue to be resected, although many patients use less. Some authorities recommend limiting the procedure so that no more than 50 percent of the patient's blood volume is lost [42], but other surgeons are more aggressive. Blood replacement during major excision and grafting in burn patients is often accompanied by transfusion of both fresh frozen plasma and platelets. Evidence for the value of fresh frozen plasma is lacking, but its use in burn patients is widespread, and transfusion services that treat such patients must be prepared to honor orders for it. The management of blood replacement in burn treatment is a prime example of a situation in which consultation between blood bank and clinician is critical.

LIVER TRANSPLANTATION
Another special case of massive transfusion occurs during liver transplantation. These patients, especially adults with preexisting coagulopathies, may use huge quantities of blood and blood products. The group at Pittsburgh found the median intraoperative blood use to be between 17 and 39 units of red blood cells per adult, depending on the diagnosis, but some used as much as 251 units [43, 44]. Patients with hepatititis or cirrhosis represented both the largest number of cases and the largest users (median, 39 units; range 7–251). As expected, all of these patients used large quantities of fresh frozen plasma and platelets. All groups who have experience with managing the blood transfusion needs during liver transplantation have developed schemes for modified crossmatching. No special blood preparation—e.g., fresh, CMV negative, washed, or ir-

Table 6-4. Expected Blood Component Use (in units) in Liver Transplantation*

	Adults			Children		
	RBC	FFP	PLTS	RBC	FFP	PLTS
During operation						
Mean	44	41	20	14	16	7
Range	3–251	2–206	0–107	2–59	2–67	0–35
During hospital stay						
Mean	71	75	58	28	38	19
Range	6–254	4–235	0–404	4–143	4–190	1–8

PLTS = platelets.
*Modified from P. Butler, L, Israel, J. Nusbacher, et al. Blood transfusion in liver transplantation. *Transfusion* 1985; 25:120–3. With permission.

radiated—is needed, nor can it be provided. It is common practice to use Rh-positive products for all but women of childbearing age or girls. Even in them, large blood needs often make it impossible to use Rh-negative blood or cells, although in children, who use considerably less (Table 6–4), an attempt should be made.

UNCROSSMATCHED BLOOD

Some transfusion situations (especially massive trauma) require the use of uncrossmatched blood. While properly crossmatched blood is undoubtedly best, rapid transfusion of uncrossmatched blood or red blood cells may be lifesaving. Every blood transfusion service must make uncrossmatched blood easily and quickly available. The protocol must include adequate documentation that an emergency exists and that uncrossmatched blood is requested, but need not include a form signed by the requesting physician. Many, or perhaps most, institutions do have request forms such as the one in Fig. 6–1 asking the physician to sign, but nobody should refuse to release uncrossmatched blood while waiting for a busy physician to sign a form. It is sufficient to note that the physician was unable to sign. Uncrossmatched blood is relatively safe in massive and acute blood loss, which should provide some reassurance to blood bankers facing frantic requests for uncrossmatched blood [45].

TRANSFUSIONS FOR NEWBORN INFANTS

Newborn infants, particularly premature ones, often present special problems when transfusion is required [46]. There are important physiologic differences between newborns and older children or adults, many of which are cited when

UNIT NO. NAME ADDRESS BIRTH DATE **(If handwritten, record name, unit no., and birth date)**	**YALE–NEW HAVEN HOSPITAL** **RELEASE FOR UNCROSSMATCHED BLOOD**

Give _____ units of UNCROSSMATCHED blood to the bearer immediately. This blood will be used as an urgent and essential part of the emergency care in the following named or identified patient _____.

I release the Blood Bank and its staff from all liability that may result from transfusion of this blood and knowingly take full responsibility, medical and legal, for any consequences or lawsuits that may ensue.

(Signed*) _____

*Signature must be legible and the complete legal signature of the responsible physician.

- -

For Blood Bank Use

Container Number(s): _____
Group and Rh: _____
Taken by: _____
Date and Time: _____
Technician: _____

F-2729 (Rev. 3/83)

Figure 6–1
One example of a release form used when uncrossmatched blood is requested.

pediatricians request special services for their patients. The following are some special problems of newborn infants that make transfusion therapy difficult:

1. Small size
2. Anemia, physiologic and iatrogenic
3. Diminished red cell production
4. Increased rate of red cell destruction
5. Presence of fetal hemoglobin
6. Increased oxygen affinity
7. Inability to increase cardiac output in response to lowered oxygen in inspired air
8. Poor heat regulation
9. Immature metabolic systems
10. Inability to mount an adequate antibody response
11. Difficulty in obtaining samples for testing
12. Incompletely developed compensatory mechanisms

By the second week after delivery, the high hemoglobin and hematocrit values found at birth begin to fall, heralding a 6- to 8-week period of physiologic anemia. In premature infants, the decline is more rapid and severe. This anemia is usually well tolerated, but can quickly become a problem if the infant is otherwise stressed. In addition, most hemoglobin in the newborn is fetal hemoglobin, which although advantageous for intrauterine life, functions less well when the infant must rely on inspired air for oxygenation. The hemoglobin-oxygen dissociation curve is shifted to the left, oxygen affinity is increased, and tissue oxygenation is less efficient (see Chap. 8).

The physiologic changes listed above are well tolerated by normal infants, but add to the difficulty of managing those who are seriously ill. Many of these patients require frequent transfusions—often, to replace blood lost through sampling for required tests. Others are transfused as part of the treatment for hypoxemia or to deal with the severe anemia sometimes seen immediately after delivery. Despite these special problems, we believe that satisfactory transfusion services can be provided without resorting to unusual, bizarre, and potentially dangerous deviations from accepted standards. On the other hand, the special needs of newborn infants often do require modification of the usual approach to adult transfusion. While some neonatologists advocate a "walking donor" program to transfuse blood freshly drawn from employees and staff, we find this approach to be unnecessary and potentially unsafe [47].

Oberman [48] has cited the major objections to a walking donor program:

1. The procedure removes control of transfusion practices from the blood bank staff.

2. Proper documentation of the donor source is often lacking.
3. Suitable compatibility testing is often waived.
4. Testing for markers of disease transmission is not done on a sample of the transfused blood.
5. The procedure makes it impossible to supply red cells, the product most often needed by the infant.
6. The amount of heparin is often excessive and poorly controlled, leading to a potential for abnormal bleeding.
7. Donor arm preparation is usually inadequate.
8. The filter, a necessary part of all transfusions, is forgotten or not used.

Institutions that treat newborn infants, especially those of low birth weight, can provide optimal transfusion therapy without resorting to such potentially unsafe practices, including the unsupervised use of a walking donor program.

Effective red cell transfusion in newborn infants includes the ability to provide a small volume of relatively fresh red cells, usually less than 7 days old. At the same time, crossmatching procedures must not require frequent additional sampling from infants who, for the most part, have become anemic because of multiple blood sampling. Finally, blood should be selected or processed in a way that will reduce the risk of CMV infection. One approach that provides these benefits is to use frozen-thawed group O red blood cells in pediatric-size packs [49]. These provide fresh red cells with high levels of 2,3-diphosphoglycerate (2,3-DPG), no donor alloantibodies, reduced risk of CMV [50], and the ability to process a routine and properly tested donation into pediatric-size units. Similar approaches with freshly drawn red blood cells and double, triple, or quadruple packs are also appropriate [51].

As in other situations, planning makes life easier. In any hospital, experience will indicate approximately how many small transfusions per week are likely to be needed, and in what volume range. An active neonatal service, treating many premature and other high-risk babies, will need transfusions of 10 to 50 ml daily, while a large pediatric surgical service may also need somewhat larger units. The transfusion service staff can allow for this by obtaining blood from its supplying bank or from its own donors in unseparated double-, triple-, or quadruple-bag sets. Although these are more expensive than regular units, they permit the utmost flexibility in separating small amounts, with or without centrifugation, and with a minimum of waste. In many cases, the community blood bank can assure a reasonable number of such blood units on a regular basis to avoid crises. In some cases, frozen-thawed red cells have been used for neonatal transfusions. These, although more expensive, can be prepared in a system that allows repeated safe transfusion of cells with high levels of 2,3-DPG from the same donor.

All things considered, we see no reason to depart from blood banking standards for neonatal transfusions, including those to small premature infants.

AUTOLOGOUS TRANSFUSIONS

Autologous transfusion, that is, transfusion of a recipient with his own blood, has many advantages, including eliminating the risks of disease transmission and alloimmunization [52]. It is a necessity in some patients who are immunized to a high-incidence blood factor, and is the method of choice in patients for whom, because of multiple or unidentified antibodies, compatible blood is difficult or impossible to find. Because of its safety, autologous blood should especially be considered for "routine" transfusions, e.g., elective plastic or orthopedic surgery.

Autologous transfusion can be accomplished by

1. Preoperative collection and storage of blood for later transfusion during surgery.
2. Phlebotomy at the start of surgery, with storage for transfusion at the end of the procedure. For all practical purposes, this approach is limited to open-heart surgery, where it is used in conjunction with hemodilution-perfusion.
3. Intraoperative blood salvage using semiautomated equipment that collects, anticoagulates, washes, and reinfuses blood shed during the procedure [52].

The usual preoperative autologous transfusion procedure involves the removal of several units of blood in the 4 or 5 weeks before surgery. Milles and co-workers have demonstrated both the safety and the practicability of this approach [53]. (See Addenda.)

The use of newer additive solutions allows storage of red cells for up to 42 days (see Chap. 8), and adds even more flexibility and safety to the procedure. When larger numbers of units are needed, one can reinfuse previously drawn red cells and remove a larger quantity of blood. This approach, known as *leapfrogging,* is useful when the motivation is high and collection of a large number of units essential, but was mainly used when blood storage was limited to 3 weeks. It is seldom necessary now [54]. While there is no absolute limit on the amount of blood that can be obtained this way, seven or eight units seems to be about the largest practical amount, and four or five is a more usual goal.

As with all situations involving blood loss, the volume is replaced quickly by fluid shifts from extravascular areas, while the red cells are replaced more slowly through erythropoiesis. Experiments in normally hydrated persons have shown that when 10 to 30 percent of the blood volume is lost acutely, fluid replacement rates are as high as 90 to 120 ml per hour for the first 2 hours, 40 to 60 ml per hour for the next 4 to 8 hours, and slower thereafter [55]. Fluid volume replacement is complete in 40 to 72 hours.

Red cell replacement is slower and depends on adequate iron stores. Even with normal or increased iron stores, full red cell replacement does not occur for at least 14 to 21 days [56]. Many physicians recommend iron supplementation as a routine for autologous transfusion patients.

Blood taken from the donor-patients and not acceptable for routine transfusion must be so labeled, and stored in the area of the blood bank refrigerator reserved for quarantined blood. If the donor-patient meets *all* standards intended to protect the recipient and does not use the blood, it is acceptable for other recipients. The unit of blood must be properly processed, stored, and labeled.

Pilot samples should be obtained from the donor-patient at the time of each venesection. They can be used for processing and for crossmatching if the unit is to be considered for a different patient.

Intraoperative Salvage

Several devices for intraoperative salvage of blood have been developed. These collect, anticoagulate, wash, resuspend, and transfuse shed red blood cells. They can be used in the operative management of trauma; peripheral vascular, cardiac, and orthopedic surgery; and gastrointestinal hemorrhage, as well as postoperatively and in other situations where the shed blood can be collected from a relatively clean operative field [57]. Patients tolerate the procedure well, although high levels of plasma hemoglobin, jaundice [58], occasional hemoglobinuria [59], and at times, disseminated intravascular coagulation occur. The procedure seems to be increasingly accepted, although questions remain about the presence of harmful material in the returned cells, the risks of infection or coagulopathy, and the immunologic competence of the shed blood [60]. The effectiveness of intraoperative blood salvage in routine cardiac surgery has been questioned. Winton and co-workers found net savings of only 105 ± 88.7 ml of red cells when 20 randomly selected patients were compared with controls, and concluded that the intraoperative blood salvage was neither cost-effective nor a useful way to decrease homologous blood use [61].

OPEN-HEART SURGERY

The continuing increase in the number and complexity of cardiac surgical procedures has, fortunately, been accompanied by a reduction in the amount of component therapy required for their support. Meticulous surgical hemostasis, autologous transfusion of washed red cells recovered from the suction apparatus, retransfusion of all blood from the oxygenator, and the acceptance of normovolemic anemia (see p. 214) have made it possible to do cardiac surgery with very little blood loss [62, 63]. Some authors have stressed the need for caution when using hemodilution in patients with myocardial ischemia, particularly when hematocrit levels go below 32 percent [64, 65]. Abnormal bleeding is occasionally seen, especially in reoperations, and in some patients, it can be a major problem. If this occurs, accurate diagnosis, especially the recognition of surgical, rather than medical, bleeding, is critical [66]. Platelet dysfunction seems to be more frequent than coagulation abnormalities, and platelet transfusions are indicated when the bleeding patient has a prolonged bleeding time or a low platelet count or sometimes even with a normal platelet count [67, 68]. Prophylactic administration of platelets is not helpful [69].

HYPERTRANSFUSION FOR THALASSEMIA OR SICKLE CELL DISEASE

Children with thalassemia or sickle cell anemia who are transfused to higher hemoglobin levels have a more normal growth rate and better general health [70, 71]. Almost all centers now treat children with either disease by hypertransfusion regimes that increase both the frequency and amount of transfusions [72]. Although such an approach inevitably increases the risks of transfusion-transmitted disease, of alloimmunization, and of iron overload, the benefits outweigh the risks. Iron overload can be decreased by using relatively fresh, rather than older, red blood cells. Some centers use only washed or frozen-thawed red cells, expecting to decrease the incidence of alloimmunization to leukocytes or platelets. Evidence for or against the value of this practice is lacking, but the routine use of these products, although inconvenient and expensive, does eliminate most allergic and febrile reactions and is indicated in patients who are prone to have them.

Any chronic transfusion program exposes the recipient to multiple blood group antigens, and thus, has the potential to increase alloantibody formation. Patients with hemoglobinopathies may make antibodies, but 90 percent of such antibodies are either to Kell or Rh antigens and present no major management problem [73]. Although the concept of preventing alloimmunization sounds attractive, in most clinical situations, the routine pretransfusion matching of multiple antigens is unnecessary for unimmunized recipients. Increased antigen matching is neither cost-effective nor necessary [74].

A major complication of any long-term transfusion program is iron overload. This can be treated with iron chelating agents, and its onset can also be delayed by selective transfusion of younger erythrocytes. Because erythrocytes become more dense as they age, centrifugation using the proper conditions can separate younger from older cells. When these younger cells, termed *neocytes,* are transfused, they have a longer mean survival in the recipient. The use of cell separators allows the preparation of neocyte concentrates, which can then be stored at 4°C or frozen for subsequent transfusion [75]. While the idea is engaging, the procedure has been disappointing when tried in settings other than the clinical experiment [76]. The cost is high, the quality of the product is inconsistent, and the long-term results are not sufficiently encouraging to justify the extra cost or complexity.

EXCHANGE TRANSFUSIONS

The primary indication for exchange transfusion continues to be hyperbilirubinemia in the newborn (see Chap. 9), but exchange is used occasionally in other cases. In the newborn, for example, it has been advocated for respiratory distress syndrome, disseminated intravascular coagulation, neonatal sepsis, and drug removal. Sickle cell disease, in both adults and children, is managed, at times, with partial exchange transfusion. This approach is most useful in treating acute complications such as pain crisis or priapism. In sickle cell patients, exchange is also advised before anesthesia or surgery, or during pregnancy. The procedure can be accomplished by alternate phlebotomy and transfusion or by automated cell separation. The latter method is somewhat more efficient and generally preferred if the equipment is available.

TRANSFUSION IN TRANSPLANT RECIPIENTS

Renal Transplantation
The original work of Opelz and Terasaki, now confirmed in many studies, has revolutionized the approach to blood transfusion in potential kidney transplant recipients [77]. Avoidance of transfusion, once the policy in most transplant centers, has been replaced by programs of intentional transfusion. This, in turn, has been associated with significant improvement in the outcome of transplantation in most, but not in all, studies. Even the advent of the immunosuppressive drug cyclosporine has not altered the recommendation for pretransplant transfusion, although there seems to be some lessening of the benefits of transfusion in cyclosporine-treated patients.

The way in which transfusion enhances transplant survival is unknown, but several mechanisms have been postulated. In one, pretransplant transfusion may result in early immunization of some persons to selected HLA antigens (see Chap. 3), thereby enabling the pretransplantation crossmatch to detect those cases where rejection of the donor organ would be most likely to occur. Preformed HLA antibody, as manifested by incompatible crossmatches, is a major contraindication to transplantation, and about 30 percent of patients who receive pretransplant transfusions become highly immunized to HLA. This "complication" of pretransplant transfusion may, in fact, be beneficial by preventing a fruitless transplant.

A second view, and perhaps one more widely held, is that the beneficial transfusion effect is related to immunosuppression induced by the transfusion, perhaps through the enhancement of suppressor T cell activity. Additional possibilities include induction of immune tolerance by some unknown mechanism, stimulation of anti-idiotypic antibody production, and depletion of reactive clones by first stimulating them by transfusion and, then, while they are actively proliferating, destroying them with immunosuppressive drugs. The possible mechanisms by which blood transfusion improves the survival of transplanted kidneys is discussed in two recent reviews [78, 79].

Opinions differ as to which component of the transfused blood is responsible for the beneficial effect, since it has been seen with leukocyte-depleted [80] and with frozen-deglycerolized red cells [81], as well as with components containing white cells. The reports are difficult to interpret, since in most studies, it has been impossible to get completely pure groups, i.e., patients in the "leukocyte-poor" subset often get some transfusions of leukocyte-containing products. The incidence of overt alloimmunization to HLA seems to be reduced in recipients who receive leukocyte-depleted products, but even these data are unconfirmed. The least-complicated approach, namely the use of simple red blood cells, gives results that are as good as any, and we recommend it.

The incidence of alloimmunization seems to be reduced when the transfused product is stored, rather than fresh [82]. This may or may not be confirmed, but the important point is that there is no reason to provide "fresh blood" for these patients.

Cytomegalovirus infection, a major cause of morbidity and mortality in patients who have had renal transplants, seems to be related to the presence of CMV in the donor kidney. There is no evidence to incriminate blood or blood products as the source and no need to provide CMV-negative components for kidney transplant recipients.

Survival of kidney grafts from living related donors is enhanced by pregraft conditioning of the recipient with several transfusions from the intended donor [83]. The optimum number of transfusions, their volume, and which portion of the blood is beneficial are not established, but one protocol uses three aliquots from a single donation, given at 2- to 3-week intervals before transplantation. This is done by drawing one unit of blood from the donor, preparing red blood cells from it, and separating the red cell unit into three aliquots using a double or triple bag. Each of these can be used for up to 42 days if an additive solution (see Chap. 8) is used, and should provide the flexibility needed to deal with any reasonable protocol. Phlebotomy 42 days before the anticipated transplant should also provide adequate time for the regeneration of the donor's red cell volume.

At times, it may be advisable to give donor-specific transfusions from an Rh-positive donor to an Rh-negative recipient. This can be done using hydroxyethyl starch to separate the red cells from the buffy coat, which is then infused [84]. Because the infused buffy coat is never completely free of red cells, Rh immune globulin may be indicated in the recipient. A full dose (i.e., 300 micrograms) should be adequate for the entire course of transfusions.

When group O kidneys are transplanted into non-O recipients, it is possible that "passenger lymphocytes" present in the kidney at the time of transplant can become engrafted into the immunosuppressed recipient. If these lymphocytes are programmed to produce anti-A or anti-B, they can, at times, produce ABO antibodies directed against the recipient's erythrocytes. This complication, marked by a positive direct antiglobulin test and even hemolytic anemia, has been reported [85]. In addition, two Rh-positive patients transplanted with kidneys from previously immunized Rh-negative donors have shown temporary Rh alloimmunization and hemolytic anemia [86].

Liver Transplantation

Transfusion problems associated with liver transplantation are related to the large amount of blood used and the frequent need for substantial clotting-factor replacement. These have been discussed under Massive Transfusion (see pp. 214–222). In terms of predicting which patient may use the largest amount of blood or factor replacement, data from Starzl's group are helpful (see p. 222) [43, 44]. They found that adult patients with hepatitis, cirrhosis, or sclerosing cholangitis used about twice as much blood as patients with carcinoma or primary biliary cirrhosis. Children used considerably less. Data from Yale University bear this out, although exceptions do occur. Nearly all adult patients who have severe coagulation abnormalities before surgery use large quantities of fresh frozen plasma during the procedure. If the surgery is successful, the coagulopathy is corrected.

Bone Marrow Transplantation

Patients undergoing bone marrow transplantation require intense, and at times prolonged, blood component support. This is because there is complete ablation of their own marrow before transplantation and a relatively long period before the engrafted marrow begins to function. In addition, they are prone to develop both graft-versus-host disease and CMV infections, and all blood products must be selected or processed with that in mind. For many, the period *before* transplantation is equally critical, since blood component therapy must be managed to minimize alloimmunization, which may later bring about rejection of the transplant. And finally, the marrow to be infused must be selected or processed to avoid immunologic complications. This may mean removal of T lymphocytes from the marrow before its infusion and, at times, extensive treatment of the recipient to remove or neutralize anti-A or anti-B before transplantation of an A- or B-incompatible marrow. In no other area is it so important for the blood bank and its medical director to be integrally involved with the day-to-day decisions about patient management. Successful bone marrow transplantation demands a complete, dedicated, well-staffed blood bank. Institutions without such facilities cannot expect to establish successful programs!

PRETRANSPLANT MANAGEMENT. Currently, marrow transplantation is done mostly for patients with aplastic anemia or acute leukemia, although the number of experimental or quasi-experimental transplants done for other diseases continues to rise. HLA compatibility is an important consideration, hence the first requirement for potential marrow candidates is complete and accurate HLA typing. This should be done early in the disease and, if at all possible, before transfusion therapy. Since marrow donors will usually be recruited from family members, they should be typed whenever marrow transplant is contemplated. Originally, marrow transplantation was done only when the intended recipient had a sibling donor who was identical to the recipient with respect to both Class I and Class II histocompatibility antigens. Newer methods of management, especially cyclosporine, have made it possible to transplant marrow successfully from other family members and even from unrelated persons. As a result, almost all patients with acute leukemia or aplastic anemia should be considered to be potential marrow recipients and—at least early in their course—should be managed accordingly [87, 88].

Because the failure of a marrow graft is often related to HLA antibodies, avoidance of all blood products before transplantation is optimal. This is usually impossible for the reason that most marrow candidates require some blood component support in the pretransplant period. It appears that patients with aplastic anemia, who are usually immunocompetent, are more liable to become immunized than patients with leukemia, who are immunosuppressed because of their disease or therapy. Thus, in patients with aplastic anemia, very sparing use of any transfusions is the goal.

In all marrow transplant candidates, it is essential to avoid using the potential marrow donor as a source of pretransplant components (e.g., platelets). If transfusions are needed, use products that are as free as possible from immunizing antigens. But even an HLA-compatible component from a donor who is a four-antigen match poses a potential risk because there are non-HLA histocompatibility antigens that cannot be detected by current methods [89]. Often frozen-deglycerolized or washed red blood cells are used, and cytapheresis products are selected for platelet support. An additional step to remove mononuclear cells may be advisable. These restrictions apply to recipients who are immunocompetent, but not necessarily to patients with malignant disease in whom there seems to be no need to restrict transfusion support in the pretransplant period [89].

PRETRANSPLANT CONDITIONING. Because the recipient's bone marrow is ablated before being replaced with donor marrow, the donor can be of any ABO group. Once the marrow graft has become established, the recipient will produce red blood cells of the donor type. The use of marrow of an ABO group different from that of the recipient does, however, pose significant management problems immediately before and during the early postgraft period. At those times, it may be difficult to decide whether to use components of the donor's or the recipient's ABO group. The goal is to minimize the possibility that A or B antibodies will interact with their respective antigens by selecting components that have the best chance of being compatible at the time they are given (see Fig. 6–2). In general:

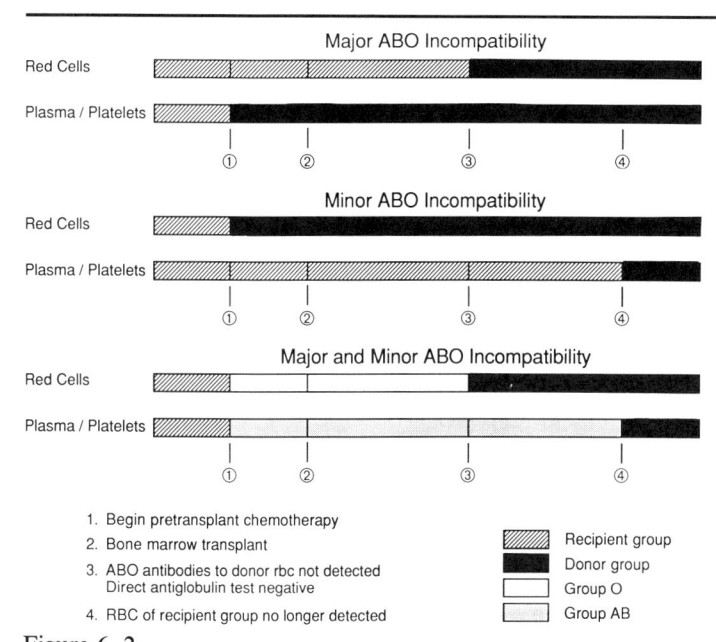

Figure 6-2
Recommended ABO blood group selection for components to be used in bone marrow transplantation. (From P. I. Warkentin, Transfusion of patients undergoing bone marrow transplantation. *Hum Pathol* 1983; 14:261-6. With permission.)

1. Red blood cells are to be of, or compatible with, the recipient's ABO group until recipient anti-A or -B is no longer detectable.
2. Plasma or plasma-containing components are to be compatible with the marrow donor's ABO group starting when the pretransplant bone marrow ablation regimen is begun.

If there is a major ABO incompatibility between donor and recipient, an important part of the pretransplant conditioning is the removal of as much of the recipient's anti-A or anti-B as possible. This has been done by plasma exchange, immunoadsorption, intentional transfusion of incompatible red cells or stroma, or some combination of these methods [90]. The goal is to deplete the recipient of ABO antibodies and, in so doing, avoid an acute hemolytic reaction when the "incompatible" marrow is transplanted. The exact level of antibody at which the transplantation of ABO-incompatible marrow becomes safe is unknown, but one recipient with an IgM titer of 32 and an IgG titer of 16 received ABO-incompatible marrow and showed negligible hemolysis [91]. ABO antibodies will return in the posttransplant period, then gradually disappear, perhaps in response to the continued immunosuppression in the recipient. Similar results have been obtained by removing the ABO-incompatible red cells from the donor marrow before it is infused [92].

Posttransplant hemolytic episodes have been reported, and at times they have been severe enough to lead to renal failure and the need for hemodialysis [90]. Patients who have a return of ABO-antibodies may have greater need for posttransplant red blood cell and platelet transfusions [90].

Minor ABO incompatibility, i.e., donor antibody against recipient red cells, is not usually a problem, although immune hemolysis has been reported.

POSTTRANSPLANT SUPPORT. Bone marrow recipients undergo a period of time between the marrow transplantation procedure and the onset of donor marrow function (see Fig. 6–1) during which intense support with platelets, red blood cells, and, at times, granulocytes is required. Because both graft-versus-host disease and cytomegalovirus infection are major problems, the components should be selected and processed to minimize these risks. For CMV-negative recipients, frozen-deglycerolized red cells or red cells from CMV-negative donors are used, and irradiation of these, as well as of all blood components for all recipients, is necessary. Whenever possible, platelets for CMV-negative recipients should be collected by cytapheresis of CMV-negative donors. Granulocytes should be similarly collected and processed. This will reduce the risk of CMV transmission and HLA alloimmunization. It is true that the necessity for these precautions is undocumented, but in bone marrow transplantation, extra care seems appropriate until the definitive studies have been done.

Transfusion in Malignant Disease

The modern management of patients with malignant diseases requires intense support with blood components. Today's chemotherapy often involves a period of bone marrow aplasia during which platelet, red cell, and, at times, granulocyte transfusions are required. The appropriate selection and use of these components in patients with malignant disease requires close and frequent liaison between the clinician and the blood bank for best results.

While most patients with solid tumors—e.g., carcinoma of the breast, lung, pancreas, prostate, etc.—will use only modest amounts of blood components, patients with lymphoma and, particularly, leukemia can be expected to use more. In leukemia especially, the need for platelet support requires early HLA typing; if this is deferred until transfusion is essential, HLA typing may be difficult or impossible. For typed patients, HLA-compatible platelets can be sought, when indicated. The use of platelet transfusions is discussed in Chapter 8.

The suggestion that blood transfusions enhance the survival of kidney grafts by inducing a state of partial immune tolerance raised the possibility that simi-

Table 6–5. Indications for Irradiated Blood Components

Absolute
Bone marrow transplant recipients
Congenital immune deficiency
Intrauterine transfusion
Questionable
Neonatal exchange transfusion after intrauterine transfusion
AIDS
Immunosuppression secondary to chemotherapy
Chemotherapy leading to lymphopenia below 500/mm^3

lar effects might be seen in other diseases. For example, *if* immune mechanisms protect against the spread of cancer cells throughout the body, and *if* transfusion is immunosuppressive, transfused patients might have an increased incidence of metastatic lesions. Such an effect has been found in patients with carcinoma of the colon and breast in whom transfusion at the time of surgery seems to be associated with an increase in the incidence of metastasis [93, 94]. The differences are small, but have been seen in more than one study, suggesting that they are significant [95]. A similar effect has been sought and not found in some cases where the transfusions were given preoperatively [96], but not in others [97, 98].

Irradiation of Blood Components
Many patients undergoing intense chemo- or radiotherapy for cancer become severely immunosuppressed. Since heavily immunosuppressed patients are at risk for graft-versus-host disease induced by transfused donor lymphocytes, it has been suggested that all components containing viable lymphocytes be irradiated before transfusion (Table 6–5) [99, 100]. Although this view is held by most physicians who treat immunosuppressed patients, not all agree [101].

The appropriate dose is not fully established, but the effects of 500 to 5,000 rad have been studied. Fifteen hundred rad will abolish mitogen-induced blast transformation by 85 percent. Mixed lymphocyte culture reactivity is eliminated by an even lower dose. No cellular damage to platelets and red blood cells has been shown, and granulocytes can withstand at least 2,000 rad without significant damage. Current consensus is that 1,500 rad is an adequate dose, and can be advised until further information is available [99]. Blood products that have been irradiated can be issued without known risk to any patients, including those who are not immunosupressed. There is no reason to discard such products if they are not used by the recipient for whom they were intended.

Multiple Antibodies

The problems encountered in transfusion of patients who have multiple antibodies can be separated into two relatively discrete areas. First, the identification of any antibodies, and second, locating blood lacking the corresponding antigens. Appropriate units can be located through a local blood supplier or by using rare-donor files such as those of the American Association of Blood Banks or the American Red Cross. In general, donors should not be bled or units thawed until it is certain that transfusion is actually intended and that the identity of the antibody or antibodies is firmly established. Frozen units may be shipped to the nearest frozen storage depot and kept there in reserve, but should be thawed only when transfusion is imminent. In the case of surgery, where blood loss may require rapid replacement, it is, at times, necessary to thaw or obtain units that in the end are not needed. One should resist the temptation to administer these anyway just because they have been thawed; unindicated transfusions should not be given.

It is worth considering that patients with multiple antibodies be transfused with washed red blood cells to prevent nonhemolytic febrile transfusion reactions that would necessitate stopping the transfusion and discarding a unit that may have been difficult to obtain. Premedication with adrenal steroids is not indicated, since there is evidence that steroids given before or during the transfusion of an incompatible unit do not influence its survival [102].

Autoimmune Hemolytic Anemia

The first step in transfusing patients with autoimmune hemolytic anemia is a careful serologic evaluation, including an attempt to identify any alloantibodies whose presence may be masked by the autoantibodies. Once a decision has been made to transfuse and the appropriate blood selected, relatively fresh red blood cells should be selected so that hemolysis from the storage lesion (see Chap. 8) is not added to possible antibody-mediated hemolysis. Although the crossmatch may appear incompatible and the intentional transfusion of apparently incompatible cells is always undesirable, most patients with acquired hemolytic anemia tolerate such transfusions without acute signs or symptoms. In some cases, transfusions may be lifesaving. If the patient's physician and the blood bank physician agree that transfusion is warranted, transfusions should be given slowly, with due regard to possible volume overload. One unit of red cells a day should be acceptable in adults [103]. One should not attempt to raise the circulating hemoglobin level to near normal values (an impossible goal) in a short period of time. In those patients who are severely anemic, small transfusions often have a beneficial value far in excess of what might be expected.

Although there is no clear evidence, it has been advised that the blood for patients with potent cold agglutinins be warmed *during* infusion [103]. As with all transfusions, only in-line blood warmers are acceptable. Another suggestion is that patients be kept warm and well covered during the transfusion.

Transfusion Techniques
Routines for the transfusion of blood vary from hospital to hospital, but patient safety is always the first consideration. No step is more important than absolute, positive identification of the donor unit and the intended recipient. The most popular system identifies each patient by a wristband worn throughout the hospital stay, bearing such information as name and hospital number. This wristband must be used to identify intended recipients, both when blood samples are drawn and when setting up the transfusion. Because identification bands may be late in arriving, special transfusion bands are used in some hospitals. These are applied at the time the sample is collected for crossmatching.

When a unit of blood leaves the blood bank, it must be identified in such a way that there can be no confusion about the intended recipient. In most places, a tag or label is fixed to the unit as it is crossmatched or issued. At the time of transfusion, identification on the patient's wristband is compared with that on the container label or tag, and transfusion is started only if they are identical. It is advisable to make a written record of this fact; patients without proper identification should not be transfused except in dire emergency. Here, the physician in charge must make the best identification possible, authorize the transfusion, and record the action in the medical record. Blood bank records should also include details of the circumstances.

Almost any peripheral vein is acceptable for transfusion, although one in the forearm is best, since the patient's arm movement need not be restricted. If it is necessary to use a vein in the antecubital space, an armboard may be required, and the patient will be unable to bend the arm while the needle is in place. Leg and ankle veins should be avoided because of the risk of thrombophlebitis.

In children, the only suitable veins may be those in the antecubital space. These are small and fragile, and great care is needed to avoid hematoma formation. Transfusion in infants is often done through scalp veins or central venous lines; special scalp-vein infusion sets are available.

Transfusion is usually given through a large needle or plastic catheter. The plastic catheter provides a secure route for the delivery of intravenous fluids and is particularly useful when the patient needs to be relatively mobile. Such catheters are nearly always used when blood is given in emergency rooms, during surgery, or whenever a reliable and stable indwelling intravenous line is required. Unfortunately, catheters tend to be associated with thrombophlebitis or sepsis, and should be replaced frequently [104]. Worse still, plastic catheters have broken loose and lodged in the right atrium. The complication rate is such that plastic catheters should be used only when the need for security and stability outweigh the potential risk. The steel needle, especially the scalp-vein needle, is better than a plastic catheter in most cases.

With either needles or catheters, careful skin preparation is required before vein puncture. Vigorous scrubbing followed by application of an iodine-containing disinfectant is advised.

Needles from 14 to 20 gauge are used for transfusion. In most cases, an 18 gauge (thin-walled 19) is used, but smaller needles are required in children or in adults with small veins. Pressure may be required to decrease transfusion time when using small needles. If massive transfusion is anticipated, needles or catheters of 14 to 17 gauge are indicated, if possible.

Transfusion can be started directly, but it is easier to manage with a Y infusion set and bag of isotonic saline connected to the other limb of the Y. When red cell transfusions are given, the higher viscosity of this component may slow the infusion rate excessively unless some modification of technique is made. This problem is avoided by allowing 50 to 100 ml of saline to flow across the Y into the red blood cell container, mixing, then proceeding with the transfusion. This is readily done without shutting off the flow through the needle, and it permits the easy flow of red cells.

Isotonic sodium chloride solutions without added glucose are the fluids of choice because they are compatible with red cells. Solutions of 5 to 10 percent dextrose in water aggregate the red cells, which may then plug the blood filter or the needle, causing difficulty during the transfusion. Furthermore, the high concentration of dextrose will make the red cells swell, which leads, in many cases, to osmotic lysis when the cells enter the recipient's circulation. The addition of small amounts of saline (e.g., 5 percent dextrose in "quarter-strength" saline solution) prevents the aggregation, but not the hemolysis.

Ringer's lactate solution is in wide use because it is more physiologic than dextrose or saline solutions. However, it contains 2.7 mEq/liter of calcium in the form of calcium chloride, which may cause clotting when mixed with anti-coagulated blood [105]. The clots may be large or small, and if the set is filled with Ringer's lactate as part of the routine for starting transfusions, the clots may plug the needle or the tubing. However convenient it may be, one should not run blood through an IV set that is already filled with Ringer's lactate unless the latter solution is first flushed out with isotonic saline.

Other solutions should not be used unless experiments have shown them to be safe when used in the intended fashion.

BLOOD FILTERS

Blood or blood products are administered through a suitable filter to avoid infusing fibrin clots or other debris. Blood administration sets have a drip chamber in the filtering unit so that the transfusionist can observe the rate of transfusion and regulate this by the number of drops per minute. At the start of the transfusion, the filter is covered so that the full filtering area is used, but not so much as to fill the entire drip chamber, because this will make it difficult to estimate the rate of transfusion.

The standard filters have a pore size of 170 μ and remove only agglutinates of platelets or white cells and the larger fibrin strands. Smaller particles, known as *microaggregates,* begin forming after a few days of blood storage (Fig. 6–3).

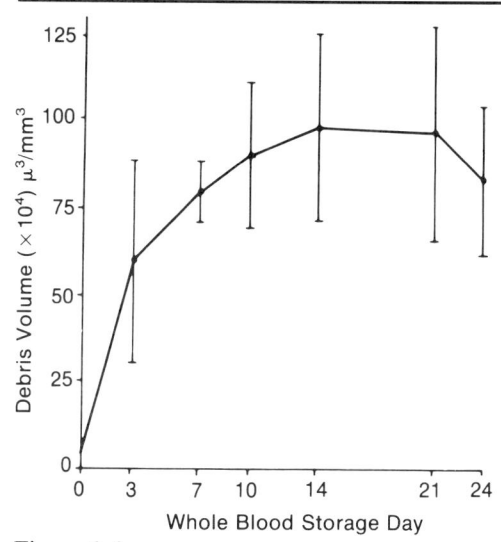

Figure 6-3
Accumulation of microaggregate debris in stored whole blood as measured by particle counting. (From A. Suehiro, H. Leinberger, J. McNamara, Counting microaggregate particles in blood. *Transfusion* 1978; 18:281–90. With permission.)

These microaggregates pass easily through regular filters and can be identified in electron micrographs of lung tissue of transfusion recipients. Some authors have suggested, not unreasonably, that this is one of the causes of the progressive pulmonary insufficiency often seen in patients who receive massive transfusions [106].

To date, evidence for such a cause-and-effect relationship is conflicting in animal experiments and lacking in the few human studies where controls or careful analysis were employed [107]. Careful reviews have concluded that there is no documentation to support the use of microaggregate filters in transfusion and that their use could not be recommended [107]. The role of microaggregate filters in the prevention of febrile transfusion reactions is discussed under Leukocyte-Poor Red Cells, Chapter 8.

Microaggregate filters of polyester screen, dacron wool, or polyurethane foam are available; the dacron wool removes particles to 40 μ. All are expensive, many clog quickly, and most slow the rate of transfusion, a particular problem in massive-transfusion situations.

In summary, the evidence at hand is insufficient to recommend widespread use of microaggregate filters except for the preparation of leukocyte-poor products. These filters offer little else to most recipients.

BLOOD PUMPS

Devices for controlling the infusion rate of intravenous solutions are now widely used in medical practice. It is not surprising that physicians and nurses have assumed that whatever is suitable for intravenous solutions is also acceptable for blood components. However, early experiences with pump-oxygenation devices intended for open-heart surgery showed that pump design could have an important effect on the hemolytic rate of pumped blood; the equipment now in use for that purpose has been designed to minimize such hemolysis. In a like manner, devices intended to speed the flow of blood in massive-transfusion situations have been designed to minimize hemolysis of red cells during pumping. In contrast, some of the newer pumps, especially those designed for pediatric use or for controlled slow infusion of medications, have small-bore passages that might be deleterious to blood components. Despite widespread use, there are, unfortunately, few data about their safety, especially in the setting of neonatal transfusion. One electromechanical infusion device is now suitable for platelet and for granulocyte transfusions [108, 109], and perhaps also for red blood cell transfusions, but this was so only after the original pump design—which caused unacceptable hemolysis—had been modified. We suggest that individuals who plan to use electromechanical infusion devices test these first to ensure that the proposed use does not lead to undue hemolysis when blood or red blood cells are pumped.

ADDITION OF MEDICATION

Medication should not be added to a unit of blood or blood product before or during the transfusion. The practice is not only dangerous, but is almost never the most effective way to administer the desired drugs. Bacterial contamination is a hazard whenever any unit of blood is entered, because blood, particularly if hanging in a warm hospital room, is a good culture medium. Some organisms grow rapidly enough to cause a severe transfusion reaction, even in the relatively short period of transfusion.

The addition of drugs to components also raises the possibility of a pharmacologic incompatibility between the drug and the component or its anticoagulant solution. For instance, calcium chloride or gluconate solutions will neutralize the anticoagulant solution and cause clotting of citrated blood. This example is, of course, self-evident, but other reactions, less apparent but equally deleterious, may occur when drugs of any kind are added to blood.

Last, but of equal importance, is the obvious fact that drugs added to blood may be given so slowly that therapeutic levels are never achieved in the patient. A good example is the once-common, but valueless, practice of adding antihistamine drugs to blood to "prevent reactions." The small amount of medication that was given during the early portion of the transfusion was totally inadequate to prevent or treat symptoms of an allergic reaction. Thus, when the patient needed the drug, most of it was still in the blood container waiting to be infused. When drugs are indicated, they should be given in adequate dose and directly to the patient, not to the blood container.

RATE OF TRANSFUSION

The rate of transfusion is governed by the clinical condition of the patient. If the patient is in acute shock from blood loss, rapid transfusion is essential. In other situations, transfusion can be given more slowly, but nothing is gained by prolonging it in most patients. A relatively slow drip, about 5 ml per minute, should be used for the first 10 to 30 minutes of the transfusion. Signs or symptoms of a transfusion reaction during this period may signal a serious incompatibility, but the slow transfusion rate will allow the blood to be stopped before a large amount of incompatible blood has been infused. If there are no signs of a reaction and if the patient is not in danger of circulatory overloading, the infusion rate should then be increased. The transfusion of a unit of red cells should be finished in about 1 to 1.5 hours; in most cases, nothing is gained by extending the transfusion time beyond this.

Even when there is danger of heart failure, red cells are usually well tolerated. A few patients with chronic anemia and an initial elevation of central venous pressure tolerate transfusion poorly and may benefit from a *modified exchange transfusion,* in which some of the patient's blood is removed while red cells are given. Since the patient is anemic, the volume removed should not exceed the volume of the transfusion. If facilities are available, the blood that has been withdrawn can be centrifuged, and the patient given back his or her own cells. This technique is seldom needed, but it may be lifesaving. At times, the use of washed, well-packed red cells will allow transfusion in patients who otherwise might go into heart failure.

INVENTORY CONTROL

In a previous edition of this book, we said that the hospital has an important role in the control of blood and component inventories. This is still true, but there is a definite trend toward increased participation by central blood banks, especially those that use automated data processing for inventory control. Several imaginative programs exist, and there is increasing interest in setting hospital inventory levels by an evaluation of past experience with complex computer models [110, 111]. In general, these programs, originally designed for the control of inventories in retail stores, determine inventory levels on the basis of demand, after setting acceptable limits for storage and outdating. Clearly, more and more blood service regions will use this approach, since at least in theory, it makes optimum use of available supplies. In areas where such programs exist or are in the planning stage, the transfusion service must participate actively, so that the unique needs and problems of a particular institution are not overwhelmed by the apparent omnipotence of the central bank and its computer. In particular, remember that shortages of beans may be acceptable in the local supermarket, but shortages of blood for treatment of trauma victims are not acceptable.

Where the hospital blood bank still controls inventory, it is important to review the levels frequently so that the smallest appropriate amount is kept on hand. Smaller hospitals, in particular, may want larger inventory than is necessary, e.g., a certain number of units of each of the major blood classifications. They may also want to keep a large amount of group O, Rh-negative red cells on hand for possible use in emergencies. When these red cells are used for recipients of other groups, it creates an excessive demand for O, Rh-negative, which consequently becomes more difficult to obtain for patients who really need it.

A unit of CPDA-1 blood has a shelf life of 35 days. If it is crossmatched three times before use (an average for many hospital laboratories), and if each time it is crossmatched it is held on reserve for 4 days, it will be unavailable for almost half of its dating period. Such a procedure increases the likelihood of the unit being outdated before it can be transfused. To prevent this, many laboratory directors have set a time limit on crossmatched blood held in reserve, usually releasing it automatically after 48 hours. This is still too long; we advise that crossmatched blood be released within 24 hours. In all except extraordinary cases, it should be possible to decide the same day whether or not to transfuse blood that has been crossmatched. In any event, because of the rapidity with which a secondary immune response may occur after transfusion, good transfusion practice requires that compatibility testing be done on freshly drawn samples whenever patients are receiving a series of transfusions. In practice, this means that a unit of blood "reserved" for such a patient should be recrossmatched at least every 2 days. Hence, it is both medically and administratively sound to release crossmatched blood that has not been used within a day. This should, of course, be understood by the physicians in the hospital. As with most rules, there will be exceptions from time to time.

Blood Ordering for Surgery

Transfusion services should establish a blood ordering policy for surgery so that the amount of blood crossmatched preoperatively and not used can be kept as small as possible. More blood is usually ordered for surgery than is needed; suitable guidelines can decrease the crossmatched-to-used ratio and, at the same time, improve blood utilization [112, 113]. An appropriate guideline indicating the usual amount of blood required for various procedures should be used. No blood should be crossmatched for procedures such as cholecystectomy, thyroidectomy, and vein stripping, or others where blood is rarely used. For such cases only a "type-and-screen" is needed. This approach is "99.9 percent" effective in preventing the transfusion of incompatible blood and is, therefore, safe, as well as economical [114].

There must, however, be a mechanism to override such a system and allow blood to be crossmatched for patients with unusual needs. Surgeons need to know that the transfusion service and its director are completely committed to prompt and safe action when a sudden unexpected need for blood arises. The entire system will fail if the technical staff are not carefully and fully instructed to release blood promptly in such cases. One approach is to do only an immediate saline crossmatch as a last check of ABO compatibility, and release the blood as "compatible by modified crossmatch." If the technical staff or the director insist that the surgeon or anesthesiologist sign a release for uncrossmatched blood, if the bag is labeled "uncrossmatched" in big letters, or if the technical staff delay or obstruct its release, the program will surely fail. We believe that the use of type-and-screen is a step forward in blood transfusion practice and deserves widespread acceptance.

Evaluation of the risks associated with this approach has shown the procedure to be safe [114]. Our experience spanning many years is identical. Clearly, the type-and-screen is safe and cost-effective and should be used widely.

References

1. International Committee for Standardization in Hematology. Standard technics for the measurement of red-cell and plasma volume. *Br J Haematol* 1973; 25:801–14.
2. Korubin V, Maisey MN, McIntyre PA. Evaluation of technetium-labeled red cells for determination of red cell volume in man. *J Nucl Med* 1972; 13:760–2.
3. Strumia MM, Colwell LS, Dugan A. The measure of erythropoiesis in anemias: 1. The mixing time and the immediate posttransfusion disappearance of T-1824 dye and of Cr^{51}-tagged erythrocytes in relation to blood volume determination. *Blood* 1958; 13:128–45.
4. Crosby WH. Misuse of blood transfusion. *Blood* 1958; 13:1198–200.
5. Friedman BA, Burns TL, Schork MA. A study of national trends in transfusion practice. Final report submitted to the National Heart, Lung and Blood Institute under terms of Contract N01 HB-9-2920. 1980.
6. Friedman BA, Burns TL, Schork MA. An analysis of blood transfusion of surgical patients by sex: a quest for the transfusion trigger. *Transfusion* 1980; 20:179–88.
7. Gould SA, Rosen AL, Sehgal LR, et al. O_2 extraction ratio: a physiologic indicator of transfusion need. *Transfusion* 1983; 23:416 (abstract).
8. Gould SA, Rice CL, Moss GS. The physiologic basis of the use of blood and blood products. *Surg Annu* 1984; 16:13–38.
9. Cosgrove DM, Thurer RL, Lytle BW, et al. Blood conservation during myocardial revascularization. *Ann Thorac Surg* 1979; 28:184–9.
10. Czer LSC, Shoemaker WC. Optimal hematocrit value in critically ill postoperative patients. *Surg Gynecol Obstet* 1978; 147:363–8.
11. Laks H, O'Connor NE, Pilon RN, et al. Acute normovolemic hemodilution: effects on hemodynamics, oxygen transport, and lung water in anesthetized man. *Surg Forum* 1973; 34:201–3.
12. Geha AS. Coronary and cardiovascular dynamics and oxygen availability during acute normo-volemic anemia. *Surgery* 1976; 80:47.
13. Lundsgaard-Hansen P. Hemodilution—new clothes for an anemic emperor. *Vox Sang* 1979; 36:321–36.

14. Heughan C, Grislis G, Hunt TK. The effect of anemia on wound healing. *Ann Surg* 1974; 179:163–7.
15. Schmidt PJ. Whole blood transfusion. *Transfusion* 1984; 24:368 (letter).
16. Grindon AJ. The use of packed red blood cells. *JAMA* 1976; 235:389.
17. Lundsgaard-Hansen P. Component therapy of surgical hemorrhage: red cell concentrates, colloids and crystalloids. *Bibl Haematol* 1980; 46:147–69.
18. Shackford SR, Virgilio RW, Peters RM. Whole blood versus packed-cell transfusions. A physiologic comparison. *Ann Surg* 1981; 193:337–40.
19. Ebert RV, Stead EA Jr, Gibson JR, II. Response of normal subjects to acute blood loss. *Arch Intern Med* 1941; 68:578–90.
20. Moss GS, Lowe RJ, Jilek J, Levine HD. Colloid or crystalloid in the resuscitation of hemorrhagic shock: a controlled clinical trial. *Surgery* 1981; 89:434–8.
21. Ring J, Messmer K. Incidence of severity of anaphylactoid reactions to colloid volume substitutes. *Lancet* 1977; 1:466–9.
22. NIH Consensus Conference. Fresh frozen plasma: indications and risks. *JAMA* 1985; 253:551–3.
23. Mannucci PM, Federici AB, Sirchia G. Hemostasis testing during massive blood replacement. A study of 172 cases. *Vox Sang* 1982; 42:113–23.
24. Counts RB, Haisch C, Simon TL, et al. Hemostasis in massively transfused trauma patients. *Ann Surg* 1979; 190:91–9.
25. Hashim SW, Kay HR, Hammond GL, et al. Noncardiogenic pulmonary edema after cardiopulmonary bypass. An anaphylactic reaction to fresh frozen plasma. *Am J Surg* 1984; 147:560–4.
26. Wilson RF, Mammen E, Walt AJ. Eight years of experience with massive blood transfusion. *J Trauma* 1971; 11:275–85.
27. Crosby WH, Howard JM. The hematologic response to wounding and to resuscitation accomplished by large transfusions of stored blood. A study of battle casualties in Korea. *Blood* 1954; 9:439–60.
28. Wilson RE, Bassett JS, Walt AJ. Five years of experience with massive blood transfusions. *JAMA* 1965; 194:851–4.
29. Cote CJ, Liu LMP, Szyfelbein SK, et al. Changes in serial platelet counts following massive blood transfusion in pediatric patients. *Anesthesiology* 1985; 62:197–201.
30. Reed DL, Ciavarella D, Heimbach DM, et al. Prophylactic platelet administration during massive transfusion. A prospective, randomized double-blind clinical study. *Ann Surg* 1986; 203:40–8.
31. Bashour TT, Ryan C, Kabbani SS, Crew J. Hypocalcemic acute myocardial failure secondary to rapid transfusion of citrated blood. *Am Heart J* 1984; 108:1040–2.
32. Olinger GN, Hottenrott C, Mulder DG, et al. Acute clinical hypocalcemic myocardial depression during rapid blood transfusion and postoperative hemodialysis. *J Thorac Cardiovasc Surg* 1976; 72:503–11.
33. Collins JA. Massive blood transfusion. *Clin Haematol* 1976; 5:201–22.
34. Mollison PL. *Blood Transfusion in Clinical Medicine*, 7th ed. Oxford, England: Blackwell Sci, 1983; 751.
35. Collins JA, Simmons RL, James PM. Acid-base status of seriously wounded combat casualties. II. Resuscitation with stored blood. *Ann Surg* 1971; 173:6–18.
36. Miller RD, Tong MJ, Robbins TO. Effects of massive transfusion of blood on acid-base balance. *JAMA* 1971; 216:1762–5.
37. Boyan CP, Howland WS. Cardiac arrest and temperature of bank blood. *JAMA* 1963; 183:58–60.

38. Arens JF, Leonard GL. Danger of overwarming blood by microwave. *JAMA* 1971; 218:1045–6.
39. Snyder EL, Bookbinder M. Role of microaggregate blood filtration in clinical medicine. *Transfusion* 1983; 23:460–70.
40. Collins JA, James PM, Bredenberg CE, et al. The relationship between transfusion and hypoxemia in combat casualties. *Ann Surg* 1978; 188:513–20.
41. Demling RH. Fluid resuscitation after major burns. *JAMA* 1983; 250:1438–40.
42. Demling RH. Burns. *N Engl J Med* 1985; 22:1389–96.
43. Butler P, Israel L, Nusbacher J, et al. Blood transfusion in liver transplantation. *Transfusion* 1985; 25:120–3.
44. Bontempo FA, Lewis JH, Van Thiel D, et al. The relation of preoperative coagulation findings to diagnosis, blood usage and survival in adult liver transplant. *Transplantation* 1985; 39:532–6.
45. Blumberg N, Bove JR. Uncrossmatched blood for emergency transfusion. *JAMA* 1978; 240:2057–9.
46. Strauss RG. Current issues in neonatal transfusions. *Vox Sang* 1986; 51:1–9.
47. Kakaiya RM, Morrison FS, Halbrook JC, et al. Problems with a walking-donor transfusion program. *Transfusion* 1979; 19:577–80.
48. Oberman HA. Replacement transfusion in the newborn period. *J Pediatr* 1975; 86:586–7.
49. Kakaiya RM, Morrison FS, Rawson JE, et al. Pedi-pack transfusion in a newborn intensive care unit. *Transfusion* 1979; 19:19–24.
50. Brady MT, Milam JD, Anderson DC, et al. Use of deglycerolized red blood cells to prevent posttransfusion infection with cytomegalovirus in neonates. *J Infect Dis* 1984; 150:334–9.
51. Konugres AA. Transfusion therapy for the neonate. In: Bell CA (ed). *A seminar on Perinatal Blood Banking.* Washington, DC: American Association of Blood Banks, 1981; 93–107.
52. Brzica SM, Pineda AA, Taswell HF. Autologous blood transfusion. *Mayo Clin Proc* 1976; 51:723–37.
53. Milles G, Langston H, Dalessandro W. *Autologous Transfusions.* Springfield, IL: Thomas, 1971.
54. Ascari WQ, Jolley PC, Thomas PA. Autologous blood transfusion in pulmonary surgery. *Transfusion* 1968; 8:111–5.
55. Moore FD. The effects of hemorrhage on body composition. *N Engl J Med* 1965; 273:567–77.
56. Finch S, Haskins D, Finch CA. Iron metabolism. Hematopoiesis following phlebotomy. Iron as a limiting factor. *J Clin Invest* 1950; 29:1078–86.
57. Popovsky MA, Devine PA, Taswell HF. Intraoperative autologous autotransfusion. *Mayo Clin Proc* 1985; 60:125–34.
58. Brewster DC, Ambrosino JJ, Darling RC, et al. Intraoperative autotransfusion in major vascular surgery. *Am J Surg* 1979; 137:507–13.
59. Due TL, Johnson JM, Wood M, Hale HW Jr. Intraoperative autotransfusion in the management of massive hemorrhage. *Am J Surg* 1975; 130:653–8.
60. Hauer JM, Thurer RL. Controversies in autotransfusion. *Vox Sang* 1984; 46:8–12.
61. Winton TL, Charrette EJP, Salerno TA. The cell saver during cardiac surgery: does it save? *Ann Thorac Surg* 1982; 33:379–81.
62. Cosgrove DM, Thurer RL, Lytle BW, et al. Blood conservation during myocardial revascularization. *Ann Thorac Surg* 1979; 28:184–9.
63. Cosgrove DM, Loop FD, Lytle BW, et al. Determinants of blood utilization during myocardial revascularization. *Ann Thorac Surg* 1985; 40:380–4.

64. Jalonen J, Meretoja O, Laaksonen V, et al. Myocardial oxygen balance during hemodilution in patients undergoing coronary artery bypass grafting. *Eur Surg Res* 1984; 16:141–7.
65. Weisel RD, Charlesworth DC, Mickleborough LL, et al. Limitations of blood conservation. *J Thorac Cardiovasc Surg* 1984; 88:26–38.
66. Mammen EF, Koets MH, Washington BC, et al. Hemostasis changes during cardiopulmonary bypass surgery. *Semin Thromb Hemost* 1985; 11:281–92.
67. Bick RL. Hemostasis defects associated with cardiac surgery, prosthetic devices, and other extracorporeal circuits. *Semin Thromb Hemost* 1985; 11:249–80.
68. Harker LA, Malpass TW, Branson HE, et al. Mechanism of abnormal bleeding in patients undergoing cardiopulmonary bypass: acquired transient platelet dysfunction associated with selective α-granule release. *Blood* 1980; 56:824–34.
69. Simon TL, Akl BF, Murphy W. Controlled trial of routine administration of platelet concentrates in cardiopulmonary bypass surgery. *Ann Thorac Surg* 1984; 37:359–64.
70. Wolman IJ. Transfusion therapy in Cooley's anemia: growth and health as related to long-range hemoglobin levels. A progress report. *Ann NY Acad Sci* 1964; 119:736–47.
71. Chaplin H Jr, Keitel HG, Peterson RE. Hematologic observations on patients with sickle cell anemia sustained at normal hemoglobin levels by multiple transfusions. *Blood* 1956; 11:834–45.
72. Propper RD, Button LN, Nathan DG. New approaches to the transfusion management of thalassemia. *Blood* 1980; 55:55–60.
73. Blumberg N, Peck K, Ross K, Avila E. Immune response to chronic red blood cell transfusion. *Vox Sang* 1983; 44:212–7.
74. Blumberg N, Ross K, Avila E, Peck K. Should chronic transfusions be matched for antigens other than ABO and $Rh_o(D)$? *Vox Sang* 1984; 47:205–8.
75. Corash L, Klein H, Deisseroth A, et al. Selective isolation of young erythrocytes for transfusion support of thalassemia major patients. *Blood* 1981; 57:599–606.
76. Pisciotto P, Kiraly T, Paradis L, et al. Clinical trial of young red blood cells prepared by apheresis. *Ann Clin Lab Sci* 1986; 16:473–8.
77. Opelz G, Terasaki PI. Improvement of kidney-graft survival with increased numbers of blood transfusions. *N Engl J Med* 1978; 299:799–803.
78. Rodey GE. Blood transfusions and their influence on renal allograft survival. In: Brown EB (ed). *Progress in Hematology,* Vol. 14. Orlando: Grune, 1986; 99–122.
79. Singal DP, Ludwin D, Blajchman MA. Blood transfusion and renal transplantation. *Br J Haematol* 1985; 61:595–602.
80. Sanfilippo FP, Bollinger RR, MacQueen JM, et al. A randomized study comparing leukocyte-depleted versus packed red cell transfusions in prospective cadaver renal allograft recipients. *Transfusion* 1985; 25:116–9.
81. Polesky HF, McCullough JJ, Yunis E, et al. The effects of transfusion of frozen-thawed deglycerolized red cells on renal graft survival. *Transplantation* 1977; 24:449–52.
82. Light JA, Metz S, Oddenino K, et al. Fresh vs. stored blood in donor specific transfusions. *Transplant Proc* 1982; 14:296–301.
83. Opelz G, Sengar DPS, Mickey MR, Terasaki PI. Effect of blood transfusions on subsequent kidney transplantation. *N Engl J Med* 1969; 280:735–9.
84. Schweizer RT, Bartus SA, Silver H, McLean RH. Kidney transplantation using donor-specific blood transfusions despite Rh incompatibility. *Transplantation* 1981; 32:345–6.
85. Mangal AK, Growe GH, Sinclair M, et al. Acquired hemolytic anemia due to

"auto"-anti-A or "auto"-anti-B induced by group O homograft in renal transplant recipients. *Transfusion* 1984; 24:201–5.
86. Ramsey G, Israel L, Lindsay GD, et al. Anti-Rh_o(D) in two Rh-positive patients receiving kidney graft from an Rh-immunized donor. *Transplantation* 1986; 41:67–9.
87. Hows JM, Yin JL, Marsh J, et al. Histocompatible unrelated volunteer donors compared with HLA nonidentical family donors in marrow transplantation for aplastic anemia and leukemia. *Blood* 1986; 68:1322–8.
88. Parkman R. Current status of bone marrow transplantation in pediatric oncology. *Cancer* 1986; 58:569–72.
89. Storb R, Weiden PL. Transfusion problems associated with transplantation. *Semin Hematol* 1981; 18:163–76.
90. Bensinger WI, Bruckner CD, Thomas ED, Clift RA. ABO-incompatible marrow transplants. *Transplantation* 1982; 33:427–9.
91. Bruckner CD, Clift RA, Sanders JE, et al. ABO-incompatible marrow transplants. *Transplantation* 1978; 26:233–8.
92. Warkentin PI, Hilden J, Kersey JH, et al. Transplantation of major ABO-incompatible bone marrow depleted of red cells by hydroxyethyl starch. *Vox Sang* 1985; 48:89–104.
93. Burrows L, Tartter P. Effect of blood transfusions on colonic malignancy recurrence rate. *Lancet* 1982; 2:662 (letter).
94. Foster RS, Foster JC, Costanza MC. Blood transfusions and survival after surgery for breast cancer. *Arch Surg* 1984; 119:1138–40.
95. Blumberg N, Heal JM, Murphy P, Agarwal MM. Association between transfusion of whole blood and recurrence of cancer. *Br Med J* 1986; 293:530–3.
96. Ota D, Alvarez L, Lichtiger B, et al. Perioperative blood transfusion in patients with colon carcinoma. *Transfusion* 1985; 25:392–4.
97. Rosenberg SA, Seipp CA, White DE, Wesley R. Perioperative blood transfusions are associated with increased rates of recurrence and decreased survival in patients with high-grade soft-tissue sarcomas of the extremities. *J Clin Oncol* 1985; 3:698–709.
98. Nathanson SD, Tilley BC, Schultz L, Smith RF. Perioperative allogeneic blood transfusion. Survival in patients with resected carcinomas of the colon and rectum. *Arch Surg* 1985; 120:734–8.
99. Leitman SF, Holland PV. Irradiation of blood products. Indications and guidelines. *Transfusion* 1985; 25:293–300.
100. Luban NLC, Ness PM. Irradiation of blood products: comment. *Transfusion* 1985; 25:301–3.
101. Lind SE. Has the case for irradiating blood products been made? *Am J Med* 1985; 78:543–4.
102. Hewitt WC, Wheby M, Crosby WH. Effect of prednisolone on incompatible blood transfusions. *Transfusion* 1961; 1:184–6.
103. Rosenfield RE, Jagathambal. Transfusion therapy for autoimmune hemolytic anemia. *Semin Hematol* 1976; 13:311–21.
104. Goldman DA, Maki DG, Rhame FS, et al. Guidelines for infection control in intravenous therapy. *Ann Intern Med* 1973; 79:848–50.
105. Ryden SE, Oberman HA. Compatibility of common intravenous solutions with CPD blood. *Transfusion* 1975; 15:250–5.
106. Ruel GJ, Beall AC, Lefrak EA, et al. Prevention of post-traumatic pulmonary insufficiency: fine screen filtration of blood. *Arch Surg* 1973; 106:386–394.
107. Snyder EL, Bookbinder M. Role of microaggregate blood filtration in clinical medicine. *Transfusion* 1983; 23:460–70.

108. Snyder EL, Ferri PM, Smith EO, Ezekowitz MD. Use of an electromechanical infusion pump for transfusion of platelet concentrates. *Transfusion* 1984; 24: 524–7.
109. Snyder EL, Malech HL, Ferri PM, et al. In vitro function of granulocyte concentrates following passage through an electromechanical infusion pump. *Transfusion* 1986; 26:141–4.
110. Hirsch RL, Brodheim E, Ginsberg FE. A computer-based blood inventory and information system for hospital blood banks as part of a regional blood-management program. *Transfusion* 1970; 10:194–202.
111. Cohen MA, Pierskalla WP. Target inventory levels for a hospital blood bank of a decentralized regional blood banking system. *Transfusion* 1979; 19:444–54.
112. Mintz PD. Expected hemotherapy in elective surgery. *NY State J Med* 1976; 76:532–7.
113. Friedman, BA. An analysis of surgical blood use in United States hospitals with application to the maximum surgical blood order schedule. *Transfusion* 1979; 19:268–78.
114. Oberman HA, Barnes BA, Friedman BA. The risk of abbreviating the major crossmatch in urgent or massive transfusion. *Transfusion* 1978; 18:137–41.

7. Complications of Transfusion

The physician deciding whether to give a transfusion has the responsibility of weighing the expected benefits against the known risks. *The physician must not take these risks too lightly.* Blood transfusion is not an innocuous minor procedure used to hasten recovery from illness and operations, and should never be a matter of routine in the replacement of even minor blood losses at surgery. In this chapter, therefore, we will point out the many risks that must be evaluated in making the clinical judgement to transfuse. These consist particularly of acute transfusion reactions and various delayed complications, such as disease transmission and alloimmunization.

In clinical usage, the term *transfusion reaction* refers to an obviously adverse response to transfusion, usually during or shortly after the transfusion and usually resulting from the combination of antigen and antibody.

Too often, lack of an overt reaction is considered a successful outcome. However, poor posttransfusion survival of tranfused blood, or failure of the patient to achieve the desired clinical effect, can occur from a multitude of causes. An antibody in a *donor's* plasma, for example, may destroy more of the recipient's own red cells than the amount of donor cells transfused, or donor red cells may be destroyed within a few days by a weak antibody in the recipient's plasma without any overt reaction. The blood bank staff must be alert not only to the possibility of obvious reactions but also to conditions that might adversely affect the outcome of the transfusion.

Hemolytic Transfusion Reactions

There are many possible causes of hemoglobinemia and hemoglobinuria at the time of blood transfusion, including some that are unrelated to blood incompatibility. Furthermore, although intravascular hemolysis is prominent in some transfusion reactions, it may be transitory, unapparent, or absent in others.

Basically, the true hemolytic transfusion reaction is caused by the in-vivo combination of an antibody with red cells possessing the corresponding antigen. Most often, and in most severe reactions, the antibody is in the patient's plasma and the antigen on the donor's red cells (*major* incompatibility). But antibody passively transferred from a donor's plasma may have a similar effect, either on the recipient's red cells (*minor* incompatibility), or on other donor red cells transfused to that patient (*interdonor* incompatibility). Severe reactions may occur in any of these situations, but are most likely when the antibody is in the recipient's plasma, because in that case, transfused red cells having the corresponding antigen are immediately surrounded by the patient's full-strength antibody under optimal conditions for interaction. In each of the other situations, the transfused antibody is diluted as it enters the recipient's circulation, and there is a large excess of antigenic sites on the recipient's red cells.

CLEARANCE OF HEMOGLOBIN

When red cells are destroyed while actually circulating in the bloodstream, hemoglobin is directly released into the plasma and becomes bound to the plasma protein *haptoglobin*. Each 100 ml of plasma can bind about 100 mg of haptoglobin in this way. The hemoglobin-haptoglobin complex, which is not excreted by the kidneys, is then cleared by the reticuloendothelial system [1]. Only when the haptoglobin is fully saturated does free hemoglobin appear in the plasma. When there is massive hemolysis, free hemoglobin appears almost at once and may be detectable in the plasma concurrently with the onset of clinical signs and symptoms [2].

Hemoglobin begins to appear in the urine when the plasma free hemoglobin (i.e., not bound to haptoglobin) reaches 25 mg/dl or more. The value for *free hemoglobin* will ordinarily be less than the result of the usual laboratory measurement of plasma or serum hemoglobin, since the latter ascertains the total amount of both free hemoglobin and that bound to haptoglobin. Reabsorption of some hemoglobin by the renal tubules results in deposits of *hemosiderin* in the tubular cells, a finding that could be important in the autopsy of a patient suspected of having suffered a hemolytic transfusion reaction. Hemosiderin may also appear in the urine following acute hemolysis, particularly if the plasma hemoglobin level is above 50 mg/dl. Hemosiderinuria would be expected to follow hemoglobinuria, and it may be worthwhile looking for it when there is a suspicion that an episode of hemolysis may have taken place within the previous week, especially if no definitive investigation was made at the time of the transfusion. A positive finding of hemosiderin in the urine undoubtedly means that there has been hemolysis. On the other hand, failure to demonstrate hemosiderin does not necessarily mean there was no hemolysis.

The time required to clear hemoglobin from the plasma by all mechanisms depends on a number of variables, and is directly related to the amount of hemoglobin being cleared. It may range from 5 hours to 12 or more. Given the initial presence of sufficient free hemoglobin in the plasma, the pattern of clearance is such that about a third of it may be passed in the urine.

The breakdown of hemoglobin produces *bilirubin,* some of which diffuses quickly into the tissues, while some appears in the plasma. Thus, there is usually *hyperbilirubinemia* after an acute hemolytic episode, with a peak at 3 to 6 hours. The amount depends on the extent and rapidity of hemolysis on the one hand, and on the rate of bilirubin excretion on the other. Since the elevated bilirubin will be of the free or unconjugated type, it would not be expected to appear in the urine unless there were already liver damage. The appearance and disappearance of these various pigments is illustrated in Fig. 7–1.

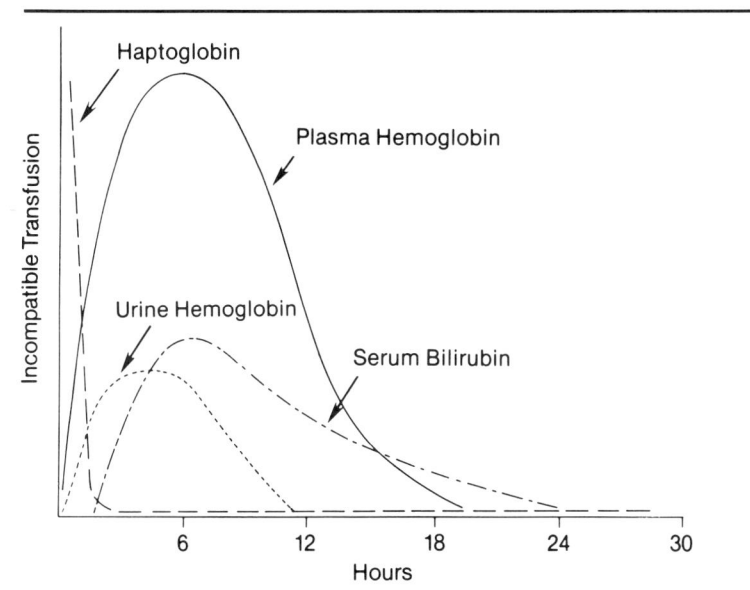

Figure 7–1
Time relationship of pigmentary changes in serum following hemolytic transfusion reaction (not to scale).

Hemolytic Transfusion Reactions Caused by Antibody in Recipient Plasma

Relation to Type of Antibody

Although it is difficult to predict the clinical reaction to incompatible red cells, certain general correlations can be made between the in vitro characteristics of the antibody and its in vivo effects. Antibodies that are readily hemolytic in vitro, predominantly of the complement-binding IgM type, are most likely to cause hemolytic transfusion reactions. This means that anti-A and anti-B are the chief culprits, since they are already present in most people and are often lytic. In the presence of strong antibodies of this type, half or more of the transfused incompatible red cells may be lysed intravascularly within minutes. In the case of weaker hemolytic antibodies, such as those of the Lewis system, the destruction is slower and little or no free hemoglobin may appear in the plasma, depending on the patient's ability to clear the destroyed or damaged red cells via the reticuloendothelial system. But despite the slower hemolysis, hemoglobinuria may occur. Both hemoglobinemia and hemoglobinuria may accompany incompatibility in the Kidd system, particularly that due to anti-

Table 7–1. Relationship Between In-Vitro Characteristics of an Antibody and Its Clinical Effect

	In-Vitro Characteristics of the Antibody	
Usual Clinical Picture (If Reaction Occurs)	Hemolytic (complement-binding IgM)	Agglutinating or Sensitizing (IgG)
Onset of reaction	Minutes	Hours to days
Site of lysis of transfused cells	Intravascular	Extravascular (spleen, liver)
Pigments found	Hemoglobinemia Hemoglobinuria Hyperbilirubinemia	Hyperbilirubinemia
Renal damage	Possible	Unlikely
Signs and symptoms	Hypotension, chills, fever, restlessness, dyspnea	Unexpected anemia or jaundice
DIC	Infrequent	Absent

DIC = disseminated intravascular coagulation.
Note: This comparison is of tendencies, not absolutes. Exceptions are to be expected.

Jk^a, although the antibody may be only weakly hemolytic in vitro or may hemolyze only enzyme-treated red cells.

Antibodies that are not hemolytic in vitro, that is, the predominantly IgG type such as the various Rh antibodies, usually cause extravascular rather than intravascular hemolysis. They *may* also cause severe transfusion reactions with hemoglobinemia and hemoglobinuria, depending on the characteristics of the antibody, the amount of incompatible blood given, and other variables. Antibodies of this type coat the transfused cells and bring about their removal from the circulation, predominantly by the spleen. The result is usually hyperbilirubinemia rather than hemoglobinemia. Most antibodies other than anti-A and anti-B react this way. For a general comparison of the effects of IgM and IgG antibodies, see Table 7–1, and for a detailed discussion of the effects of antibody on red cells, see Mollison [2].

Clinical Signs and Symptoms
There is a difference in clinical signs and symptoms between hemolytic transfusion reactions characterized by predominantly intravascular as opposed to extravascular hemolysis. This distinction, however, is by no means clear-cut, and correlation between the behavior of an antibody in vitro and in vivo is not perfect. The immediate cause of the clinical signs and symptoms in hemolytic transfusion reactions is uncertain. In the case of antibodies that are hemolytic in vitro, the clinical effects may be due to products released by the action of

complement on the red cells. Hemoglobin in and of itself is probably not the cause, since hemoglobinemia alone does not induce a clinical reaction.

In the case of a reaction caused by a strong hemolytic antibody, such as anti-A or anti-B, the reaction usually begins with the first few milliliters infused. Symptoms may include a burning sensation along the course of the vein being used for the transfusion, flushing of the face, fever and headache, pain in the lower back, and often an oppressive feeling in the chest. Shock may be a prominent feature. With a nonhemolytic (e.g., Rh) antibody, chills and fever often predominate and the other signs and symptoms may not occur. In general, the clinical picture is characterized by its variability. However, any unusual symptoms in a patient receiving a transfusion merit investigation and should be regarded as indicating a reaction until proved otherwise. Severe reactions without obvious clinical symptoms may occur under anesthesia, often manifesting themselves first as abnormal oozing of blood, or as hemoglobinuria.

The abnormal bleeding may be due to the liberation of thromboplastic substances from damaged red cells, followed by fibrinogen consumption and hypofibrinogenemia. Since the patient may in fact need more transfusions, recognition of the nature of the reaction is extremely important [3].

Renal failure sometimes follows incompatible transfusions accompanied by extensive intravascular hemolysis. Whether this serious complication is caused by some undefined toxic effect of hemoglobin or by shock accompanying the initial transfusion reaction is uncertain [4]. Some combination of factors seems more probable, since renal failure by no means invariably follows a hemolytic reaction, and hemolysis not caused by blood group incompatibility rarely produces such a result. On the other hand, renal failure does not ordinarily occur in connection with extravascular destruction of red cells. Oliguria and anuria following transfusion are not necessarily caused by transfusion; renal failure may be a complication of trauma, hemorrhage, collapse, and other conditions for which transfusions are given, particularly when blood volume restoration has been inadequate. Incompatible transfusion may, of course, produce effects additive to the foregoing.

Problems of Identification

Most serious reactions involve incompatibility in the ABO system, and more often than not the error is one of identification, rather than of laboratory technique. Most errors are immediately obvious on investigation, but sometimes considerable detective work is required to get all the details. The two most deadly, and most common, errors are (1) improper identification of recipient blood samples, usually because the sample taken from one patient has been identified with the name of another; and (2) transfusion of blood into the wrong recipient. In both cases, all laboratory procedures may have been carried out perfectly, but this offers no protection against such errors, which are not related to laboratory work. Mistakes in identification are particularly prone to occur when orders for blood for more than one patient are being handled at a time, and in emergencies, such as accidents involving several people, especially if the victims are all in the same family. Detection of one mistake should immediately lead to efforts to find another, because the usual error is switching the specimens and labels between two patients. A similar problem occurs when the identification tags or labels on blood containers are inadvertently exchanged on issuance.

Examination of accounts of fatal transfusion reactions reported to the FDA [5–8] shows that most of them were caused by classic red cell incompatibility, in turn due to clerical errors of identification. Many occurred in operating rooms or intensive care units where someone failed to carry through elementary patient and blood identification procedures. One estimate of the fatality rate is about one per million units transfused [7]. Such a figure does not seem impressive until one realizes that every one of those deaths was caused by a preventable human error.

Problems with Laboratory Tests

Red cell incompatibility sufficient to cause a reaction is ordinarily detectable by a properly done crossmatch. Therefore, once it has been determined that a true hemolytic reaction has occurred, and that there was no mixup of specimens or blood units, laboratory error or inadequacy must be sought. There can be many causes: inadequate incubation, failure to see hemolysis in vitro, failure to see agglutination, failure to add antiglobulin serum (and the other causes of false-negative antiglobulin tests), failure to make use of an antiglobulin crossmatch; but most important, use of the wrong samples for the crossmatch, or occasionally, failure to do a crossmatch at all, such as might occur in emergencies.

Delayed Hemolytic Reactions

In some patients who are already immunized to certain blood group antigens, the antibody may be so weak as to be undetectable by either antibody screening tests or by regular crossmatching. If such a patient is given apparently compatible blood that happens to possess the corresponding antigen, a secondary antigenic stimulus is provided [9]. The resulting antibody response may be very rapid and may cause a reaction, with partial or complete elimination of the transfused antigen-positive donor cells several days after the transfusion. Certain Rh antibodies, particularly anti-E or anti-c, and antibodies of the Kidd system, are prone to cause delayed hemolytic reactions. Although most such reactions are relatively mild, they are occasionally severe.

Salama and Mueller-Eckhardt reported that such delayed hemolytic reactions were regularly associated with strong complement deposition on the patient's own red cells as well as on those of the incompatible donor, and that the responsible alloantibody may often be eluted from circulating red cells long after the transfused red cells have disappeared [10]. These findings are at odds with those of most other observers and remain to be explained [11].

Unexpectedly Mild Reactions

On occasion, for reasons that are not always apparent, a patient receives incompatible blood, yet fails to exhibit the usual signs and symptoms of a transfusion reaction or has only trivial or transitory effects [12, 13]. Sometimes this condition may be related to an initially low level of antibody in the recipient's plasma. For example, a group A patient with a low titer of agglutinating anti-B might tolerate an incompatible transfusion of group B blood better than would another patient having a higher titer of high-affinity anti-B. Antigen-antibody reactions that are weak in vitro (e.g., those with A_2 or D^u antigens) cannot be relied on to behave the same way in vivo, and severe clinical reactions may occur regardless of the antigenic reactivity if the recipient's antibody is a clinically potent one.

Decreased Survival of Transfused Red Cells Without Demonstrable Antibody

An occasional patient is encountered in whom transfused, apparently compatible red cells survive poorly even in the absence of any demonstrable blood group antibody [14]. There may be no overt reaction. Such an occurrence may well be caused by antibodies undetectable by the usual techniques; a compatible crossmatch does not always ensure normal survival of transfused red cells.

HEMOLYTIC TRANSFUSION REACTIONS CAUSED BY ANTIBODY IN DONOR PLASMA

Minor Incompatibility

Cases have been reported of hemolysis of the recipient's red cells, even on rare occasions, with anuria, following transfusion of donor blood containing antibodies directed against an antigen on the recipient's red cells. This has been particularly noted among group A recipients transfused with group O donor whole blood having strong incomplete or hemolytic anti-A. It is because of the possibility of this type of reaction that the use of group O whole blood is not advised in emergencies with patients who have not yet been typed.

In transfusing platelet concentrates or many units of cryoprecipitated antihemophilic factor where the ABO type is often disregarded, it is possible to give appreciable amounts of ABO-incompatible plasma. This can and often does cause coating of the recipient's red cells, and it may lead to a positive direct antiglobulin test, with or without a fall in the hemoglobin level, that is, a temporary alloimmune hemolytic process [15].

Minor incompatibility may also occur as a result of irregular donor antibodies of other blood group systems, but the reactions are inclined to be mild or even inapparent. High-titer donor antibodies, particularly anti-D or anti-K, may result in a positive direct antiglobulin test with deleterious effects on a recipient's red cells [16].

Interdonor Incompatibility

The half-life of passively transferred IgG antibody is 22 to 26 days, and at any time during the persistence of such a transfused antibody, further transfusion with donor red cells having the antigen could result in the destruction of some or all of the new donor cells [17]. This is an unlikely event, since it occurs only with multiple transfusions of whole blood and requires the presence of an antibody missed by routine screening.

HEMOLYSIS UNRELATED TO BLOOD GROUP INCOMPATIBILITY

In addition to the occasional hemolytic reaction for which no explanation can be found, hemolysis of either donor or recipient red cells can take place concurrently with transfusion in a variety of circumstances.

Faulty Storage of Blood

Excessive fluctuation of storage temperature may damage red cells, and blood is not considered transfusable if its temperature during storage or transportation has exceeded 10°C. Excessive warming of whole blood or red blood cells by any technique (e.g., placing bags in hot water, or exposure to microwaves with their characteristic spot-overheating) can cause extensive hemoglobinemia if the blood is subsequently transfused [18]. Blood stored in poorly regulated refrigerators may partially freeze with resulting hemolysis.

Faulty Transfusion Procedure

Exposure of stored blood or red blood cells to dextrose solutions (e.g., 5 or 10 percent dextrose in water, or dextrose in 0.45 or 0.225 percent saline) for even 15 minutes can damage the red cells. We have seen definite hemolysis in the plasma of a patient when red blood cells were transfused after having been resuspended and then allowed to hang for 15 to 30 minutes in 5 percent dextrose in 0.45 percent saline. Other work has shown decreased survival of red cells incubated for as little as 15 minutes in 5 percent dextrose in water [19]. We have also seen instances of lack of response to transfusion when red cells were given through the same tubing with such solutions. There is more contact between red cells and fluid in the intravenous tubing than most people realize.

Injection of blood under pressure can cause rupture of red cells and detectable hemolysis, particularly in the case of older, stored blood. However, the amount of hemolysis is only slight and the old concept that hemolysis is worse with small-bore needles seems not to be true [20].

Conditions in the Patient

Clinical conditions unrelated to transfusion can cause hemolysis. *Glucose 6-phosphate dehydrogenase (G-6-PD) deficiency* in the recipient's red cells makes them susceptible to hemolysis by certain drugs that may be used in treatment (e.g., primaquine and some sulfonamides). If the patient happens to receive a transfusion at or about the same time, such hemolysis may be misinterpreted as due to incompatible blood. The reverse situation may also occur: donor blood deficient in this enzyme may be hemolyzed by trigger drugs given to the recipient.

Myoglobinemia and *myoglobinuria* sometimes occur in patients with ischemic musculature after temporary clamping of the aorta in major vascular surgery. *Water* used to irrigate the urinary bladder during transurethral prostatectomy may enter the circulation and cause hemolysis. This has been thought to precipitate renal failure in patients whose kidneys are already damaged. Substantial hemolysis has been caused by the accidental infusion of water instead of electrolyte solutions, with and without concurrent blood transfusion.

Depending on mechanical and other variables, artificial heart valves and total artificial heart implants can cause ongoing red cell destruction that requires more or less continuous blood replacement.

MANAGEMENT OF HEMOLYTIC REACTIONS

Diagnosis

Patients receiving transfusions must be watched with care, but also with common sense. Chills and fever, for example, are important early signs of incompatibility, but a patient who was feverish before transfusion might well remain so during and after transfusion. Most important is the sudden onset of any of the signs and symptoms already described, such as chills, fever, flushing, back or chest pain, or shock, especially in the earlier stages of the transfusion. At these stages, a blood sample may show hemoglobinemia or a positive direct antiglobulin test. Most other laboratory procedures—such as measurement of hemoglobin, bilirubin, or haptoglobin, or more detailed serologic investigation—are retrospective. In patients under *general anesthesia,* shock or the development of a bleeding tendency may be the only indication of incompatibility. In all cases, the evidence must be carefully evaluated to determine whether it is really related to blood incompatibility. For example, shock at surgery is more likely to be caused by unrecognized bleeding.

Treatment

As soon as a hemolytic reaction is suspected, the transfusion must be stopped, since serious consequences are proportional to the amount of incompatible blood given [5, 21]. If there is evidence of hemolysis, or even if there is only a strong suspicion that an incompatible unit has been given, it is best to begin treatment at once, without waiting for clinical or laboratory confirmation of the diagnosis. Although it is commonly thought that incompatible transfusions cause death by renal failure, in fact, death is usually brought about by shock and hypotension. Nevertheless, renal failure is a severe complication and should be prevented at all costs. It is usual to refer patients suspected of having suffered a hemolytic reaction to a nephrologist for immediate treatment. The details of therapy are beyond the scope of this book, but the principal steps are as follows:

1. Stop the blood transfusion that appears to be at fault.
2. Maintain blood volume with intravenous electrolyte infusion, supplemented with mannitol or furosemide, but do not give vasopressor drugs.
3. Maintain a urinary flow of 1 to 3 ml per minute. If diuresis ensues, maintain volume with intravenous fluids. Otherwise, suspect renal tubular necrosis and restrict fluid intake.

Other Forms of Transfusion Reaction

Allergic Reactions

Allergic reactions are usually manifested as hives (urticaria)—itchy, pale, irregular, slightly raised skin lesions of various size—appearing during transfusion. There may be only one or two, or many. The frequency of such reactions is usually given as 1 to 3 percent of all transfusions. More serious variants of allergic reactions, such as facial or glottal edema, or asthma, are fortunately rare. More rarely still, pulmonary edema and infiltrates may occur, by either active or passive routes [22, 23]. A few allergic reactions may be caused by passive transfer of donor antibodies to the recipient, in which case the onset of the reaction may be delayed until the patient is exposed in some other way to the antigen. Such delayed manifestations are unlikely to be reported as transfusion reactions.

A few anaphylactic reactions are associated with immunization to IgA in IgA-deficient recipients [24, 25]. Although reported cases are few, the route of immunization seems to have been transfusion in most, but not all, cases. In a random population, about 1 in 700 healthy people will have a deficiency of IgA, and can therefore produce the corresponding antibody [24]. An unknown number of other people who have normal IgA levels can develop anti-IgA of limited specificity and are at risk for the same type of reaction.

Patients with common variable immunodeficiency, who require gamma globulin replacement therapy, paradoxically can make anti-IgA and have been reported to suffer anaphylactic reactions to even minuscule amounts of IgA in therapeutic immunoglobulin preparations [26].

Treatment

The transfusion should be stopped as soon as the reaction is detected, and an adequate dose of an antihistamine drug should be administered, preferably parenterally. Although it is always possible that such an allergic reaction may progress to cause more serious effects despite appropriate medication, this does not usually happen. Most physicians consider it reasonable to restart the transfusion if urticarial symptoms subside quickly after antihistamine administration. In the case of more severe manifestations, such as anaphylaxis, more vigorous and specific therapy will be needed [27].

Prevention

Anyone who is to have elective blood transfusions should be questioned about a history of allergy. If there is such a history, an adequate dose of antihistamine may be given by mouth or parenterally 15 or 20 minutes before the start of the transfusion. The same applies if the patient has had previous allergic transfusion reactions. It is unsound practice, either therapeutically or prophylactically, to add antiallergic medication to the blood itself, since the amount and rate at which medication enters the patient will be inadequate.

IgA-deficient patients with anti-IgA can have severe reactions to very small amounts of IgA. When time permits, it is better for such patients to receive blood or components from IgA-deficient donors, registries of whom are maintained by the American Association of Blood Banks (AABB) and by the American National Red Cross, as well as by some large blood banks. In the case of red blood cells, an alternative is to remove plasma proteins by thorough washing or by the use of frozen-thawed red cells (see Chap. 8).

Febrile Reactions

Febrile reactions are characterized by chills and varying degrees of fever (usually defined as a rise of at least 1°C) during transfusion, and must be distinguished from febrile episodes unrelated to transfusion, and from simple chills due to the effects of drafts, air conditioning, etc. on scantily covered patients. The reaction usually begins an hour or so after the start of the transfusion. Fever may be accompanied by headache, flushing, tachycardia, and discomfort; it is transitory, usually not lasting for more than an hour or so.

The incidence of reported febrile reactions is probably less than 2 percent of transfusions, but it varies considerably in different patient populations and is higher in women. More reactions of this type would probably be recorded if patients' temperatures were routinely taken during transfusions. Many febrile reactions are caused by recipient antibodies directed against donor leukocyte antigens [28], in which case immunization is the result of previous transfusion or pregnancy. A few of them may have other causes, such as reactions to ill-defined plasma factors, perhaps serum protein allotypes, and passive transfer of leukocyte antibodies. The almost universal use of disposable blood containers and tubing has virtually eliminated the febrile reactions to pyrogenic products of bacterial growth, which were once common.

Treatment
Since the signs and symptoms may be indistinguishable from the early evidences of a hemolytic transfusion reaction, the transfusion must be stopped at once and investigation instituted for a possible hemolytic reaction. Symptomatic treatment is appropriate, including antipyretic medication. If the fever subsides, and there is no evidence of hemolysis or blood mixup, it may be possible to restart the transfusion from the same unit of blood. More often, however, by the time the investigation is finished, the unit will probably have been hanging at room temperature long enough for bacterial growth to have become a risk, and restarting is inadvisable.

Prevention
One general suggestion is to keep blood recipients properly covered and comfortably warm during transfusion. Chilliness and shivering are thus prevented and not reported as a transfusion reaction. An antipyretic drug may be given shortly before transfusion to patients known to have occasional febrile reactions. For patients with bleeding tendencies, an antipyretic other than aspirin, such as acetaminophen, should be used. There is no convincing evidence that antihistamines have any therapeutic or prophylactic value. In patients who regularly have febrile reactions, yet require continued transfusions, some method of removing white cells and platelets should be tried empirically. Without this, it may even be impossible to transfuse a full unit of red cells before fever strikes and the transfusion has to be stopped. Present-day techniques of washing red cells or of making leukocyte-poor preparations (see Chap. 8) are sufficiently effective to prevent most reactions of this type.

Some transfusionists have recommended that we should consider washing all red cell transfusions to prevent febrile and allergic transfusion reactions [29]. In view of the much higher cost of washed preparations, and the fact that most patients do not have such reactions, we do not consider that recommendation justified. A simpler and less costly method of preventing febrile (but not allergic) reactions is that of centrifugation of the red cells followed by microaggregate filtration [30].

CIRCULATORY OVERLOAD

Transfusion of whole blood to patients with already increased plasma volumes or with incipient heart failure may cause a feeling of tightness in the chest and a dry cough; the process may progress to pulmonary edema if the transfusion is continued. It seems that we are seeing more of this type of reaction nowadays, particularly in patients with complex disease processes that require frequent transfusions of multiple blood components. It is all too easy to lose track of the amount of fluid in each component transfused.

Treatment consists of stopping the transfusion, or at least slowing it, and placing the patient in a sitting position. Treatment for incipient pulmonary edema should then be instituted.

Prevention lies in the avoidance of whole blood transfusions, or of giving excessive numbers of any components, in patients with severe anemia or increased plasma volume. If transfusion is essential, red blood cells may be given slowly (100 ml per hour), preferably with the patient in a sitting position, although prolonged transfusions introduce the additional risk of bacterial growth. Better expedients are to remove as much plasma as possible after hard centrifugation, or to wash the red cells in saline; in either case, almost all the plasma is removed. Another option is to divide a unit of red cells in two and give one half at a time. Washed or centrifuged and resuspended red cells can usually be given at more or less normal rates to patients with heart failure, but careful bedside observation is still vital.

Embolism

Although various forms of embolism (i.e., particles or foreign material in the blood vessels) may occur during transfusion, the principal variety we are concerned with is *air embolism*. This used to occur in connection with rapid pressure infusion of blood from glass bottles. The virtually universal use of plastic bags has all but eliminated this hazard, although it is possible for air to enter a plastic blood bag if the infusion set is changed during transfusion, or if someone erroneously attempts to vent the bag. If the amount of air is large, the recipient's blood becomes frothy and cannot be pumped properly by the heart. The victim becomes cyanotic and dyspneic and goes into shock, sometimes with cardiac arrest.

Immediate treatment consists of lowering the patient's head and turning the *right* side up. This will permit the air to collect in the right atrium, keeping the pulmonic valve clear and allowing the air to escape harmlessly a little at a time. If cardiac arrest occurs, treatment will have to be more drastic and may be unsuccessful.

Prevention consists of avoiding air in intravenous lines and paying particular attention to this when changing infusion sets.

Cold Blood

It is now well known that the rapid transfusion of large quantities of ice-cold blood may cause the recipient's heart to stop. This complication seems to be predominantly a problem in extensive surgery accompanied by massive blood transfusion, but it also happens occasionally in exchange transfusion in babies. It does not apply to adults receiving 3 or 4 units of blood at the usual rates of transfusion.

Complications caused by rapid transfusion of cold blood may be prevented by warming the blood to not more than 37°C as it passes through the delivery tubing on its way to the patient's vein. Methods of warming blood are discussed in Chapter 6.

CONTAMINATED BLOOD COMPONENTS

Some bacteria, usually gram-negative pseudomonads, coliforms, and achromobacters, can grow in blood at refrigerator temperatures and produce deadly endotoxins. Transfusion of such infected blood results in a catastrophic reaction characterized by shaking chills, severe hypotension, and pain in the abdomen and extremities, often with vomiting and bloody diarrhea [31]. The shock syndrome is peculiar in that it is accompanied by a dry, flushed skin, and by fever. Symptoms appear after a latent period of about 30 minutes and may follow transfusion of as little as 50 ml. Although they are not common nowadays, reactions to contaminated blood still occur [5]. Bacterial contamination of platelet concentrates stored at ambient temperature has been a factor in limiting storage of such products to 5 rather than 7 days (see Chap. 8).

Treatment

If not recognized and treated at once, the reaction is usually fatal. Treatment cannot, therefore, await the completion of laboratory procedures to identify the organisms. Treatment of septic shock is a medical emergency and the details are beyond the scope of this book. It includes the immediate administration of broad-spectrum antibiotics, such as gentamicin and cephalothin, by the most rapid route possible, supplemented with appropriate fluid replacement, respiratory support, vasopressors to maintain blood pressure and urinary output, and corticosteroids [32].

Prevention

The utmost care is required in the maintenance of aseptic blood collection techniques. Since a rise in temperature will immediately accelerate the growth of any contaminating organisms, blood should *never* be allowed to stand unnecessarily at room temperature (including unduly prolonged transfusion) or, worse still, to reach higher temperatures. This is one of the main reasons for the often-repeated admonitions not to warm containers of blood before transfusion, which would promote rapid growth of any bacteria in the event of subsequent delay. Blood that has exceeded 10°C before transfusion is best considered unusable. In other words, to guard against the possibility of bacterial infection, it is best to regard all stored blood as potentially contaminated. Since organisms growing at low temperatures usually also cause some hemolysis of stored blood, all blood units must be carefully inspected before release. The observer must look for signs of hemolysis at the cell-plasma interface, for discoloration, or for any other unusual appearance.

CITRATE TOXICITY

Citrate is rapidly metabolized, mainly by the liver, and excreted in the urine; therefore, attainment of toxic levels depends on either very rapid transfusion of large quantities of citrated blood or impaired function or circulation of the liver [33]. Citrate effects a reduction in ionized calcium in the blood, and can cause muscular tremors and even cardiac arrhythmia. The whole matter of citrate toxicity is unsettled, since the apparent effects occur in patients receiving massive transfusions under circumstances already conducive to cardiac arrest and death. However, in *hemapheresis* of even normal, healthy donors, we have seen citrate effects ranging from mild circumoral paresthesias to tetany and cardiac arrhythmia, which has made us a great deal less skeptical about the reality of citrate effects.

Citrate toxicity applies not only to whole blood transfusions, but also to large plasma infusions, such as might occur in the setting of plasma exchange using normal plasma as the replacement medium (see Chap. 10). Citrate effects in transfusion are covered in more detail in Chapter 6.

BLEEDING TENDENCY

When patients receive massive amounts of stored blood (i.e., amounts approaching or exceeding their total blood volume in a short period of time), *thrombocytopenia* may result because of the loss of platelet viability in stored blood. Such patients may subsequently develop a bleeding tendency, and their platelet counts may then remain low for several days, probably reflecting the rate at which new platelets are provided by the marrow (see also Chap. 6).

Similar problems occur in cardiovascular surgery, when patients have endured prolonged periods of time on extracorporeal circulation. In that situation, there appears to be partial activation of platelets with release of alpha granule contents and prolongation of the bleeding time. Such a defect may occur even when the platelet counts are above $100,000/mm^3$ [34]. Extensive bleeding may also occur in repeat cardiothoracic operations, probably as a result of large, highly vascular raw surfaces.

Platelet defects or deficiencies are usually manifested by continued oozing of blood from wounds and cut surfaces. Bear in mind that continued brisk or localized bleeding is more likely to be caused by an unrecognized bleeding vessel, and that incomplete neutralization of heparin may also cause bleeding. In these cases, platelet transfusions are not likely to help.

Treatment

Platelet transfusions are usually corrective. In this kind of situation, surgeons may request "fresh" whole blood, but there is no evidence that even the most freshly collected blood is as effective as platelet concentrates. Furthermore, with the testing now required (e.g., for HBsAg, ALT, and anti-HIV), very recently collected blood is seldom as available as platelet concentrates. Since it obviously pays to be prepared, surgeons should notify the blood bank in advance when they anticipate massive transfusions, prolonged pump times in heart surgery, or other potential bleeding problems, so that adequate supplies of platelets will be available.

Graft-Versus-Host Disease

Graft-versus-host disease (GVHD) occurs when immunologically competent lymphocytes are introduced into an immunoincompetent host (recipient) who is different with respect to histocompatibility antigens. The incoming lymphocytes cannot be destroyed by the recipient, and recognizing the host as foreign, they attack the host tissues. GVHD occurs in allogeneic bone marrow transplantation, and following nonirradiated transfusions of cellular blood components to patients with depressed immune function from almost any cause, whether disease or therapy [35]. It may also rarely occur following intrauterine fetal transfusions or exchange transfusions in premature newborns.

The effects of GVHD usually begin in about 1 or 2 weeks, producing fever, skin rash, diarrhea, pancytopenia, and hepatitis. Death often results. Sometimes the engrafted donor lymphocytes can be identified by HLA typing or cytogenetic testing. Treatment has not generally been successful. Fortunately, some cases of GVHD are mild or transitory [36].

Prevention

GVHD is caused by immunocompetent donor lymphocytes, capable of spontaneous division. It can be prevented by total removal of lymphocytes from transfused blood components or by inactivating the lymphocytes by irradiation (see Chap. 6).

Electrolyte Toxicity

The plasma potassium gradually increases in stored blood and can become a risk to patients who are already hyperkalemic—those with significant renal impairment, for instance. Transfusion of excessive potassium to such patients may be avoided by the use of reasonably fresh (less than a week in storage) red blood cells [37]. This decreases the amount of potassium transfused in the plasma and provides fewer effete red cells. Older blood contains a larger proportion of red cells destined for rapid destruction in the recipient, which involves greater release of red cell potassium. Plasma ammonium also increases during blood storage and could be risky to a patient with advanced liver disease. Here, too, the use of red blood cells or reasonably fresh blood is preferable.

Table 7-2 summarizes the more usual transfusion reactions and their causes.

Table 7-2. Common Forms of Transfusion Reactions

Reaction	Cause
Hemolytic, immediate	Major incompatibility
	Minor incompatibility
	Interdonor incompatibility
	Nonimmune factors
Hemolytic, delayed	Secondary antibody response
Allergic	Allergen in donor plasma
Anaphylaxis	Idiosyncratic response (IgA, other)
Febrile	Antibodies to donor WBC, platelets, plasma
Overload	Excess volume infusion
Embolism	Usually air in transfusion set
Cardiac arrhythmia	Cold blood or citrate effect (rapid massive transfusion)
Respiratory	Leukocyte antibodies
Bleeding tendency	Massive transfusion (thrombocytopenia)
Electrolyte toxicity	Excess K or NH_3 in older stored blood
Graft-v-host	Donor lymphocytes, immunocompromised recipient

Investigation of Suspected Transfusion Reactions

A suspected reaction cannot be investigated if the blood bank does not know about it. Physicians and nurses must be on the alert for untoward signs or symptoms in patients receiving blood and must make them known promptly to the blood bank. The need for reporting reactions may have to be emphasized from time to time; failure in this regard should be considered a serious breach of the customary standards of patient care. It is better to have a few reports of inconsequential symptoms than to miss the early opportunity for investigating and treating a true reaction.

A standardized investigational procedure should be used for any or all suspected transfusion reactions, even those tentatively classified as febrile, allergic, etc., without real suspicion of immune hemolysis. At the time a reaction occurs, nobody can be sure of its nature; it may be serious or trivial, and only further investigation can tell which.

In the *immediate investigation,* all that is necessary is to determine whether the patient received the blood intended for that patient, whether the proper blood was selected, and whether there is evidence of hemolysis. This can be done quickly and simply in most cases, without going into a detailed serologic investigation, such as would be appropriate if there were a strong suspicion of hemolysis. Such a simplified approach conforms fully to federal regulations and AABB standards.

BLOOD SAMPLES, CONTAINERS, AND RECORDS

To be able to carry out retrospective investigation of a suspected transfusion reaction, it is essential to keep all *pilot samples* (tube segments) from transfused units and all *patient samples* used for crossmatching properly stoppered and refrigerated for at least a week after transfusion and, if possible, even longer. A period of 2 weeks is not unreasonable and is occasionally useful, since some transfusion reactions are not reported on time or are delayed in onset. This may be a luxury, however, and many blood banks may not have the space available for storage of samples for more than the required week.

Some blood banks also save the containers themselves for a day or so, so that serologic typing of the small amounts of residual blood can be rechecked against the blood in the pilot sample.

LABORATORY PROCEDURES AND INVESTIGATION

The most important immediate step is for the laboratory to check the clerical records, to make absolutely sure that the blood the patient received was indeed the blood intended for that patient. Most of the time, this check will tell the story. The second, and equally important, step is to check a freshly collected blood sample, taken from the patient at the time the reaction is reported. Care is necessary in the collection, so as not to cause mechanical hemolysis. The sample is spun, and the supernatant examined for a pink color. In the absence of excessive bilirubin or other abnormal pigments, hemoglobin becomes visible as a pink tinge in the plasma at levels of 20 to 25 mg/dl. A carefully collected specimen of normal plasma or serum should not have more than 2 or 3 mg of hemoglobin/dl. Visual comparison of the pretransfusion and posttransfusion serums may at once reveal a telltale difference in color.

Although one could argue that repeat ABO and Rh typing and a direct antiglobulin test are superfluous in allergic and most febrile reactions, these tests are routine in many blood banks. In more significant reactions, such procedures at an early stage may reveal incompatible red cells that will have been completely removed from the circulation within a few hours. Any evidence of incompatibility or hemolysis at this time must be communicated at once to the patient's physician and to the blood bank physician, since the information may be essential for proper treatment. Serum from the specimen taken at this time may also be used for other laboratory procedures that might be indicated if there should be evidence of an incompatible transfusion. In case of completely negative findings, and lacking real clinical suspicion of incompatibility, it may be possible to restart a unit that was not completely transfused.

Definitive Investigation

If there is evidence of hemolysis, incompatibility, or a serious reaction, further investigation is carried out on the patient's blood collected at the time of the reaction, the donor pilot sample, the blood remaining in the container, if available, and the patient's pretransfusion blood sample. In addition to ABO and Rh typing and the direct antiglobulin test, this may include crossmatching and a repeated antibody screening test. A minor crossmatch may be included if the circumstances warrant it. Microscopic observation should be part of the testing, so as to detect possible mixed cell populations. Any discrepancies with the results previously reported must normally be resolved before further transfusions involving red cells are undertaken. An exception is made in clinically urgent situations, in which crossmatch-compatible blood may be given under careful observation.

A full investigation and scrutiny of all laboratory work records are essential, and the technologists who did the work must be questioned in detail at the earliest moment. If an error is discovered, *no alterations may be made in the work records*. Notes may be added, but they must be clearly dated and identified as additions. It is worth emphasizing that even the best laboratory procedures may fail to detect serologic incompatibility. Some blood group antibodies, particularly some of the less-common Rh antibodies and those of the Kidd system, may be so weak as to be undetectable in the pretransfusion crossmatch or may require special techniques for their detection (see Chap. 5). Despite in vitro weakness, certain of these can cause serious immediate or delayed transfusion reactions. Therefore, failure to find an antibody in preliminary investigation of apparent hemolysis calls for further testing by the most sensitive methods with suitable test cells, comparing the pretransfusion sample with samples taken at the time of the reaction and even continuing with additional samples over the ensuing 2 or more weeks. Consultation with a specialized laboratory may be advisable, if for no other reason than to provide impartial confirmation or to assist in the interpretation of complicated findings.

The procedures outlined above are intended to provide clinical or laboratory evidence of hemolysis or incompatibility, and are indicated only when the immediate investigation suggests hemolysis, or when there is significant clinical suspicion of it. To do so much testing in the absence of such evidence would introduce unnecessary extra work and costs not based on clinical reality. It is also important to keep in mind that not all hemolysis is caused by incompatibility, as discussed earlier in this chapter.

See Table 7–3 for an outline of recommended procedures in the investigation of suspected incompatibility.

Records

A full and scrupulously detailed record must be kept of all phases of the investigation; it should remain on file as long as legally necessary. All these records should be reviewed by the blood bank physician. The conclusions should be reported to the physicians and noted in the patient's medical record. In the United States, fatal reactions must be reported to the FDA immediately. Any serious reaction, particularly if litigation seems likely, should also be reported

Table 7–3. Schedule of Investigation of Reported Transfusion Reactions

A. All reported reactions
   1. Specimens needed
      a. Pretransfusion blood of recipient
      b. Posttransfusion blood of recipient
   2. Investigation (letters refer to specimens listed above)
      Check donor and patient identification and crossmatch report
      Repeat ABO and Rh typing (b, and donor bag, if indicated)
      Direct antiglobulin test (b, if indicated)
      Examine for visible hemolysis (b); if necessary, compare (b) with (a)
   If these procedures reveal no evidence of incompatibility or hemolysis, and there is no additional information to arouse suspicion, no further investigation is needed. Otherwise, proceed as follows:
B. If there is evidence of hemolysis or incompatible transfusion*
   1. Specimens needed
      a. Pretransfusion blood of recipient
      b. Posttransfusion blood of recipient
      c. Pilot samples of donor blood
      d. Blood from container implicated in reaction (if available)
      e. Posttransfusion urine
   2. Immunologic investigation
      Repeat ABO, Rh, and direct antiglobulin test (a, c, d)
      Repeat crossmatch (a, b, c; d, if indicated) (major; minor only if indicated)
      Repeat antibody screen (a, b, c) (special, sensitive techniques if necessary)
      Identification of any unexpected antibody or incompatibility
   3. Other procedures as indicated
      Serum haptoglobin (a, b)
      Bacteriologic smear and culture (d)
      Serum urea and bilirubin (a, b)
      Urine hemoglobin (e)
      Urine hemosiderin (e)
   4. Investigation of nonimmune causes of hemolysis (see pp. 256–257)

*The procedures and specimens listed are generally applicable. Different approaches may be needed for particular cases.

to the appropriate authorities in the hospital. The blood bank staff, especially physicians, should notify their own insurance carriers if these are different from the ones used by the hospital.

Disease Transmission

Viral Hepatitis

Transmission of hepatitis by blood or plasma is one of the most serious complications of blood transfusion and constitutes a risk to the life and health of blood recipients as well as a legal hazard to physicians. There are at least four major types of viral hepatitis:

1. *Infectious, or type A, hepatitis,* caused by hepatitis A virus (HAV)
2. *Serum, or type B, hepatitis,* caused by hepatitis B virus (HBV)
3. *Delta hepatitis,* caused by hepatitis delta virus (HDV) *plus* HBV
4. *Non-A, non-B hepatitis,* which is probably more than one disease.

The clinical form of posttransfusion hepatitis (PTH) varies from severe, fatal liver necrosis to very mild or clinically silent disturbance of liver function, detectable only by sensitive laboratory procedures (subclinical or anicteric hepatitis, or *"transaminitis"*). The more severe forms are associated with HBV; and non-A, non-B form generally produces a milder disease, but one more likely to lead to a lingering chronic active hepatitis or cirrhosis. Very little posttransfusion hepatitis in adults is caused by HAV [38], although sporadic outbreaks have occurred in intensive care nurseries [39].

Present overall mortality from icteric hepatitis B (not just transfusional) is estimated at about 1 to 3 percent [40]. Mortality from transfusion-associated hepatitis a few years ago was found to range from zero (below 20 years of age) to about 12 percent (over 60) [41]. Regardless of mortality, posttransfusion hepatitis is a serious, crippling illness, leading to heavy hospitalization costs, social and economic losses, and human suffering. Table 7–4 compares three major types of viral hepatitis.

Hepatitis delta virus is a defective RNA virus with a capsule of HBsAg. It cannot replicate without the presence of HBV [42, 43]. Infection with HDV is generally more severe than with HBV alone. Pockets of HDV infection have occurred in various parts of the world, including the United States, and an asymptomatic carrier state apparently exists. With respect to PTH from delta virus, screening for HBsAg provides a high degree of safety, though not absolute. One hazard is to existing carriers of HBV: if they are exposed to HDV they are at risk of fulminant hepatitis. It has been recommended that blood products for transfusion to such carriers be screened for high ALT levels, and any derivatives be prepared from single donors or small pools [43].

Abbreviations commonly used for hepatitis and its various markers are as follows:

Anti-HAV: Antibody to hepatitis A virus
Anti-HBc: Antibody to hepatitis B core antigen
Anti-HBe: Antibody to hepatitis B e antigen
Anti-HBs: Antibody to hepatitis B surface antigen
Anti-HDV: Antibody to hepatitis delta virus
HAV: Hepatitis A virus
HBcAg: Hepatitis B core antigen
HBeAg: Hepatitis B e antigen
HBsAg: Hepatitis B surface antigen
HBV: Hepatitis B virus
HDV: Hepatitis delta virus
NANB: Non-A, non-B

Table 7-4. Characteristics of Three Types of Viral Hepatitis*

	Type A	Type B	Type Non-A, Non-B
Nucleic acid	RNA (single stranded)	DNA (double stranded)	Unknown
Class	Enterovirus	Hepadna	Unknown
Incubation period (days)	15–45	45–150	20–70
Mode(s) of transmission	Fecal-oral	Percutaneous Oral-oral Venereal Perinatal	Percutaneous Perinatal Fecal-oral
Transfusion-related hepatitis (%)	0	5–10	90–95
Sporadic hepatitis (%)	30	50	20
Progress to chronic hepatitis (%)	0	About 10	10–40
Asymptomatic carrier state	No	Yes	Yes
Chronic liver disease (%)	0	50	50
Associated with hepatocellular carcinoma	No	Yes	Unknown
Preexposure prophylaxis			
Active	None available	Vaccine	None available
Passive	ISG	HBIG	ISG

ISG = immune serum globulin; HBIG = hepatitis B immune globulin
*Slightly modified from Vyas and Blum [43]. With permission.

Incidence

Data reporting the incidence of PTH are most accurate and complete when based on an active, preferably prospective follow-up of all patients who receive transfusions. Otherwise, a large number of cases will be misdiagnosed or unreported. Some comparisons of hepatitis frequency before and after the institution of testing for HBsAg can be found in a 1978 review [45].

In prospective studies of transfused patients that were designed to detect anicteric and asymptomatic, as well as icteric, forms of hepatitis, attack rates ranged from 5 percent of transfused patients to 35 percent or even more. The reasons for this variability are not always clear, but it appears to be strongly related to the source of the transfused blood [46, 47]: patients receiving blood only from commercial paid donors had a hepatitis incidence nearly six times that of patients receiving all their blood from volunteer donors [40]. It also appears that the socioeconomic status of patients and donors may play a role [48, 49] (obviously, it is not the transfer of money that makes a blood donation infective). In the past, it appeared that some detectable evidence of hepatitis occurred in about 8 to 10 percent of transfused patients [43], although this may have changed with the current donor screening relating to AIDS and the addition of testing for anti-HIV, ALT, and possibly anti-HBc (see pp. 272–274).

When consideration is limited to reported icteric hepatitis, the incidence will seem much lower. Goldfield and his associates took this more pragmatic approach [41], and analyzed the PTH incidence for the state of New Jersey. For the 10 years 1967 through 1976, they found that the clinical hepatitis incidence in transfused patients declined steadily from 0.5 percent in 1967 to 0.14 percent in 1976, during which time the proportion of commercial blood used fell from 33 to 0.1 percent. Of course, the same period also saw the institution of required testing for HBsAg, but since this affects primarily the transmission of hepatitis B, the likelihood is that the reduction in hepatitis was largely due to the elimination of commercial blood donations. However, commercial paid donors are not the only ones implicated in a high infectivity rate. One source of voluntary donors (an institution for military recruits) was associated with a sixfold increase in hepatitis transmission. Goldfield also observed that 40 percent of PTH occurred in patients who had received only one or two units of blood.

Transmission

Although minute amounts of serum from an infected person may transmit hepatitis, the likelihood that a recipient will contract the disease appears to be greater in proportion to the number of units of blood or plasma received.

Much is still unknown about the transmission of hepatitis. A carrier state exists, in which some apparently healthy people are able to transmit the disease, and the carrier condition may persist for years [40, 43, 47]. Since blood donors implicated in hepatitis transmission have usually never knowingly had hepatitis, the carrier state must be associated with subclinical, as well as overt, hepatitis. Perhaps 10 percent of those who get hepatitis B and more than a third of those who contract NANB hepatitis become carriers [43, 47, 48].

The chronic carrier of HBV who has no obvious disease and is not immunosuppressed probably transmits the disease only through blood donation, or by some other means based on exchange of less-obvious amounts of blood or plasma (e.g., shared needles in drug abuse). Those who are immunosuppressed (such as renal dialysis patients) or who have subclinical or chronic active hepatitis may be more infectious and can probably transmit the virus by various body secretions and mucous membrane contact [48].

Hepatitis Antigens and Antibodies

HBV is a 42-nm sphere (also called a *Dane particle*) with a shell 7-nm thick, containing the surface antigen (HBsAg). This particle also has a complex core, which includes the core antigen (HBcAg) as well as "e" (HBeAg) [50], a DNA polymerase, and a ring of DNA that is about 70 percent double stranded and 30 percent single stranded [40, 43]. The corresponding antibodies are anti-HBs,

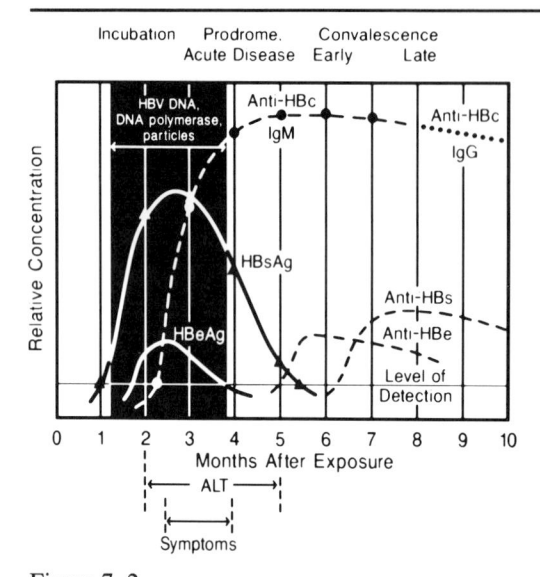

Figure 7-2
Clinical and serologic changes in a case of acute hepatitis B after exposure to infection. (Modified slightly and redrawn from F. Blaine Hollinger, Serologic evaluation of viral hepatitis. *Hospital Practice* 1987; 22:101–14. With permission.)

anti-HBc, and anti-HBe. When HBeAg is present along with HBsAg, the blood is more than 30,000 times as infectious [43]. HBeAg probably reflects active viral replication.

The surface antigen usually appears during an attack of hepatitis B. In the normal course of events, this disappears from the serum on recovery, after which anti-HBs and anti-HBc appear [43]. Anti-HBs does not indicate infectivity for HBV; in fact, its appearance may mark resolution of the carrier state, since persistence of HBsAg usually goes along with that (Fig. 7–2). IgM anti-HBc usually indicates a recent HBV infection.

Hepatitis Testing
The clear association of HBsAg with PTH led to the requirement for regular testing for this antigen in every blood donation (see Chap. 4). Obviously, there is no absolute measure of infectivity of donor blood, since virus dose and recipient susceptibility are also involved, but retrospective testing of blood that had already been given showed the high correlation between the presence of HBsAg in donor blood and the occurrence of hepatitis in a recipient. This was initially evident with comparatively insensitive test procedures (agar gel diffusion and counterelectrophoresis). With more sensitive procedures, more potentially infective bloods are detected and more cases of hepatitis prevented.

Federal regulations require that all donor blood be tested for HBsAg by radioimmunoassay (RIA) or some other test method of equivalent sensitivity, e.g., ELISA. Still more sensitive procedures for detecting HBsAg would probably reach a point of diminishing returns, with greater test complexity and expense, and the likelihood of more false-positives and consequent donor loss. Testing at the current level of sensitivity certainly reduces the incidence of hepatitis B, but does not eliminate it.

Additional Hepatitis Testing

Posttransfusion hepatitis A is rare, and type B has been significantly reduced by testing for HBsAg. About 90 to 95 percent of PTH is now NANB type, and the seriousness of this problem is indicated by the fact that as many as 40 percent of the patients afflicted develop chronic disease. The figures on NANB hepatitis incidence vary in different geographic locations, and also according to whether or not hepatitis associated with cytomegalovirus is included in the NANB category. The diagnosis of an NANB PTH is difficult: it requires the exclusion of other known viruses, of routes of exposure other than transfusion, of hepatotoxic medications, and of other liver diseases.

ALANINE AMINOTRANSFERASE. Thirty or so years ago, it was noted that some donors associated with PTH had elevated serum transaminase levels. The advent of testing for specific hepatitis markers discouraged the use of nonspecific tests, such as ALT (formerly known as serum glutamic pyruvic transaminase, SGPT). However, interest in ALT screening has revived in recent years for several reasons: first, increasing consciousness of the prevalence of NANB hepatitis; second, realization of the serious long-term effects of NANB infection; and, third, an increasing public unwillingness to accept any preventable risk, no matter what the cost of prevention. Recent work showed an association between elevated donor ALT levels and NANB PTH, and predicted a reduction of about 30 percent in this disease by the elimination of donor blood with increased ALT [51, 52]. This reduction has not yet been confirmed in practice [53]. Moreover, the relationship between ALT levels and PTH is loose: 70 percent of PTH is not prevented by such screening, and about 70 percent of donors with elevated ALT were not associated with PTH.

In addition to the 70 percent false-negatives and 70 percent false-positives mentioned above, the test result is susceptible to many physiologic and pathologic variables of such nature that 80 percent of donors with elevated results will have normal results on a subsequent test [54]. This makes it difficult to give a donor a valid explanation for an elevated ALT level. Finally, there will probably be a loss of 1 to 3 percent of donor units.

ANTI-HBC. A relationship also exists between antibody to the core proteins of HBV in the donor and the development of some forms of NANB hepatitis in the recipient [55]. Although no controlled clinical trial has been carried out, it has been estimated that testing for this marker in donor blood could effect a 43 percent reduction in NANB PTH [56]. In both series, not all donors with anti-HBc also had elevated ALT levels, so the two markers behave as independent variables. It is worth mentioning that the latter study [56], and some of the other analyses relating hepatitis to the occurrence of laboratory abnormalities in donors [55], are based on prospective studies that were done before the initiation of voluntary self-exclusion of certain donor groups in connection with AIDS, the same donor groups that are a hazard with respect to hepatitis transmission.

Prevention of Hepatitis

Increased concern over transfusion-transmitted diseases in general, and about the chronic consequences of NANB PTH in particular, have aroused renewed interest in surrogate tests that might reduce the incidence of this complication. Despite the cost, the nonoverlap of the anti-HBc and high-ALT groups, and the other concerns mentioned above in connection with ALT testing, the FDA Blood Products Advisory Committee, in February, 1986, recommended that both ALT and anti-HBc procedures be applied to donor blood [57]. This recommendation has been widely adopted.

Prevention of Hepatitis: Further Steps

In our opinion, the most effective, and most neglected, measure of prevention is the avoidance of transfusions that are not absolutely essential. A sizeable proportion of today's transfusions would probably be better not given, on the basis of known hazards contrasted with dubious or borderline clinical benefit. However, even the best efforts of blood bankers have been unable to convince some of our clinical colleagues of this truism.

Surveillance of PTH must continue, and any donor group that is found to produce a high rate of infectivity should be excluded. The formerly prevalent commercial blood banks have been by now almost completely eliminated as a source of regular blood components, although, in the form of plasmapheresis stations, they continue to supply plasma for fractionation. Male homosexuals have been shown to have a high hepatitis rate, and are presently requested to exclude themselves voluntarily because of the likelihood of the AIDS carrier state as well (see Chap. 1). The effectiveness of such self-exclusion is good, but not complete. Because of the high incidence of hepatitis among hemodialysis patients, most blood banks exclude the staff of dialysis units as blood donors.

Hepatitis can be transmitted by any blood component that contains even traces of plasma, including washed or frozen-thawed red blood cells [58, 59]. The virus also survives the manufacturing processes used in the preparation of antihemophilic factor and factor IX concentrates. It is not transmitted by properly manufactured albumin or plasma protein fraction. Non-A, non-B hepatitis transmission has been associated with some lots of intravenous immune serum globulin [60].

Hepatitis B immune globulin is effective in reducing the incidence of HBV infection after exposure in some clinical settings, including that of accidental needlestick exposure to potentially infective blood [61]. For those likely to incur repeated exposures, such as laboratory workers, hepatitis B vaccine will provide a more lasting protection.

The avoidance of unnecessary transfusions and the exclusion of donor groups known to have an increased incidence of hepatitis infectivity will both help reduce the incidence of NANB PTH. The adoption of ALT and anti-HBc screening may also be useful, but that remains to be seen.

CYTOMEGALOVIRUS

Cytomegalovirus, which is widely distributed in the population, can be transmitted by transfusion. Recipients who become infected this way may show only a rise in the titer of antibody, or a syndrome clinically resembling infectious mononucleosis, or a mild form of hepatitis [62]. This occurs 2 to 7 weeks after transfusion, and was described originally as a "postperfusion syndrome" in patients who had undergone open-heart surgery. It may also be classified as a form of posttransfusion hepatitis. In cardiovascular surgery, some 20 to 30 percent of blood recipients develop clinically unapparent CMV infection and form antibody to CMV [63]. Seroconversion is proportional to the volume of blood transfused, and seems to be unrelated to whether the blood was fresh or stored. Attempts to isolate the virus from the leukocyte fraction of donor blood have usually been unsuccessful [63, 64].

CMV infection seems to be relatively innocuous in immunocompetent patients, although the virus itself has some immunodepressive effect. But it may cause significant, even fatal, illness in immunocompromised patients, especially transplant recipients and premature newborns. In such patients, transfused blood products are by no means the only possible source of CMV; indeed, many of the infections probably occur through reactivation of virus already possessed by the patient or acquired in transplanted organs. The main population at risk appears to be those who do not have anti-CMV, although reactivation of latent virus, or reinfection with another strain, may occur in seropositive patients. When such patients receive seronegative blood products, or transplanted organs from seronegative donors, the risk is minimal. It appears also that frozen-thawed red blood cells [65] and, presumably, other leukocyte-depleted blood products are equally safe.

Particular concern attaches to premature newborns, especially those below 1,250 gm birth weight, since CMV is sometimes fatal in this group [66]. We recommend the use of seronegative blood transfusions in this situation if the babies are seronegative, and probably also in seropositive infants who require multiple transfusions [63]. Seronegative pregnant women that need transfusions, including intrauterine, should probably also receive blood from seronegative donors. CMV is, however, ubiquitous, and the premature newborn is potentially exposed to many environmental sources of the virus. Appropriately selected blood products should thus be only part of a comprehensive program of infection control, as for all immunocompromised patients.

ACQUIRED IMMUNODEFICIENCY SYNDROME

AIDS is associated with everything needed to gain wide public attention: sex, blood, illicit drugs, and untimely death. The initial observations were in young homosexual men and intravenous drug abusers, leading some to proclaim the disease an instrument of divine retribution. Its association with blood transfusion was tentative and inferential at first, largely based on a few cases not belonging to any known risk group and having a history of transfusions [67–70]. A further clue was the occurrence of AIDS in hemophiliacs being treated by antihemophilic factor concentrate. The relationship is no longer in question.

The infective agent responsible for AIDS is a retrovirus, the human immunodeficiency virus (HIV, now the preferred term). It has also been known as human T-cell lymphotropic virus type III (HTLV III), or lymphadenopathy-associated virus (LAV), or AIDS-related virus (ARV).

Incidence

As of August 1985, 194 cases of transfusion-associated AIDS (TAA) had been reported to the U.S. Centers for Disease Control [70]. In 47 of these cases, at least one of the donors belonged to a high-risk group (five patients received blood from more than one high-risk donor). Two donors were implicated in two cases of TAA each. In a few cases, donor-recipient pairs have each developed AIDS after the transfusion. One patient had no high-risk donor identified, and the investigation of the remaining ones is incomplete. (See Addenda.) Bearing in mind that about 5 million patients receive transfusions annually in the United States, the incidence is obviously low. It cannot be calculated accurately because the time over which the cases of TAA have been acquired is uncertain, and the exact number of patients transfused per year is not known. Furthermore, the incubation period of the disease is long (a mean of about 31 months from transfusion to diagnosed disease in adults, 21 months in children) [70].

Recipients at highest risk seem to be hemophiliacs, with a frequency of about one case of overt AIDS per 300 patients [69], and a higher incidence of cases with lymphadenopathy or immunologic abnormalities such as a decreased ratio of T4 to T8 lymphocytes [71]. The latter observation is commonly associated with AIDS or AIDS-like syndromes (e.g., AIDS-related complex), but its exact significance in hemophiliacs is uncertain.

It appears that infants are more susceptible to TAA than adults, and have a shorter incubation time for the disease. The first reported transfusional case was in an infant [67], and infants make up about 10 percent of TAA, although they receive only about 2 percent of transfusions. The reasons for this disproportion are unknown, but the receipt of multiple small transfusions to make up for iatrogenic blood losses may have something to do with it, as may the relative immaturity of infants' immune systems.

Transmission

It became apparent early that AIDS is an infectious disease, probably caused by a virus. From the observations in hemophiliacs, it appeared that the agent was being transmitted in antihemophilic factor concentrate, and soon afterwards, cases began appearing in connection with other blood components. Since even those donors who later came down with AIDS had been in apparently good health at the time of the blood donations that infected a recipient, there is obviously a prodromal infectious stage during which virus can be transmitted, and probably a chronic carrier state as well.

The AIDS virus is a singularly fragile retrovirus, surviving poorly outside the body and easily killed by environmental exposure and simple disinfection. It is present in many body fluids, particularly blood and semen. Transmission, therefore, requires close and intimate contact with exchange of body fluids, as in sexual intercourse and the sharing of needles in illicit intravenous drug use. A further possibility exists that one or more cofactors may be required for the development of disease. The likelihood of infection of casual contacts, even within a household or in a medical care environment, is very low, in sharp contrast to hepatitis. The presence of antibody does not indicate immunity, but may in fact herald infectivity.

Prevention

For reasons given at the outset of this section, AIDS has attracted a great deal of public attention. Widespread publicity attended the first transfusion-associated case, and blood banks were subjected to extraordinary pressure to "do something" at a stage when facts were too few to permit rational, scientific judgment. We have described earlier the process by which the existing screening and testing system (summarized in Table 7–5) was reached [72].

GENERAL METHODS. AIDS transmission is more likely in blood donations from certain high-risk groups, specifically the following: homosexual or bisexual men; intravenous drug abusers; people with AIDS, AIDS-related complex, or a positive test for anti-HIV; hemophiliacs (who are not likely to be blood donors themselves); and the sexual partners of any of the foregoing. On the basis of recommendations of the FDA supported by the American Association of Blood Banks, the Red Cross, and the Council of Community Blood Centers, since 1983, all such persons have been asked to exclude themselves voluntarily from blood donation. *Homosexual* or *bisexual men* are defined as those who have had any sexual contact with another man since 1977. The FDA also advises the

Table 7–5. Current Steps in the Prevention of Transfusion-Associated AIDS

1. General public information programs
    Nature of AIDS
    Infectivity in relation to behavioral patterns
    Groups and behaviors at risk
    Activities and contacts that are not at risk
2. Information for blood donors
    Blood donation not a risk to donor
    Predonation information as to risk activities
    Opportunity for confidential self-exclusion
    Opportunity to designate blood donation "not for transfusion"
3. Predonation health evaluation
    Questions referable to signs and symptoms of AIDS or related conditions
    Examination of veins for needle tracks
4. Testing, specific
    Anti-HIV
5. Testing, surrogate
    Hepatitis markers (HBsAg, anti-HBc)
    Other

exclusion of entrants since 1977 from localities in which heterosexual spread of AIDS is common (such as central Africa and Haiti), and (as of November, 1986) also male or female prostitutes and those who have consorted with prostitutes.

Self-exclusion is accomplished in two ways. The first is partly a function of campaigns to educate the public as to who ought not to donate, and partly the result of the widespread publicity that has surrounded TAA from the beginning. The second method is by the provision of information about AIDS to would-be donors at the time they present themselves for donation. This is usually in the form of a leaflet or brochure (Fig. 1–4, Chap. 1, is one example). Generally, the donor must certify in some way, preferably in writing, that he or she has read and understood the information and is eligible to donate blood. To avoid embarrassment to those who should disqualify themselves and to promote truthfulness, the setting must be such that donors can do this in confidentiality without attracting attention. A further opportunity for self-exclusion can be provided by a postdonation questionnaire or telephone access, whereby the donor can indicate whether or not the blood should be used for transfusion, identifying it only by donation number.

How effective has self-exclusion been? Based partly on the concept that those considering blood donation are, for the most part, responsible citizens, and perhaps partly on wishful thinking, most blood bankers had the impression that the system was working well [73]. However, the introduction of testing for anti-HIV in 1985 brought about a change, in that it provided a motive for worried members of the high-risk groups to donate blood in order to get the results of the antibody test. This did indeed happen, despite the efforts of public health authorities and blood banks to prevent it by education and the establishment of alternative test sites [74]. Also, of the first 41 antibody-positive Red Cross donors who were contacted and interviewed, 36 turned out to be members of high-risk groups, 30 of them homosexual or bisexual men [75]. These donors had not excluded themselves because they did not originally view themselves as members of defined risk groups. Despite these worrisome observations, and the feelings of some that donor questioning should ask point-blank about sexual preference [76], most authorities believe that the self-exclusion procedure is already direct enough and that it makes a useful contribution to the safety of blood recipients.

The donor's medical history questionnaire provides another general method of screening out donors who might have symptoms of AIDS or its prodromal stages. Appropriate questions must be included (see Fig. 1–3, Chap. 1).

Other approaches to donor selection have been proposed. The first is the selection by a patient of friends or relatives as blood donors, i.e., "directed donations" (see Chap. 1). While there is no doubt that this makes the patient feel better about receiving transfusions, there is no evidence whatever that directed donations make any contribution to patient safety, nor is there any logical reason why they should do so. Despite some feelings to the contrary, there is also no evidence that directed donations carry any additional risk. Another approach is to limit blood donation to women, which would doubtless cause a severe reduction in the available blood supply. A third proposal, by a California women's organization to the American Blood Commission, is to require labeling of all blood donations as male or female [77].

Autologous donation and transfusion, to the extent that it prevents exposure to homologous blood, obviously reduces all transfusion risks, including that of TAA. The use of autologous blood has increased with the AIDS scare, but not to the extent that might have been expected. The use of this system should be encouraged.

TESTING OF DONOR BLOOD. When TAA first began to appear, there were suggestions that donor blood be tested for various surrogate markers. Some blood banks implemented such procedures as helper-suppressor T lymphocyte ratio or anti-HBc testing. Other candidate tests included circulating immune complexes, thymosin alpha-1, beta-2-microglobulin, and acid-labile alpha interferon [69, 72]. Most authorities felt that such procedures would be costly and ineffective, that they were poorly standardized and difficult to adapt to blood bank use, and that they would eliminate too many donors, thereby endangering the nation's blood supply. The consensus was to await a more specific test. When the test for anti-HIV was made available in the spring of 1985, it was adopted almost immediately by the vast majority of blood banks, although it is not yet a federally-required procedure.

The initial results of testing for anti-HIV indicate that about 0.17 percent of donors are repeatably positive by the basic ELISA procedure [75]. Of those, some 23 percent were confirmed by the more specific Western blot test. In that Red Cross series, all donors had been given the opportunity for self-exclusion, and the overall prevalence of confirmed positivity was 38 per 100,000 donations [75]. Rates of positivity vary in different parts of the country.

The elimination of HIV-seropositive blood units will undoubtedly reduce the incidence of TAA, although that will take a few years to demonstrate. We do not really know the significance of anti-HIV in persons not belonging to a high-risk group. False-positives do occur (e.g., some tests give positive reactions in persons with anti-HLA DR4), and false-negatives have been seen as well—possibly in the early stages after exposure to the virus and before seroconversion [78, 79]. (See Addenda.)

Certainly, we have inadequate understanding of the test and its implications to explain the significance of results to seropositive donors. There is little doubt that this will cause distress and that it will have some effect on blood donations. Already some 34 percent or so of the general public irrationally fear that they might contract AIDS from *donating* blood [80]. (See Addenda.) Moreover, we have already seen that some people in high-risk groups have donated blood to obtain test results [74]; it is also possible, or even probable, that others will refrain from donating either because they do not want the test results or because they lack faith that confidentiality of records will be maintained.

Obviously, a great deal more research is needed on AIDS and its relationship to blood transfusion, and continued observation will have to be maintained on the results of serologic testing and its effects on the blood supply and on blood donors. The likelihood is that TAA will continue to increase before a mitigating effect of serologic testing can be seen. Table 7-5 lists the current steps in the prevention of TAA.

Investigating Former Recipients: The "Look-Back"

Definitive testing of donors for anti-HIV began only in March, 1985, and detected as positives some who had donated blood previously. Because of concern that some of the earlier recipients may have received infectious blood, and might themselves have, in effect, become AIDS carriers, the major blood banking organizations (American Red Cross, American Association of Blood Banks, Council of Community Blood Centers) decided to launch a program to locate such recipients for testing and counseling. This is called the *look-back* procedure, and has now been carried out on a national scale. The details vary, but in general, the donations from each donor found to be seropositive are being traced back in time until two consecutive seronegative recipients are found, or until 1977. Because of the importance of the procedure to public health, every effort is made to persuade recipients to be tested, but obviously they cannot be compelled to do so, and some have refused.

Preliminary results as of November, 1986, indicate that about 60 percent of the transfusion recipients will have died in the interim. Of the remainder, about half have seroconverted and a few have clinical AIDS [81]. Seroconversion is less likely for transfusions received in the late 1970s or early 1980s than in the later years before testing was instituted. (See Addenda.)

Malaria

Since the plasmodia that cause malaria reside in the carriers' red cells and may sometimes be found in those cells years after infection, transmission of this disease by transfusion of blood or red cell–containing components is always a possibility. In the United States, malaria is rare, however, and the likelihood of transfusional malaria is likewise scant [82]. Despite increased travel and population shifts such as the post-Vietnam war emigration, only a few cases of malaria per year are associated with transfusion. It is, however, a dangerous disease, the more so because it is unexpected and easily misdiagnosed in this country. When properly applied, the present standards of donor selection (see Chap. 1) are adequate to safeguard the vast majority of patients, and the low frequency of the disease does not justify additional laboratory procedures.

Syphilis

Transmission of syphilis by transfusion is rare because the treponemas do not survive storage at refrigerator temperatures for more than 4 or 5 days. Refrigerated storage of blood and components therefore controls this hazard. However, the remaining potential risk with the use of fresh or unrefrigerated blood components such as platelets [83, 84] does not seem to have resulted in any increase in transfusional syphilis, of which few present-day transfusionists have ever seen a case.

Serologic testing for syphilis in donor blood is still required by the FDA, although not by AABB standards. Such tests detect an occasional unsuspected case of syphilis in a donor, but do not protect against transfusion transmission, which would occur only from donors in an early, spirochetemic phase of the disease, before seroconversion. Continuation of serologic testing is clearly not justified on the basis of its efficacy in preventing syphilis, or for case finding, since almost all the seropositives turn out to be biologic false-positives, thus a source of embarrassment to donors and a nuisance to blood banks. Moreover, it causes a loss of substantial numbers of blood units. The transfusion of seropositive blood components can make a recipient temporarily seropositive, but no harm has been shown from this. In the present climate of opinion regarding transfusion safety, we are pessimistic about the likelihood that the serologic test for syphilis will soon be abandoned.

Other Diseases

Babesiosis is a malaria-like disease caused by a protozoan microorganism, *Babesia microti* or *B. bovis,* that normally parasitizes domestic or wild animals [85]. The vector is a hard tick, usually of the genus *Ixodes*. The few human cases are caused by the bite of an infected tick and are most often seen in the northeastern United States during summer, particularly in the area around Long Island Sound. As with malaria, occasional transfusion-associated cases of babesiosis are seen, rarely severe [86]. There is no practical screening test for donor blood, and it is common practice to defer donors from endemic areas, at least during the summer season.

On rare occasions, *brucellosis* has been reported to be transmitted to a patient by donor blood, and in South America this has also been the case with the trypanosomes of *Chagas' disease*. Theoretically, of course, any disease characterized by the presence of any sort of microorganism in the blood could be transmitted by transfusion, but in fact, the persons so afflicted would rarely feel well enough to donate blood. The exceptions are the various carrier conditions, the most important of which have already been discussed. (See Addenda.)

Hemosiderosis

The human body is remarkably efficient at conserving iron and loses only about 1 mg per day. Therefore, the transfusion of large amounts of blood to persons who are not chronically bleeding provides a plentiful source of exogenous iron. This accumulates in the tissues and can cause transfusional hemosiderosis. The average unit of blood contains about 250 mg of iron. Since excessive iron may cause dysfunction of many organs and tissues, it constitutes a danger to those who must have large numbers of transfusions over a long period of time (such as patients with hypoplastic anemia or thalassemia). Although iron chelation therapy is possible [87], there is little opportunity in the blood bank of preventing iron overload other than keeping transfusions to as few as possible and using relatively fresh red blood cells (less than a week in storage) for such patients, to minimize premature red cell breakdown and thus decrease the frequency of transfusions.

Another method is the selective transfusion of young red cells, that is, predominantly reticulocytes, so-called neocytes [88] (see Chap. 6).

Table 7–6 summarizes the various diseases that may be transmitted by blood transfusion.

Blood Group Immunization

Persons vary greatly in the ability to make antibodies on exposure to foreign blood group antigens. In general, recipients make antibodies only to antigens they do not possess themselves. The likelihood of immunization depends on (1) the immunogenicity of the antigen concerned, (2) its frequency, (3) the recipient's capability for antibody formation, and (4) other unknown considerations.

Immunogenicity

Certainly, some blood group antigens are much more capable than others of inducing antibody formation. Judging from the regularity with which injection

Handwritten annotations: CJ Disease; B19 Parvovirus; HTLVI; Lyme Disease; Yersinia

Table 7–6. Diseases Transmissible by Transfusion

Disease	Cause	Screening or Prevention
Viral		
Hepatitis	HAV, HBV, NANB, HDV	HBsAg, ALT, (anti-HBc) Risk-group exclusion
Cytomegalovirus infection	CMV	Anti-CMV
AIDS	HIV	Anti-HIV Risk-group exclusion
Treponemal		
Syphilis	*Treponema pallidum*	Serologic test
Protozoan		
Malaria	*Plasmodium* sp.	Geographic and exposural exclusion
Chagas' disease	*Trypanosoma cruzi*	Serologic test (endemic areas)
Babesiosis	*Babesia microti* and ticks	Geographic and seasonal exclusion
Bacterial		
Sepsis	Cryophilic bacteria	Asepsis, refrigeration
Brucellosis	*Brucella* sp.	Exclusion on history
Other		
Graft-v-host disease	Lymphocytes	Irradiation of components
Hemosiderosis	Exogenous iron	Minimize number of transfusions Neocytes

of ABO-incompatible blood raises the titer of anti-A or anti-B and changes the form of the antibody toward the incomplete or hemolytic variety, A and B are highly immunogenic. Transfusion of one unit of Rh-positive blood to an Rh-negative recipient causes formation of anti-D in about 80 percent of cases; thus D is also highly immunogenic [89]. All other common blood factors are of appreciably lower immunogenicity than A, B, and D. The Lewis, M, N, and P antigens appear to have a low immunogenicity, in that antibodies related to these systems do not, as a rule, result from obvious exogenous stimulation.

FREQUENCY

The development of blood group antibodies depends on not only the immunogenicity of the antigen but also the likelihood of exposure to the antigen. D antigen is important not only because of its potency but also because 15 percent of white persons lack it, and they would have an 85 percent chance of receiving Rh-positive blood in any transfusion if this factor were not regularly considered in blood selection. On the other hand, about 90 percent of persons are K (Kell)-negative, and they would have only about a 10 percent chance of exposure to K on a random basis. Other factors may also have a high degree of immunogenicity but seldom cause antibody formation because of their even lower incidence. Among the high-incidence antigens, Vel appears to be definitely immunogenic, but Vel-negative persons are very rare. The importance of the various blood group systems with regard to antibody formation is discussed in Chapter 3. Ethnic variations in antigenic frequency have little effect on transfusion hazards [90].

INDIVIDUAL CAPACITY FOR ANTIBODY FORMATION

Those who regularly study cases of blood group immunization are impressed with the unpredictability of antibody responses. Obviously, red cells have many antigens, and any person who lacks one of them may, under appropriate circumstances, make an antibody to it. But given equal opportunity for immunization, why does a person produce an antibody to one antigen and not to another carried on the same red cells? In some cases, antibodies develop to an antigen considered to have low immunogenicity, such as Jk^a, but not to a more immunogenic one, such as E or c. There is little doubt that some people make antibodies more readily than others, and there may also be processes of selectivity in the antibody response to different antigens. Diminished antibody responses are found in persons with malignancy of the lymphocytes and plasma cells, and also in hypogammaglobulinemia.

WHITE CELL AND PLATELET ANTIBODIES

Both transfusion and pregnancy can give rise to antibodies directed against leukocytes and platelets, some of whose antigens are held in common [91]. In fact, it appears that platelet and white cell antigens are much more immunogenic than those of red cells, because some patients can receive blood transfusions for years and never make red cell antibodies, while at the same time making one or more white cell or platelet antibodies. In general, immunization to HLA or to platelet-specific antigens increases in proportion to the number of transfusions given, although some patients do not seem to form such antibodies. The result is shortened survival of transfused platelets, and sometimes also febrile transfusion reactions. Although further platelet transfusions are not absolutely precluded in such a case, they may become ineffective, since the antibody formation causes refractoriness to platelet transfusions (see Chap. 8). When patients such as leukemics become unresponsive to platelet transfusions in this way, it may be necessary to select related or HLA-compatible donors for platelet apheresis (see Chap. 3). In addition, passively transferred leukocyte or other antibodies in donor plasma can cause severe febrile and other reactions in recipients [23].

Posttransfusion Purpura

Posttransfusion purpura is a rare, but serious, complication of transfusion, characterized by the sudden onset of purpura and profound thrombocytopenia about a week after a transfusion [92]. Other than thrombocytopenia and a prolonged bleeding time, tests of coagulation give normal results. In virtually every case, investigation reveals an antibody to a high-frequency platelet antigen, usually anti-PL^{A1}; the patient's platelets lack the corresponding antigen, and the donors implicated have it. The pathogenesis of this complication thus involves alloimmunization, but the reason why the antibody attacks the patient's own platelets is unknown. Possibilities include the adsorption of immune complexes onto the patient's platelets, or the adsorption of PL^{A1} antigen that was either free in the transfused blood or released from destroyed, transfused platelets [93].

Awareness and recognition of the syndrome are important in management. The condition is usually self-limiting. Therapy is not well established, but possibilities include high-dose steroids, removal of the antibody by intensive plasma exchange, and (possibly) blockage of the reticuloendothelial system with intravenous immune globulin.

Neonatal Thrombocytopenia

Neonatal thrombocytopenia results when a mother is immunized to fetal platelet antigens, usually, as in posttransfusion purpura, PL^{A1} (see Chap. 3) [94]. In this case, the mother's antibody attacks fetal platelets, not her own, causing purpura in the newborn. Treatment consists of transfusion of PL^{A1}-negative platelets to the baby. The most convenient way of obtaining such platelets is by platelet apheresis of the mother, although of course they can also be obtained from other PL^{A1}-negative donors.

Neonatal Neutropenia

Neutropenia may occur in the newborn as a result of alloimmunization of the mother to neutrophil antigens; indeed, most of the neutrophil-specific antigens and antibodies have been discovered because of this occurrence (see Chap. 3) [95].

Immunosuppressive Effects of Transfusion

Transfusions have a generally immunodepressive effect on the recipient, which improves the outcome of renal transplants, but may have adverse effects on the progress of malignant tumors. This is discussed in greater detail in Chapter 6.

References

1. Javid J. Human haptoglobins. *Curr Top Hematol* 1978; 1:151–92.
2. Mollison PL. *Blood Transfusion in Clinical Medicine*, 7th ed. Oxford, England: Blackwell, 1983; Chaps. 12, 13.
3. Goldfinger D. Acute hemolytic transfusion reactions. A fresh look at pathogenesis and considerations regarding therapy. *Transfusion* 1977; 17:85–98.
4. Schmidt PJ, Holland PV. Pathogenesis of acute renal failure associated with incompatible transfusion. *Lancet* 1967; 2:1169–72.
5. Honig CL, Bove JR. Transfusion associated fatalities: review of Bureau of Biologics reports. *Transfusion* 1980; 20:653–61.
6. Myhre BA. Fatalities from blood transfusion. *JAMA* 1980; 244:1333–5.
7. Schmidt PJ. Transfusion mortality, with special reference to surgical and intensive care facilities. *J Fla Med Assoc* 1980; 67:151–3.
8. Camp FR Jr, Monaghan WP. Fatal blood transfusion reactions. An analysis. *Am J Forensic Med Pathol* 1981; 2:143–50.
9. Pineda AA, Taswell HF, Brzica SM. Delayed hemolytic transfusion reaction. An immunologic hazard of blood transfusion. *Transfusion* 1978; 18:1–7.
10. Salama A, Mueller-Eckhardt C. Delayed hemolytic transfusion reactions: evidence for complement activation involving allogeneic and autologous red cells. *Transfusion* 1984; 24:188–93.
11. Chaplin H Jr. The implication of red cell-bound complement in delayed hemolytic transfusion reactions. *Transfusion* 1984; 24:185–7.
12. Buchholz DH, Bove JR. Unusual response to ABO incompatible blood transfusion. *Transfusion* 1975; 15:577–82.
13. Young LE, Platzer RF, Yuile CL, et al. Recovery of group O recipient after transfusion of two liters of group A blood. *Am J Clin Pathol* 1947; 17:777–82.
14. van der Hart M, Engelfriet CP, Prins HK, van Loghem JJ. A haemolytic transfusion reaction without demonstrable antibodies in vitro. *Vox Sang* 1963; 8:363–70.
15. Pierce RN, Reich LM, Mayer K. Hemolysis following platelet transfusions from ABO-incompatible donors. *Transfusion* 1985; 25:60–2.
16. Bowman HS, Brason FW, Mohn JF, et al. Experimental transfusion of donor plasma containing blood group antibodies into incompatible normal human recipients: II. Induction of isoimmune hemolytic anemia by transfusion of plasma containing exceptional anti-CD antibodies. *Br J Haematol* 1961; 7:130–45.
17. Zettner A, Bove JR. Hemolytic transfusion reaction due to interdonor incompatibility. *Transfusion* 1963; 3:48–51.
18. Mohandas N, Greenquist AC, Shohet S. Effects of heat and metabolic depletion on erythrocyte deformability, spectrin extractability and phosphorylation. In: Brewer GJ (ed). *The Red Cell*. New York: A. R. Liss, 1978.
19. Jones JH, Kilpatrick GS, Franks EH. Red cell aggregation in dextrose solutions. *J Clin Pathol* 1962; 15:161–2.
20. Eurenius S, Smith RM. Hemolysis in blood infused under pressure. *Anesthesiology* 1973; 39:650–1.
21. Tovey GH. Management of haemolytic transfusion reaction. *Vox Sang* 1963; 8:257–61 (editorial).
22. Byrne JP, Dixon JA. Pulmonary edema following blood transfusion reaction. *Arch Surg* 1971; 102:91–4.
23. Popovsky MA, Moore SB. Diagnostic and pathogenetic considerations in transfusion-related acute lung injury. *Transfusion* 1985; 25:573–7.
24. Pineda AA, Taswell HF. Transfusion reactions associated with anti-IgA anti-

bodies: report of four cases and review of the literature. *Transfusion* 1975; 15:10–15.
25. Vyas GN, Holmdahl L, Perkins HA. Serologic specificity of human IgA and its significance in transfusion. *Blood* 1969; 34:573.
26. Burks AW, Sampson HA, Buckley RH. Anaphylactic reactions after gamma globulin administration in patients with hypogammaglobulinemia. *N Engl J Med* 1986; 314:560–4.
27. Kelly JF, Patterson R. Anaphylaxis. Course, mechanisms, and treatment. *JAMA* 1974; 227:1431–6.
28. de Rie MA, van der Plas-van Dalen CM, Engelfriet CP, von dem Borne AEGK. The serology of febrile transfusion reactions. *Vox Sang* 1985; 49:126–34.
29. Goldfinger D, Lowe C. Prevention of adverse reactions to blood transfusion by the administration of saline-washed red blood cells. *Transfusion* 1981; 21:277–80.
30. Meryman HT, Hornblower M. The preparation of red cells depleted of leukocytes. Review and evaluation. *Transfusion* 1986; 26:101–6.
31. Braude AI. Transfusion reactions from contaminated blood. *N Engl J Med* 1958; 258:1289–93.
32. Sprung CL, Caralis PV, Marcial EH, et al. The effects of high-dose corticosteroids in patients with septic shock. A prospective, controlled study. *N Engl J Med* 1984; 311:1137–43.
33. Ludbrook J, Wynn V. Citrate intoxication. A clinical and experimental study. *Br Med J* 1958; 2:523–8.
34. Harker LA, Malpass TW, Branson HE, et al. Mechanism of abnormal bleeding in patients undergoing cardiopulmonary bypass: acquired transient platelet dysfunction associated with selective alpha-granule release. *Blood* 1980; 56: 824–34.
35. Weiden P. Graft-v-host disease following blood transfusions. *Arch Intern Med* 1984; 144:1557–8.
36. Cohen D, Weinstein H, Mihm M, Yankee R. Nonfatal graft-versus-host disease occurring after transfusion with leukocytes and platelets obtained from healthy donors. *Blood* 1979; 53:1053–6.
37. Simon GE, Bove JR. The potassium load from blood transfusion. *Postgrad Med* 1971; 49:61–4.
38. Hollinger BF, Khan NC, Oefinger PE, et al. Posttransfusion hepatitis type A. *JAMA* 1983; 250:2313–7.
39. Noble RC, Kane MA, Reaves SA, Roeckel I. Posttransfusion hepatitis A in a neonatal intensive care unit. *JAMA* 1984; 252:2711–5.
40. Hoofnagle JH. Type A and type B hepatitis. *Lab Med* 1983; 14:705–16.
41. Goldfield M, Bill J, Colosimo F. The control of transfusion-associated hepatitis. In: Vyas GN, Cohen SN, Schmid R (eds). *Viral Hepatitis*. Philadelphia: Franklin Institute Press, 1978.
42. Rosina F, Saracco G, Rizzetto M. Risk of post-transfusion infection with the hepatitis delta virus: a multicenter study. *N Engl J Med* 1985; 312:1488–91.
43. Vyas GN, Blum HE. Hepatitis B virus infection. *West J Med* 1984; 140:754–62.
44. Nishioka NS, Dienstag JL. Delta hepatitis: a new scourge? *N Engl J Med* 1985; 312:1515–6.
45. Vyas GN, Cohen SN, Schmid R (eds). *Viral Hepatitis*. Philadelphia: Franklin Institute Press, 1978.
46. Aach RD, Lander JL, Sherman LA, et al. Transfusion-transmitted viruses: interim analysis of hepatitis among transfused and nontransfused patients. In: Vyas GN, Cohen SN, Schmid R (eds). *Viral Hepatitis*. Philadelphia: Franklin Institute Press, 1978.

47. Gitnick G. Non-A, non-B hepatitis: etiology and clinical course. *Lab Med* 1983; 14:721–6.
48. Purcell RH. The viral hepatitides. *Hosp Pract* 1978 (July); 13:51–63.
49. Seeff LB, Wright EC, Zimmerman HJ, et al. Posttransfusion hepatitis, 1973–1975: a Veterans Administration cooperative study. In: Vyas GN, Cohen SN, Schmid R (eds). *Viral Hepatitis*. Philadelphia: Franklin Institute Press, 1978.
50. Tabor E, Goldfield M, Black HC, Gerety RJ. Hepatitis Be antigen in volunteer and paid blood donors. *Transfusion* 1980; 20:192–8.
51. Aach RD, Szmuness W, Mosley JW, et al. Serum alanine aminotransferase of donors in relation to the risk of non-A, non-B hepatitis in recipients. *N Engl J Med* 1981; 304:989–94.
52. Alter HJ, Purcell RH, Holland PV, et al. Donor transaminase and recipient hepatitis. Impact on blood transfusion services. *JAMA* 1981; 246:630–4.
53. Alter HJ. Posttransfusion hepatitis: clinical features, risk and donor testing. In: Dodd RY, Barker LF (eds). *Infection, Immunity, and Blood Transfusion*. New York: A. R. Liss, 1985.
54. Polesky HF, Hanson M. Transfusion-associated hepatitis: a dilemma. *Lab Med* 1983; 14:717–20.
55. Stevens CE, Aach RD, Hollinger BF, et al. Hepatitis B virus antibody in blood donors and the occurrence of non-A, non-B hepatitis in transfusion recipients. An analysis of the transfusion-transmitted viruses study. *Ann Intern Med* 1984; 101:733–8.
56. Koziol DE, Holland PV, Alling DW, et al. Antibody to hepatitis B core antigen as a paradoxical marker for non-A, non-B hepatitis agents in donated blood. *Ann Intern Med* 1986: 104:488–95.
57. American Association of Blood Banks. FDA advisory panel recommends surrogate testing for NANB. *AABB Blood Bank Week* 1986, 3(8):1.
58. Alter HJ, Tabor E, Meryman HJ, et al. Transmission of hepatitis B virus infection by transfusion of frozen-deglycerolized red blood cells. *N Engl J Med* 1978; 298:637–42.
59. Haugen RK. Hepatitis after the transfusion of frozen red cells and washed red cells. *N Engl J Med* 1979; 301:393–5.
60. Weiland O, Mattson L, Glaumann H. Non-A, non-B hepatitis after intravenous gammaglobulin. *Lancet* 1986; 1:976–7.
61. Centers for Disease Control. Postexposure prophylaxis of hepatitis B. *JAMA* 1984; 251:3210–5.
62. Sandler SG, Grumet FC. Posttransfusion cytomegalovirus infections. *Pediatrics* 1982; 69:650–2.
63. Adler SP. Neonatal cytomegalovirus infections due to blood. *CRC Crit Rev Clin Lab Sci* 1985; 23:1–14.
64. Jackson B, Orr H, Jordan C, McCullough J. Non-detection of cytomegalovirus (CMV) in the peripheral blood of CMV seropositive healthy blood donors by DNA-DNA hybridization. *Transfusion* 1985; 25:472 (abstract).
65. Brady MT, Milam JD, Anderson DC, et al. Use of deglycerolized red blood cells to prevent posttransfusion infection with cytomegalovirus in neonates. *J Infect Dis* 1984; 150:334–9.
66. Yeager AS, Grumet FC, Hafleigh EB, et al. Prevention of transfusion-acquired cytomegalovirus infections in newborn infants. *J Pediatr* 1981; 98:281–7.
67. Amman AJ, Cowan MW, Wara DW, et al. Acquired immunodeficiency syndrome in an infant: possible transmission by means of blood products. *Lancet* 1983; 1:956–8.

68. Curran JW, Lawrence DN, Jaffe H, et al. Acquired immunodeficiency syndrome (AIDS) associated with transfusion. *N Engl J Med* 1984; 310:69–75.
69. Perkins HA. Transfusion-associated AIDS. *Am J Hematol* 1985; 19:307–13.
70. Peterman TA, Jaffe HW, Feorino PM, et al. Transfusion-associated acquired immunodeficiency syndrome in the United States. *JAMA* 1985; 254:2913–7.
71. Evatt BL, Ramsey RB, Lawrence DN, et al. The acquired immunodeficiency syndrome in patients with hemophilia. *Ann Intern Med* 1984; 100:499–504.
72. Bove JR. Transfusion-transmitted diseases: current problems and challenges. *Prog Hematol* 1986; 14:123–47.
73. Pindyck J, Waldman A, Zang E, et al. Measures to decrease the risk of acquired immune deficiency syndrome by blood transfusions: evidence of volunteer blood donor cooperation. *Transfusion* 1985; 25:3–9.
74. Perkins JT, Micelli C, Janda WM. Does antibody screening of donors increase the risk of transfusion-associated AIDS? *N Engl J Med* 1985; 313:115–6 (letter).
75. Schorr JB, Berkowitz A, Cumming PD, et al. Prevalence of HTLV III antibody in American blood donors. *N Engl J Med* 1985; 313:384–5 (letter).
76. Miller PJ, O'Connell J, Leipold A, Wenzel RP. Potential liability for transfusion-associated AIDS. *JAMA* 1985; 253:3419–24.
77. Council of Community Blood Centers. Blood from female donors safer, says California women's group. *CCBC Newsletter* 12/27/85–1/3/86; pp. 2–3.
78. Curran JW, Morgan WM, Hardy AM, et al. The epidemiology of AIDS: current status and future prospects. *Science* 1985; 229:1352–7.
79. Mayer KH, Stoddard AM, McCusker J, et al. Human T-lymphotropic virus type III in high-risk, antibody-negative homosexual men. *Ann Intern Med* 1986; 104:194–6.
80. Berkman EM. News release. Washington, DC: American Association of Blood Banks, January 9, 1986.
81. American Association of Blood Banks. Looking back on "look-back" finds search incomplete; about half of those identified are infected. *Blood Bank Week* 1986; 3(44):2–4.
82. Guerrero IC, Weniger BC, Schultz MG. Transfusional malaria in the United States, 1972–1981. *Ann Intern Med* 1983; 99:221–6.
83. van der Sluis JJ, Onvlee PC, Kothe FCIIA, et al. Transfusion syphilis, survival of Treponema pallidum in donor blood. I. Report of an orienting study. *Vox Sang* 1984; 47:197–204.
84. Walker RH. The disposition of STS-reactive blood in a transfusion service. *Transfusion* 1965; 5:452–6.
85. Gombert ME, Goldstein E, Benach JL, et al. Human babesiosis. Clinical and therapeutic considerations. *JAMA* 1982; 248:3005–7.
86. Marcus LC, Valigorsky JM, Fanning WL, et al. A case report of transfusion-induced babesiosis. *JAMA* 1982; 248:465–7.
87. Propper RD, Cooper B, Rufo RR, et al. Continuous subcutaneous administration of deferoxamine in patients with iron overload. *N Engl J Med* 1977; 297:418–23.
88. Propper RD, Button LN, Nathan DG. New approaches to the transfusion management of thalassemia. *Blood* 1980; 55:55–60.
89. Mollison PL. *Blood Transfusion in Clinical Medicine,* 7th ed. Oxford, England: Blackwell Sci, 1979, 353.
90. Giblett ER. A critique of the theoretical hazard of inter- versus intraracial transfusion. *Transfusion* 1961; 1:233–8.
91. Issitt PD. *Applied Blood Group Serology,* 3rd ed. Miami, FL: Montgomery Scientific Publ., 1985, 432–4.

92. Moore SB. Post-transfusion purpura: a brief review. *Ir Med J* 1985; 78:365–7.
93. Kickler TS, Ness PM, Herman JH, Bell WR. Studies on the pathophysiology of posttransfusion purpura. *Blood* 1986; 68:347–50.
94. von dem Borne AEGK, van Leeuwen EF, von Riesz E, et al. Neonatal alloimmune thrombocytopenia: detection and characterization of the responsible antibodies by the platelet immunofluorescence test. *Blood* 1981; 57:649–56.
95. Lalezari P. Neutrophil antigens: immunology and clinical implications. In: Greenwalt TJ, Jamieson GA, *The Granulocyte: Function and Clinical Utilization*. New York: A. R. Liss, 1977, 209–25.

8. Blood Components, Fractions, and Derivatives

The skillful and intelligent use of blood components and derivatives is one mark of today's well-trained physician. Whole blood is a complex mixture of formed elements, proteins, and electrolytes, each with a different and important function. The indiscriminate transfusion of such a mixture is seldom justified, since most patients can be treated more effectively and safely with one of the available blood components. Moreover, modern transfusion therapy requires physicians to make optimal use of every blood donation. In most cases, that goal is best accomplished when each donor serves more than one patient. This can be achieved by increasing the use of component therapy and by selecting the proper component *and only the proper component* for each indication.

With modern techniques and equipment, whole blood can be separated into its individual constituents. Many of these are of unknown clinical importance. Others are used only in research, and some—plasma, red blood cells, immunoglobulins, and serum albumin, for example—are in daily use and have become vital therapeutic modalities (Table 8–1). *Blood components* are prepared from a single donation of blood by simple physical separation methods such as centrifugation, and are generally transfused without further processing. *Blood fractions or derivatives* are prepared by complex physical and chemical processes that use the plasma from many donors as the starting material. Modern equipment—refrigerated centrifuges and plastic bags, in particular—has made blood component preparation practical for almost every blood bank. Blood fractionation, on the other hand, is still a complex manufacturing process beyond the scope of most blood banks and of this book.

Red Blood Cells

PREPARATION

Blood component preparation begins with the separation of plasma from whole blood, leaving a unit of red blood cells available for use in routine blood bank operation. Without an adequate program to utilize this material for transfusion, a blood component program will be wasteful and unsatisfactory. Indications for red cell transfusion are discussed in Chapter 6.

Red cells for transfusion can be prepared by centrifugation or sedimentation of whole blood. Neither centrifugation nor sedimentation has a deleterious effect on the cells, and the plasma may be removed by either method at any time before the expiration date of the blood. In either case, the technique, equipment, and preservative solution must be adequate to maintain sterility and preserve metabolic integrity. Under these conditions, the cells have a posttransfusion recovery equivalent to that of whole blood. If the plasma is

Table 8–1. Official Names for Some Blood Components and Derivatives According to the FDA

Official Name	Other Names
Whole Blood	Blood, whole blood
Red Blood Cells	Red cells, "packed cells"
Fresh Frozen Plasma	FFP
Liquid Plasma	Plasma, single-donor plasma, bank plasma
Plasma	Plasma, single-donor plasma, bank plasma
Plasma Protein Fraction (Human)	PPF
Albumin (Human)	Albumin, normal serum albumin, serum albumin, salt-poor albumin
Platelets	Random-donor platelets, platelet concentrate, platelets
Platelets, Pheresis	Single-donor platelets, apheresis platelets
Cryoprecipitated AHF	Cryoprecipitate, cryo
Antihemophilic Factor (Human)	AHF, factor VIII concentrate
Factor IX Complex	Factor IX concentrate
Anti-Inhibitor Coagulant Complex	Activated factor IX, factor VIII bypassing activity (FEIBA®)
Immune Globulin (Human)	Immune globulins, gamma globulin
$Rh_o(D)$ Immune Globulin (Human)	Rh immune globulin
Source Plasma	Apheresis plasma
Recovered Plasma	Bank plasma

removed by a method that does not have the potential to contaminate the red cells, the expiration date remains the same as that of the original whole blood or, when additive solutions are used (see pp. 299–300), becomes whatever is specified for the particular additive solution. When there is a possibility of contamination, for example, if the contents may have been exposed to room air, the red blood cells are considered usable for only 24 hours.

STORAGE

Blood banking, as we know it today, depends on the safe, efficient, and prolonged storage of blood, particularly of the red cells. The prime consideration in blood storage is to establish and maintain conditions allowing transfusion of red cells that will survive and function normally *after* infusion into the recipient. The preservation of other components—fibrinogen, platelets, or antihemophilic factor, for example—is also important, but red cell preservation is central to all aspects of blood storage and is the area of most concern in the evaluation of blood preservation.

The adequacy of red cell storage is related to maintenance of normal cell metabolism and is evaluated by posttransfusion survival (viability) studies. Functional considerations, particularly the ability of the red cell to bind and release oxygen appropriately, are of equal importance. Red cell metabolic pathways are described in detail in textbooks of biochemistry and hematology and will not be repeated here. During storage, there is a critical relationship between glucose metabolism, adenosine triphosphate (ATP) production, and the energy needed for red cell viability. While there is good correlation between ATP levels during storage and red cell viability, the correlation is not good enough to be used as the sole indicator of acceptable storage conditions. As a result, any new approach to red cell storage must be evaluated by experiments that show adequate survival of erythrocytes at the end of the proposed storage time. Adequate survival has been defined arbitrarily as a mean of 75 percent survival after 24 hours of storage. There are no criteria for functional characteristics; red cells that are viable at 24 hours are presumably adequate as to function. The best method for determining poststorage survival is debatable, with some favoring the more complex double-label method, and others a single-labeling technique [1, 2]. If experiments are carefully controlled, either approach seems acceptable, although a double-label technique offers some increase in accuracy [3]. This is especially true in cases where the early loss of red cells is expected to be large. Red cells damaged during storage are removed within several hours after transfusion, while those cells that survive for 24 hours have an essentially normal life span.

Functional Characteristics of Stored Red Cells

The most critical function of red cells is oxygen transport: the uptake of oxygen in the lung, its transport around the body, and its ultimate delivery to the tissues [4]. This physiologic function is mediated by a remarkable reversible equilibrium between hemoglobin and oxygen. The maintenance of this normal oxygen-hemoglobin interaction is one major goal in red cell preservation.

Oxygen constitutes about 20 percent of the inspired air and, under normal conditions, exerts a partial pressure (PO_2) in the lungs of about 107 mm Hg. At this pressure, the equilibrium favors oxyhemoglobin formation, so that hemoglobin becomes fully saturated with oxygen (Fig. 8–1A).

In the tissues, oxygen tension is approximately 40 mm Hg, a level at which hemoglobin is only about 70 percent saturated with oxygen. Thus, the normal response is that hemoglobin, which arrives at the tissue completely saturated with oxygen, will unload about one-quarter of it. As the partially saturated hemoglobin returns to the lung, where the PO_2 is 107 mm Hg, oxygen will be taken up to saturate the hemoglobin again. The hemoglobin saturation at various partial pressures of oxygen is shown in Fig. 8–1A. The sigmoid shape of the curve indicates an important functional characteristic of the hemoglobin-oxygen relationship: Over a wide range of higher partial pressures, the hemoglobin molecule can be fully saturated, thus facilitating oxygen uptake in the

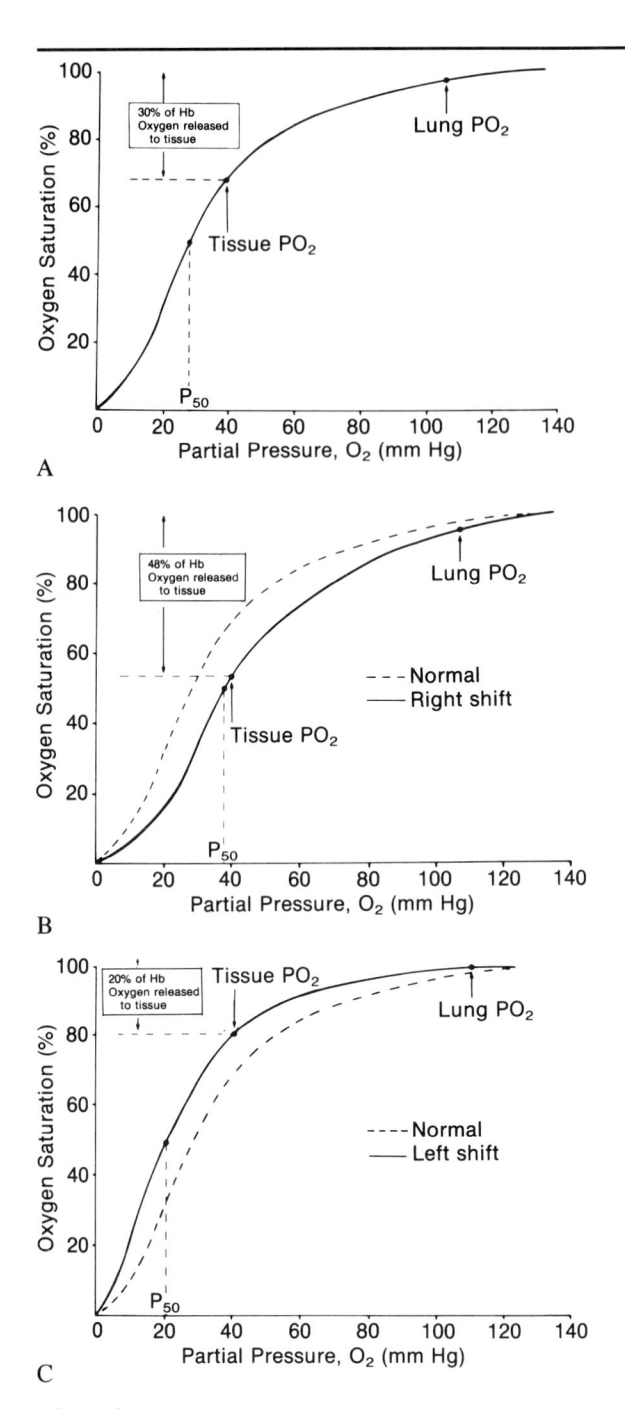

Figure 8–1
(A) The normal oxygen dissociation curve of hemoglobin. Note the high saturation at partial pressures of oxygen usually associated with the lung and the release of about 30 percent of bound oxygen at usual tissue PO_2 levels. The P_{50} value is the partial pressure at which oxygen saturation is 50 percent. (B) Oxygen dissociation curve showing a right shift. Note the increased ability to release oxygen at the PO_2 value normally found in tissue. The P_{50} value is also increased. (C) Oxygen dissociation curve showing a left shift. Oxygen release is inhibited at normal tissue PO_2 levels.

lung. In the range of partial pressures found at the tissues, the curve falls rapidly, indicating that, in tissue, a relatively small decrease in PO$_2$ will be the stimulus for the unloading of large quantities of oxygen. The general shape of the curve is fixed; it can shift to the right or left with respect to a point on the abscissa, however, depending on many variables, including pH, PCO$_2$, alterations in hemoglobin structure, and the presence of 2,3-DPG.

A useful way to describe the degree of right or left shift in the curve is in terms of the *P$_{50}$ value*, the partial pressure of oxygen at which 50 percent of the hemoglobin is saturated with oxygen. A curve that has shifted to the right has a higher P$_{50}$; this represents a situation in which the hemoglobin can release a larger amount of oxygen at any given partial pressure of oxygen (Fig. 8–1B). A left shift is just the reverse; here, oxygen is more tightly bound, and a less-than-normal amount is released at any particular partial pressure of oxygen (Fig. 8–1C). In terms of blood storage and transfusion, conditions leading to a right shift of the curve are theoretically more advantageous than those leading to a left shift.

OXYGEN RELEASE AND 2,3-DIPHOSPHOGLYCERATE. The concentration of 2,3-DPG in the red cell is most important in determining the oxygen-release function of hemoglobin [5]. Storage conditions that maintain or enhance the 2,3-DPG concentration theoretically provide for better posttransfusion oxygen exchange by a right shift of the curve. In this regard, citrate phosphate dextrose (CPD) solution is better than the old acid citrate dextrose (ACD) solution or the newer CPD adenine-1 (CPDA-1) solution.

Whether transfusion with red cells that have a low level of 2,3-DPG is less effective clinically is still not established. It seems logical that impaired oxygen delivery to tissues should be disadvantageous, and experiments in animals have shown the expected effects. Rats exchange-transfused with blood low in 2,3-DPG showed about a 10 percent decrease in work performance [6]; rats with low levels of 2,3-DPG and anemia had a mortality rate from controlled hemorrhage that was twice that seen in those with normal levels [7]; and oxygen consumption in isolated dog hindlimbs was greater when the perfused blood had normal 2,3-DPG levels [8].

Studies in humans are far more difficult to evaluate, since so many compensatory mechanisms are operating. In addition, both 2,3-DPG and P$_{50}$ levels that are abnormal immediately after transfusion return to normal within 24 hours [9]. Assigning significance to the clinical studies in humans is difficult. It appears that massive transfusion with cells depleted in 2,3-DPG may be disadvantageous, but only in selected patients, especially those with anemia, coronary artery disease, or the inability to increase cardiac output in response to stress [10]. In other cases, the supposed advantages, if any, of transfusing blood containing normal or high levels of 2,3-DPG are unconfirmed.

Red cells with increased levels of 2,3-DPG and abnormally high P$_{50}$ values can be prepared by rejuvenating stored cells with a solution containing pyruvate, inosine, glucose, and phosphate [11]. These cells are then frozen, and upon thawing and transfusion, lead to improved oxygen delivery. Transfusion of these "super cells" to baboons lessened the demand for increased blood flow that otherwise would have been needed to ensure adequate tissue perfusion after hemorrhage [12]. In humans undergoing coronary artery bypass surgery, transfusion of rejuvenated cells led to improved myocardial performance, suggesting that in some patients, artificially decreasing oxygen affinity by transfusing cells with abnormally high levels of 2,3-DPG could be of value [13]. Other studies have not shown a beneficial effect, and the issue remains in doubt [14].

RED CELL VIABILITY. In blood preservation, it is essential to establish conditions that will allow red cell viability after transfusion of the stored component. The maintenance of red cell viability as measured by posttransfusion red cell survival is so important that it has become the key determinant in evaluating new methods of blood storage. The effectiveness of blood preservation and storage is appraised by measuring the proportion of stored red cells that survive in the circulation for 24 hours after transfusion. In almost all cases, cells that survive 24 hours will remain viable and circulate for the remainder of their expected life span. Current regulations regarding anticoagulant solutions and storage periods (permissible dating) are based on the long-established concept that at least 75 percent of the transfused red cells should be present in the recipient's circulation 24 hours after transfusion. To be acceptable, preservatives and storage routines must be at least this effective.

Factors Influencing Red Cell Recovery

COLLECTION. The abrupt change in environment that takes place when red cells are collected into the acidic and hypotonic anticoagulant solution is responsible for irreversible damage to some of the cells. The damage has been termed the *lesion of collection* and affects, for the most part, cells drawn at the start of the donor bleeding [15]. These red cells, in contrast to those drawn toward the end of phlebotomy, deteriorate more rapidly on storage, and their recovery is about half that found for the mean of the entire collection. The lesion of collection is also responsible for the fact that, even in unstored blood, the recovery is 95, rather than the expected 100, percent.

TEMPERATURE. Among the first studies done when blood storage became practical were those seeking optimum storage temperature. From the evidence accumulated, 4°C (now 1 to 6°C) was chosen, with additional data showing that temperatures up to 10°C were acceptable. Deterioration was accelerated at 15°C or higher. Current standards require storage at controlled and monitored temperatures between 1 and 6°C, with occasional elevations to 10°C (e.g., during transportation) being considered acceptable.

The need to prepare platelets before refrigeration of the blood has prompted a recent reevaluation of the effect of delayed refrigeration on the storage characteristics of the blood [16, 17]. Delaying refrigeration increases the loss of 2,3-DPG over this period. Once the blood is refrigerated, however, the *rate* of loss is the same as that seen with blood that has been refrigerated immediately after collection [17]. Federal regulations allow a delay of up to 6 hours before refrigeration.

ANTICOAGULATION SOLUTIONS. The most important factor influencing red cell recovery after blood storage is the anticoagulant solution used. It is for this reason that most investigations are directed toward improving the anticoagulant solution rather than toward altering the containers or refrigeration. All solutions in current use are both anticoagulants and red cell preserving mediums, but it is common to refer to them as anticoagulants, forgetting their equally important function in preservation. The various changes that take place in blood during the storage period are related both to the storage time and the nature of the anticoagulant solution. These changes, known as the *storage lesion,* are similar for blood collected into all of the licensed anticoagulant solutions.

ANTICOAGULANT CITRATE DEXTROSE. For years, the standard anticoagulant-preservative solution used in the United States was ACD. Two critical ingredients, dextrose and sodium citrate, were used in the original formula, described by Robertson in 1918 [18]. Because solutions of sodium citrate and dextrose became yellow when mixed and autoclaved, Loutit, Mollison, and Young replaced some of the sodium citrate with citric acid, expecting that the lower pH would result in less discoloration on autoclaving [19]. This is indeed what happened, along with an unexpected improvement in the posttransfusion survival of the stored cells. These investigators were the first to evaluate carefully the posttransfusion viability of cells stored at different temperatures and in different preservative solutions. They advised use of a solution containing 100 ml of 2 percent trisodium citrate and 20 ml of 15 percent glucose for the preservation of 420 ml of blood, a formula almost identical with that of ACD solution, formula B. This solution is no longer used for blood collection, having been replaced first by ACD formula A, next by CPD, and now by CPDA-1 (Table 8–2).

CITRATE PHOSPHATE DEXTROSE. CPD solution was developed by Gibson and his associates to obviate some of the deleterious effects of ACD [20]. In particular, a higher pH and a more isotonic solution were desired. Several mixtures con-

Table 8–2. Formulas for CPD and CPDA-1 Solutions*

Ingredient	CPD	CPDA-1
Trisodium citrate (gm)	1.66	1.66
Citric acid (mg)	206	206
Dextrose (gm)	1.61	2.01
Monobasic sodium phosphate (mg)	140	140
Adenine (mg)		17.3

*Total volume is 63 ml for each solution. Amounts listed are for the collection of 450 ± 45 ml of blood.

taining various concentrations of citrate, dextrose, and phosphate were studied before the formula given in Table 8–2 was chosen.

Studies on blood collected into CPD solution showed that the recovery and the survival of red cells were as good or better than those with ACD, and that red cell function, particularly as measured by the rate of fall of 2,3-DPG, was better. For these reasons, CPD replaced ACD as the anticoagulant of choice, even though the hoped-for 28-day storage period was not approved by the FDA.

CITRATE PHOSPHATE DEXTROSE ADENINE-1. Many chemicals, including adenine, guanine, hypoxanthine, inosine, and uridine, have been added to preservative solutions in an attempt to improve storage. Because the red cell is dependent on ATP as an energy source, the availability of adenine appears to be critical in the maintenance of high ATP levels. Simon and his associates showed originally that the addition of 0.75 μmole of adenine per milliliter of blood improved survival of stored red cells, and several formulations of CPD-adenine have since been tried [21]. A solution containing 0.5 μmole of adenine per milliliter of blood, used successfully in Sweden since 1965, was found to be acceptable for all transfusions, including massive transfusion and exchange transfusion in the newborn. Because of concern about potential adenine toxicity, the solution used in the United States contains 0.25 μmole of adenine per milliliter of blood—half the amount in the Swedish formulation. In addition, extra glucose has been added to allow for 35 days of storage.

Adenine itself appears to be nontoxic, although about 10 percent of the material is converted in vivo to 2,8-dioxyadenine, which is relatively insoluble. Individuals given 10 mg of adenine per kilogram of body weight show no toxic effect; at 15 mg/kg some patients show renal deposits of 2,8-dioxyadenine but no evidence of toxicity [22]. This dose is equivalent to the amount of adenine in 60 units of blood (0.25 μmole adenine) or, since not all of the adenine is intracellular, 120 units of red blood cells.

Clinical reports suggest that blood collected in CPDA-1 is well tolerated and safe, although there are concerns that the CPDA-1 solution provides levels of nutrients that are barely adequate for 35 days of storage, particularly when plasma is removed and the collection stored as red blood cells. Because of this, several new anticoagulant solutions have been developed, but currently these are not in use.

ADDITIVES. In 1974 Högman presented a new approach to the storage of red cells for transfusion when he prepared a protein-poor medium and showed that red cells stored in it had acceptable survival despite increased in vitro hemolysis during storage. The hemolysis was attributed to a chymotrypsin-like enzyme from human leukocytes and could be prevented either by addition of synthetic enzyme inhibitors or by removal of the buffy coat [23, 24]. He postulated that hemolysis was prevented when plasma was in the solution, because plasma normally contained inhibiting enzymes. These observations laid the groundwork for the preparation and widespread use of several additive solutions for red cell storage (Table 8–3). In practice, blood is collected into a multiple container system, one container of which contains the additive solution (Fig. 8–2). After collection, the whole blood unit is centrifuged and plasma plus buffy coat expressed into the empty satellite container for further processing into platelets and plasma. The additive solution (see Table 8–3) is then expressed into the red cells, which can be stored for up to 42 days. Advantages include the following:

1. An additional 7 days of storage time for the red cell preparation
2. Increased yield of plasma from each collection
3. A red blood cell preparation with better storage characteristics and an improved flow rate at the time of transfusion
4. Removal of an unwanted and potentially dangerous buffy coat

Added expense, both for the bags themselves and for the processing involved, has prevented more widespread use of the system, although some blood banks have found that the *extra* plasma that can be harvested from the red blood cells more than adequately compensates for the added cost of preparation.

OTHER ANTICOAGULANTS. In experimental situations, blood can be collected through an *ion exchange resin* that removes almost all the cations, including calcium. Blood so collected is useful for serum production and, on occasion, for research.

Disodium dihydrogen ethylenediaminetetraacetate is a strong chelating (binding) agent that effectively prevents blood coagulation by decalcification. Earlier reports that blood collected into EDTA was advantageous for platelet survival have been discounted, and EDTA solution is no longer used.

Table 8–3. Composition of Additive Solutions Currently Available in the United States

	AS-3 (Nutricel®, Cutter®)	AS-1 (Adsol®, Fenwal®)
Primary Bag	63 ml CP2D*	63 ml CPD*
Additive Bag		
Volume (ml)	100	100
Dextrose (mg)	1,100	2,200
NaCl (mg)	410	900
Citric acid (mg)	42	
Sodium citrate (mg)	558	
Monobasic sodium phosphate (mg)	276	
Adenine (mg)	30	27
Mannitol (mg)		750

*Formula for CPD is in Table 8–2. CP2D is identical, except that the dextrose content is twice as high, i.e., 3.22 gm.

Containers with *heparin* solution (originally 300 to 450 USP units heparin per 100 ml of blood) are no longer available.

Inhibition of Clotting

Blood for transfusion must be collected in a way that interferes with normal blood clotting so that the blood remains fluid. Anticoagulant solutions in use today do this by binding calcium, a critical element for coagulation. In the absence of free (ionic) calcium, clotting does not take place.

CPD and CPDA-1 solutions use the citrate ion as a calcium-binding agent. The reaction is as follows:

$$3\ Ca^{++} + 2\ Na_3\ citrate \rightarrow Ca_3\ citrate + 6\ Na^+$$

The CPD and CPDA-1 solutions in current use give a final concentration of 0.31 gm of citrate* per 100 ml of blood, considerably more than is required. This increased amount of citrate provides reserve calcium-binding capacity so that almost no clotting takes place during the storage period. It does mean, of course, that each blood transfusion is also a transfusion of a small amount of citrate ion that is available to bind the recipient's calcium. The potential complications are discussed in Chapter 7.

*The figures used for concentrations of citrate ion are only approximate, since they do not take into account the fact that citrate salts are not 100 percent ionized in bank blood.

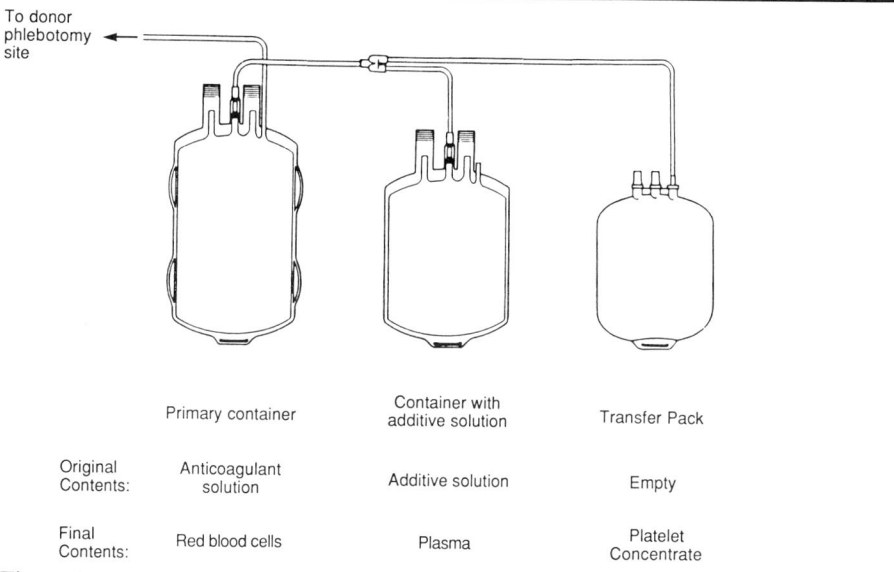

Figure 8-2
Typical blood container arrangement for use with additive solutions.

	Primary container	Container with additive solution	Transfer Pack
Original Contents:	Anticoagulant solution	Additive solution	Empty
Final Contents:	Red blood cells	Plasma	Platelet Concentrate

Posttransfusion Survival
The posttransfusion survival of red cells collected into CPD or CPDA-1 solution varies with storage time. There is a loss of about 5 percent of the red cells, even when the blood has not been stored; this is attributed to the lesion of collection (see p. 296). As blood is stored, more and more cells lose their ability to survive after infusion. The changes are gradual and affect about 5 to 10 percent of the cells each week, so that in currently used solutions, the 24-hour survival is between 72 and 92 percent (mean, 78 percent) after 35 days of storage [16].

There is a wide variation in the ability of red cells from different donors to withstand normal blood bank storage conditions. One manifestation of this is seen in posttransfusion studies, where the recovery of stored red cells from normal individuals ranges from 50 to 95 percent.

Breakdown Products
As blood is stored there is continual metabolic activity, which results in changes in both the red cells and the plasma. These changes, known collectively as the storage lesion, become more pronounced with time. Some of the characteristics of stored blood are shown in Table 8-4.

Table 8-4. Storage Lesion in a Typical Unit of CPDA-1 Red Blood Cells

	Days Stored at 4°C					
	0	7	14	21	28	35
Hematocrit (%)	75	—	—	—	—	75
pH (at 37° C)	7.04	6.92	6.80	6.65	6.58	6.55
*Plasma glucose (total mg)	284	211	165	131	99	78
*Plasma hemoglobin (total mg)	26	38	73	143	247	334
*Plasma K (total meq)	0.3	4.1	5.4	6.2	6.7	7.2
*Plasma Na (total meq)	12.1	8.8	7.8	7.1	6.6	6.2
*Plasma ammonia (total µg)	90	442	683	882	1123	1399
*Total citrate (gm)	0.43	—	—	—	—	0.43

*These values represent total amounts present in a *unit* of CPDA-1 red cells, assuming 70 ml of plasma per unit of RBC. Original data from Fenwal Laboratories, Deerfield, IL.

HYDROGEN ION CONCENTRATION. CPD and CPDA-1 solutions have a pH of about 5.6. When mixed with blood in the recommended proportions, they provide considerable buffering, so that the pH of the blood-anticoagulant mixture is about 7.1 immediately after the drawing. As can be seen from Table 8-4, there is a gradual fall in pH during the storage period, caused by the lactic acid derived from continued red cell metabolism [25].

POTASSIUM. The concentration of potassium is 3.5 to 5.0 mEq per liter in normal plasma, and 100 mEq per liter inside normal red cells. During blood storage, there is a slow, but constant, leakage of potassium from the cells into the surrounding plasma [26]. In some patients, particularly those who have severe kidney disease where even small amounts of potassium can be dangerous, relatively fresh or washed red blood cells may be indicated. After transfusion, intracellular potassium that had been depleted from the red cells during storage is reconstituted by inflow from the patient's plasma. As a result, hypokalemia can be seen after massive transfusion of stored blood (see Chap. 6).

OTHER ELECTROLYTES. No electrolyte changes of importance other than those of hydrogen ion and potassium take place during blood storage [25, 27]. Because CPD acts as an anticoagulant by binding calcium, it should be obvious that bank blood is totally free of ionic calcium.

HEMOGLOBIN. As blood is stored, another manifestation of cellular injury is the accumulation of free hemoglobin in the plasma. This pigment is liberated from damaged cells, at times, in large enough quantity to give a pink color to the supernatant plasma. On the other hand, a clear supernatant does not always mean absence of free hemoglobin. During storage, the red cells settle to the bottom of the container, where they remain unless the blood is mixed. Should there be red cell damage during this time, the liberated hemoglobin does not rise through the settled cells to color the supernatant plasma. Only after mixing and resettling can one be sure that significant hemolysis is absent. The finding of hemoglobin-tinged plasma is, in itself, far less important than consideration of the nature of the cellular damage that caused it. Cellular damage sufficient to destroy a few cells may render almost all the remaining cells nonviable. In such a case, transfusion would invariably lead to a severe hemolysis. But this is not always the case. For example, high levels of supernatant hemoglobin are seen after the storage of red cells in CPDA-1 for 35 days, but their survival is acceptable. On the other hand, hemolysis sometimes may be seen with bacterial contamination of the stored blood, and a severe reaction will follow transfusion of such blood. Visible hemolysis in the plasma of whole blood indicates a dangerous unit that should not be transfused. In red blood cells, a similar generalization cannot be made.

FROZEN RED CELLS

As with so many other important events in medical history, it was chance observation that led to the first successful freezing of blood. Anyone who has seen the marked hemolysis after a blood sample has been frozen and thawed is well aware of the damage that freezing and thawing produce. Polge, Smith, and Parkes reported in 1949 that glycerol had the capacity to protect fowl spermatozoa from the damage usually associated with freezing and thawing [28]. Smith then noted that red cells in the sperm seemed unaffected by the freezing and thawing and did further experiments to show that the protective effect of glycerol extended to the red cells. Within the year, there were reports that red cells frozen in glycerol survived well in rabbits and in humans. The importance of these early discoveries can be appreciated when one realizes that glycerol is used today in a method only slightly different from that described in the first reports.

The hemolysis seen after freezing and thawing is caused by the formation of ice crystals inside the cells, which in turn, leads to excessive concentrations of solutes in tiny intracellular pools. These lakes of hypertonic fluid irreversibly damage the cell membrane so that hemolysis accompanies thawing. Protection against this damaging effect is the goal of all cell-freezing processes and can be achieved by several methods.

In the most widely used process, glycerol in *high* concentrations (approximately 40 percent) is used as the cryoprotective agent and the cells are stored at $-80°C$. In the less widely used *low*-glycerol method, the final concentration of glycerol is closer to 15 percent, with the freezing and storage temperature at about $-196°C$, the temperature of liquid nitrogen.

Low-Glycerol Method

The very low temperature of liquid nitrogen, $-196°C$, makes it possible to freeze erythrocytes almost instantaneously. The freezing is too fast for ice crystals to form; hence, pools of hypertonic fluid do not build up within the cell, and 90 percent of the cell water is converted to ice without significant hemolysis. If, in addition, the cells to be frozen are first suspended in a hypertonic fluid, some intracellular water is removed by diffusion, the cells shrink, and there is improved viability after thawing. Many *extracellular* additives will serve, including the sugars glucose, maltose, sucrose, and lactose, or such macromolecular substances as albumin, dextran, hydroxyethyl starch, and polyvinylpyrrolidone (PVP). Similar results can be obtained with the use of a mannitol-glycerol mixture. In this case, the glycerol crosses the cell membrane and becomes an *intracellular,* as well as an extracellular, additive. Because liquid nitrogen ensures rapid freezing, low concentrations of glycerol (28 percent in the additive fluid; 14 percent final concentration) are effective, and the method is called the *low-glycerol rapid-freeze technique.*

High-Glycerol Method

Glycerol, as mentioned above, easily crosses the red cell membrane. With concentrations of glycerol between 50 and 80 percent in the additive solution, cells can be frozen and stored at higher temperatures in the *high-glycerol slow-freeze technique* [29]. Blood to be frozen is taken into the usual anticoagulant solution, and the plasma removed by centrifugation. The red cells are then mixed with a solution containing glycerol. One mixture in common use is 400 ml of a solution containing 6.2 M glycerol, 0.14 M sodium lactate, 5 mM potassium chloride, and 5 mM sodium phosphate to 250 ml of red cells. Glycerol concentrations that are too high cause some hemolysis of cells, while too little glycerol results in inadequate protection. The glycerol quickly diffuses across the red cell membrane so that the final concentration becomes about one-half of the starting concentration.

The glycerolized red cells are then simply placed in a mechanical freezer at temperatures below $-70°C$. Most freezers used for this purpose maintain $-85°C$, and at this temperature, red cells are well preserved for many years, although federal regulations allow only 10 years of storage.

Thawing and Deglycerolization

When a unit of frozen red cells is needed, it is removed from the freezer and thawed at about 40°C. After this, the glycerol must be removed in such a way that both intracellular and extracellular concentrations decrease equivalently; otherwise, osmotic hemolysis will ensue. Mollison and Sloviter, according to one of the first reports, used the method of dialysis through a semipermeable membrane [30]. It was effective, but too slow to be practical, and was soon replaced by a method of sequential washing of the glycerolized cells with

Table 8–5. Characteristics of a Frozen Red Cell Program

Advantages
- Fewer febrile and allergic transfusion reactions
- Possible lower incidence of alloimmunization to HLA
- Long-term storage for rare-donor units, for autologous transfusion, and for inventory control
- High levels of 2,3-DPG in transfused blood
- Ability to store rejuvenated, outdated red cells
- Lower incidence of hepatitis (unproved)

Disadvantages
- High cost
- Short postthaw dating
- Increased red cell loss in processing
- Increased processing time in emergency

glycerol solutions of decreasing concentrations. This method is still used for deglycerolizing small volumes of cells for in vitro work, but the number of centrifugations required makes it too cumbersome for transfusion-size units. The method can be modified for use in any one of several cell washers.

Advantages and Disadvantages

Thousands of transfusions of frozen-thawed red cells have been given, and there is no doubt that the approach is safe, practical, and has some advantages (Table 8–5). Selected studies show that as much as 10 percent of the red cells may be lost in the freezing and thawing process, and an additional 10 to 15 percent do not survive for 24 hours after transfusion [31]. Thus, even in a research setting, losses may be as high as 25 percent. One evaluation in a more routine operation showed higher losses, 20 and 25 percent, respectively, making the overall loss closer to 40 percent [32]. This is considered high by current standards. In addition, that study showed over 5 percent of units to be contaminated with bacteria, although transfusion of these did not cause obvious complications. About 3 percent of units are lost from causes other than outdating, mostly from mechanical failure in the cell processors or broken plastic [32]. One cannot escape the conclusion that red cell losses are too high for routine use of frozen red cells.

The washing associated with deglycerolization probably reduces the incidence of posttransfusion hepatitis [33], but does not eliminate it [34, 35].

A major logistic problem impeding the expansion of frozen red cell programs is the federal regulation that frozen-thawed red blood cells outdate 24 hours after the thawing and deglycerolization procedure. The concern is, of course, that these cells are processed in an open system and therefore have a high risk of bacterial contamination. There is a mounting body of evidence that a longer postthaw period may be safe, but federal regulations remain unchanged [36].

The washing associated with deglycerolization produces a product that has almost no white blood cells and less microaggregate debris. Because of this, the incidence of febrile transfusion reactions is decreased, as is the frequency of alloimmunization to HLA. Previously, the latter had been considered a major advantage in patients awaiting kidney transplantation, and large quantities of frozen-thawed red cells were used for such patients. Recent evidence has changed this view, and frozen-thawed red cells are now rarely used for patients in dialysis units.

The application of blood freezing procedures to rejuvenate (see p. 295) and freeze outdated red cells with high levels of 2,3-DPG has not become widely accepted [11].

The many advantages of a large-scale frozen red cell program are offset by several disadvantages. The first—a 24-hour postdeglycerolization expiration time—leads to serious logistic problems and the potential for high loss through outdating. The second is cost: The procedure requires a large investment in equipment, supplies, and labor, and doubles or triples the cost of a unit of red cells. One program, for example, would need five additional persons to process about 8,000 units per year [37]. For that blood bank, the cost of a unit of red blood cells would increase by 80 percent were only frozen red cells to be used. Finally, the time needed to thaw and deglycerolize a unit of red cells makes it impossible to deal effectively with emergent situations.

While we do not dispute the advantages of frozen-thawed red cells, serious cost-benefit considerations make it unlikely that national use will increase much beyond the current low level. The only absolute indication is the storage of rare-donor blood for immunized recipients. The rejuvenation and freezing of blood units that are about to outdate is possible, but has not been widely adopted. There may be some justification for the use of frozen-thawed red cells as a ready source of blood that is high in 2,3-DPG and probably free from the risk of CMV transmission, as is useful in transfusion of low–birth weight infants. Few other indications seem valid [38].

LEUKOCYTE-POOR RED CELLS

Leukocyte-poor red cells can be prepared by a number of methods including washing, filtration, or the use of reconstituted frozen red cells (Table 8–6). If filtration is used, it is usually necessary to chill and centrifuge units before filtration to obtain optimal results. When the ultimate in white cell removal is indicated, frozen-thawed red cells (see below) may be the product of choice, but these are unnecessary in most clinical circumstances [39].

Many transfusion reactions, particularly in patients who have had previous transfusions or a pregnancy, are caused by antibodies to donor leukocytes (see Chap. 7). Thus, reactions to leukocyte antibodies can usually be prevented by

Table 8-6. Efficiency of Various Methods for the Preparation of Leukocyte-Poor Red Blood Cells

Method	WBC Removed (%)	RBC Lost (%)
Reconstituted frozen red cells	91–97	5–15
Washing	90–93	10–13
Filtration	75–100	5–20

use of leukocyte-poor red blood cells. In most cases, reactions will be minimal or absent if the number of leukocytes in the donor unit is reduced to 10^9 or less [40]. We do not advocate the administration of leukocyte-poor red cells until patients have had at least two reactions, since most people who have one reaction will not have a second after transfusion of regular red cells [41].

A second indication for the transfusion of leukocyte-poor red cells is to reduce alloimmunization to donor HLA antigens. Because preformed HLA antibodies are associated with acute rejection of transplanted organs and because the prevalence of such antibodies is a function of the number of previous transfusions and their leukocyte content, it would seem logical to attempt to remove leukocytes and platelets from blood intended for patients awaiting organ transplant. In fact, this is not usually the case. In kidney transplantation, there is evidence that transfusion with leukocyte-containing components *improves* graft survival (see Chap. 3). In liver and heart transplantation, rejection has not been clearly shown to be caused by HLA antibodies, so that persons awaiting these organs need not receive leukocyte-poor transfusions. Only for patients awaiting bone marrow transplantation is there a reasonable indication for leukocyte-poor components, and this possibly only for those patients with aplastic anemia. Data are lacking as to whether leukocyte-poor components are of any value in marrow transplant candidates.

Clinicians may request leukocyte-poor red cells for patients with leukemia or lymphoma who are not bone marrow transplantation candidates in an attempt to prevent HLA alloimmunization [42]. There, as yet, is no evidence that leukocyte depletion of blood components is of value, probably because such patients are immunosuppressed and also receive many other leukocyte-containing components [43, 44].

Finally, leukocyte-poor red cells may be requested for immunosuppressed patients with the goal of preventing graft-versus-host disease. If this is to be achieved, it will be by irradiation of the components, because total leukocyte removal cannot be achieved by available methods (see Chap. 6).

In summary, we recommend leukocyte-poor red cells predominantly to prevent repeated febrile transfusion reactions, sometimes to prevent HLA alloimmunization before bone marrow transplantation, and for little else.

Table 8–7. IgA Concentrations of Blood Products*

Blood Product	IgA Concentration (gm/L)
Plasma Protein Fraction	0.254
Albumin (20%)	0.008
Immune Globulin—normal	6.695
Immune Globulin—anti-tetanus	4.150
Immune Globulin—anti-Rh(D)	4.860
Factor IX Complex	0.536
Factor VIII Concentrate	0.649
Washed red blood cells	0.00248
Frozen-thawed red cells	0.000117

*Modified from P. L. Yap, A. D. Pryde, D. B. L. McClelland. IgA content of frozen-thawed-washed red blood cells and blood products measured by radioimmunoassay. *Transfusion* 1982; 22:36–8. With permission.

Washed Red Cells

Washing of red cells is an effective way to remove leukocytes, platelets, microaggregate debris, and plasma. Using the proper conditions, it is possible to remove up to 90 percent of the leukocytes with a loss of about 10 to 15 percent of the red cells. Washed red cells avoid most febrile and allergic transfusion reactions and are well received by transfusionists because of their excellent flow characteristics. The extra cost and time involved in washing (compared with filtration methods) are difficult to justify unless there are specific reasons for *plasma* removal, for example, IgA deficiency [45]. Even washed red cells contain substantial amounts of IgA, so increased washing volumes or frozen-thawed red cells may be required for patients with IgA deficiency (Table 8–7).

Frozen-Thawed Red Blood Cells

Frozen-thawed red cells* are the best leukocyte and plasma-free preparation available, although the adequacy of leukocyte removal is related to the manner in which cells are washed and reconstituted [46]. During the freezing, thawing, and removal of the cryoprotective agent, almost all identifiable leukocytes are also removed.

Frozen-thawed red cells also have the advantage of a reduced risk of transmitting CMV infection [47]. For this reason, and because when frozen shortly after collection they have a high level of 2,3-DPG, they have been used for transfusion of newborn infants despite the cost and inconvenience (see Chap. 6).

*The official FDA term to be used for labeling this product is *Red Blood Cells Deglycerolized*, but we will use the term *frozen-thawed red cells* throughout this book.

Table 8-8. Plasma Products as Defined by the FDA

Proper Name	Method of Collection	Storage Temperature	Dating Period
Plasma	Separated from whole blood or by plasmapheresis	−18°C or colder	5 years
Fresh Frozen Plasma	Separated from whole blood and frozen solid within 6 hours	−18°C or colder	5 years
Liquid Plasma	Separated from whole blood within 26 days after phlebotomy (40 days, if CPDA-1 is used)	1–6°C	26 days from date of collection (40 days if CPDA-1 is used)
Source Plasma*	Plasmapheresis	−20°C if intended for manufacture into injectable products	10 years
Recovered Plasma*	Separated from whole blood	Not yet established by the FDA	Not yet established by the FDA

*Intended to be used only for further manufacturing.

Plasma and Plasma Products

Today, plasma, whether harvested from a single donation of whole blood or obtained by plasmapheresis, is almost always frozen promptly after collection and used later as fresh frozen plasma or as the starting material for processing into various blood derivatives. The FDA has given the various types of plasma specific names depending on the method of collection and storage and the intended use (Table 8–8). Some of these, e.g., fresh frozen plasma, are important blood components used daily in clinical practice, while others, e.g., recovered plasma, are intended only for further processing. Plasma is a valuable resource and should be prepared from as many blood donations as possible, hence the continued emphasis on red cell, rather than whole blood, transfusion in patients who do not need to receive plasma.

Plasma and Liquid Plasma

Plasma and Liquid Plasma are two blood components prepared by removing the plasma from a unit of whole blood at any time up to 5 days after its expiration date. If stored at −18°C or colder, the product is labeled *Plasma*; if stored at 1 to 6°C, it is called *Liquid Plasma*. Neither product has widespread clinical use, and it is rare for either to be seen in blood bank practice. Because of logistic difficulties, some blood banks prepare Plasma rather than Fresh Frozen Plasma and issue it in lieu of Fresh Frozen Plasma (see below), although levels of the labile coagulation factors V and VIII are lower. Both Liquid Plasma and Plasma are often shipped to fractionators to be used as starting materials for blood derivative production. Plasma is no longer recommended for use as a volume expander in blood loss or shock.

Fresh Frozen Plasma

Since the last edition of this book, there has been an unprecedented and, for the most part, unexplained increase in the use of fresh frozen plasma [48]. This profligate use, documented in several studies and recognized by all who prepare or issue blood components, has been ascribed by some to the decreased availability of whole blood and to the desire of physicians to reconstitute whole blood from red cells and fresh frozen plasma. Others have been unable to show this correlation, but almost everyone agrees that current patterns reflect overuse, with much of the plasma being given without appropriate indications. A 1984 Consensus Development Conference, sponsored by the National Institutes of Health, concluded that the dramatic increase had occurred despite a "... paucity of definitive indications for its use" [49].

Fresh Frozen Plasma is defined as plasma that has been separated from Whole Blood and frozen solid within 6 hours after phlebotomy. Federal regulations require that it be stored at −18°C or colder; the expiration date is 12 months from phlebotomy. These requirements ensure that fresh frozen plasma will have high levels of the labile coagulation factors V and VIII. Recent evidence suggests that relatively good yields of both Factor V and VIII can be obtained even if the plasma is frozen as late as 24 hours after phlebotomy [50]. Federal regulations, however, have not changed; to be labeled *Fresh Frozen Plasma*, the product must be frozen solid within 6 hours after phlebotomy. If there is a longer delay, it is known as *Plasma*.

Fresh frozen plasma must be thawed with agitation in a waterbath at 37°C. Because this procedure takes approximately 30 minutes and introduces the possibility of bacterial contamination, various workers have proposed that fresh frozen plasma may be thawed in a microwave oven. With current technology, this is not acceptable, since adequate thawing of the entire unit will almost surely produce hot spots and consequent protein denaturation in some areas [51]. Modified microwave ovens may be acceptable, but only when careful monitoring and experimental protocols are in effect [52]. *Fresh frozen plasma cannot be thawed safely in a regular microwave oven.*

To obtain the best yield of labile coagulation factors, fresh frozen plasma should be transfused as soon as possible after thawing. Storage for up to 24 hours at 1 to 6°C is acceptable, but not desirable [53].

Table 8-9. Indications for the Administration of Fresh Frozen Plasma

---

Bleeding or preparation for surgery in patients with deficiencies of coagulation proteins for which specific factor concentrates are unavailable or undesirable, e.g., factor XI

Bleeding or preparation for surgery in patients with multiple coagulation-protein deficiencies

Rapid reversal of coumarin-type drug effect

Antithrombin III deficiency in patients who are refractory to heparin

Protein-losing enteropathy in infants

Thrombotic thrombocytopenic purpura, usually in conjunction with plasma exchange

C1-esterase inhibitor deficiency in patients who have life-threatening edema

---

There are relatively few well-documented and universally accepted indications for fresh frozen plasma (Table 8-9), and most studies show that only a minor amount of the fresh frozen plasma produced is used for patients meeting the criteria. Most of it is given either to patients who have multiple coagulation-factor defects associated with liver disease but are not bleeding, or to patients who are receiving massive transfusion. In neither group is there adequate documentation of effectiveness.

Patients with severe liver disease have low levels of all vitamin K–dependent clotting proteins and almost always have prolonged prothrombin and partial thromboplastin times; abnormal bleeding is common, but this is usually gastrointestinal hemorrhage from bleeding varices rather than diffuse bleeding caused by the coagulopathy. In such patients, clinicians have a natural urge to attempt the restoration of normal *laboratory values* by administering fresh frozen plasma. But this product, given in any but massive doses, rarely has a measurable effect on the coagulopathy or on the bleeding, and its value is at best debatable.

If plasma is to be used at all, it should be given in adequate doses—at least four units in an adult—and its effects followed by measuring the prothrombin time or the partial thromboplastin time. Assuming a plasma volume of about 3,000 ml in an anemic man, five units of fresh frozen plasma (approximately 1,000 ml) are needed to raise circulating levels of any factor from zero to about 33 percent of normal. Since it is commonly agreed that levels above 30 percent are adequate in most cases, this dose should be effective. In our experience, it rarely is, and patients with liver disease usually continue to have abnormal laboratory test results and bleeding, despite the administration of fresh frozen plasma.

Similar considerations apply in massive transfusion, except that several studies have documented that fresh frozen plasma given prophylactically does not prevent the onset of abnormal bleeding [54, 55]. Massive blood replacement does lead to dilution of clotting factors, and replacement of these might help, at

Table 8–10. Characteristics of Microvascular Bleeding*

Bleeding from mucous membranes
Catheter site and puncture-wound bleeding, persisting after pressure
Continuous oozing from raw tissue
Generalized petechiae
Increasing size of ecchymoses

---

*Modified from R. L. Reed, D. Ciavarella, D. M. Heimbach, et al. Prophylactic platelet administration during massive transfusion: a prospective, randomized, double-blind clinical study. *Ann Surg* 1986; 203:40–8. With permission.

least in theory. Recommendations such as "2 or 3 units of fresh frozen plasma for every 10 to 15 units of whole blood or red blood cells" are widely quoted, but there is no evidence that these are valid. Recent studies advise the use of platelets, rather than fresh frozen plasma, in the microvascular bleeding (defined in Table 8–10) associated with massive trauma, and remind clinicians that each platelet transfusion is also a transfusion of 400 to 600 ml of plasma with some coagulation factors [56, 57].

In both liver disease and massive transfusion, fresh frozen plasma should be reserved for the treatment of *bleeding* associated with documented abnormalities of coagulation. There is no evidence that prophylactic treatment is useful except in anticipation of an invasive procedure.

Because of the tremendous increase in demand for fresh frozen plasma, several studies have reevaluated the levels of various coagulation proteins in plasma products prepared with less rigorous standards than those applied to fresh frozen plasma. For example, after storage at 4°C, levels of factor VIII* in plasma are 77 percent at 12 hours and 69 percent at 24 hours when compared to the 6-hour (100 percent) value [58]. Factor V is even less labile and remains at near 100 percent in plasma stored at 4°C for as long as 14 days. In another study, plasma from blood that had been held at 4°C for 18 to 20 hours before separation showed a 50 percent loss of factor VIII but no change in factor V [50]. Both studies suggest that plasma, rather than fresh frozen plasma, may be adequate for almost any patient, except one with disseminated intravascular coagulation, since factor VIII levels are almost never reduced to the point at which they become a problem in other patients.

SOURCE PLASMA

Source Plasma is plasma collected by plasmapheresis and intended for further manufacturing use. Specifics about the collection, testing, storage, and shipping of Source Plasma are contained in the U.S. Code of Federal Regulations.

---
*Values for factor VIII refer to factor VIII:C, the coagulant activity of the factor VIII molecule.

Blood Fractions or Derivatives

Blood fractions or *derivatives* (either term is acceptable) are prepared by large-scale processing of plasma using some combination of physical and chemical methods. About 75 percent of the 15 million liters of plasma used annually for the fractionation process is source plasma collected by plasmapheresis from paid donors. This plasma is pooled into batches of from 2,000 to 10,000 liters so that every derivative prepared from the pool includes contributions from many donors. A well-recognized hazard accompanying these large pool sizes is the transmission of infectious diseases, especially hepatitis and AIDS, by those derivatives that cannot be sterilized during processing (see Chap. 7).

Nearly all current fractionation methods depend on the selective precipitation of proteins from plasma mixed with cold ethanol as temperature and pH are changed. This approach is known as *Cohn fractionation*. In this process, 2,000 to 10,000 liters of plasma are pooled and treated sequentially in the cold with various concentrations of ethanol and buffers to precipitate fractions containing different plasma proteins.

Fibrinogen, or fraction I, the first material precipitated, is harvested at $-3°C$, in an 8 percent ethyl alcohol concentration at pH 7.2. After this precipitate is removed, the conditions are changed to $-5°C$, 25 percent ethyl alcohol, and pH 6.9, at which point fraction II plus III precipitates. This contains immunoglobulins, thrombin, prothrombin, and factor IX. Material harvested several steps later (fractions IV and V) contains albumin and about 12 percent alpha and beta globulins. Additional processing of this fraction leads to plasma protein fraction and albumin.

Plasma Protein Fraction

Plasma protein fraction (PPF), a useful plasma volume expander, is heat treated for 10 hours at 60°C to inactivate both the hepatitis viruses and HIV. The protein concentration is 5.0 ± 0.3 gm/dl, about 88 percent of which is albumin, some in the form of dimers or large polymers. The sodium concentration is 130 to 150 mEq/liter; there is less than 2 mEq/liter of potassium and some residual citrate [59]. Since anti-A and anti-B are not present, there is no risk of hemolysis when plasma protein fraction is used in recipients of groups A, B, or AB. At one time, hypotensive reactions were seen, especially when the material was administered rapidly. These appear to have been caused by increased prekallikrein activator and, because of this, manufacturers recommend that Plasma Protein Fraction be administered at a rate less than 10 ml per minute. All coagulation factors, including fibrinogen, are absent, so this fraction cannot be used to treat coagulation defects. Plasma Protein Fraction is commercially available from several manufacturers and may be stored at room temperature for 3 years.

Albumin

Albumin is prepared by the same methods as Plasma Protein Fraction but requires several additional purification steps. The final product is 96 percent albumin, some of which exists as dimers or other polymers. Stabilizers such as sodium acetyltryptophanate or sodium caprylate, or both, are present, and the sodium content is between 130 and 160 mEq/liter [59]. The term *salt-poor* was originally used to differentiate this material from an earlier product produced for the military and containing 300 mEq/liter of sodium, but that term is obsolete. Both 5 and 25 percent solutions of albumin are available. Albumin has many advantages over plasma, including freedom from risk of transmitting hepatitis, lack of blood group antibodies, and good storage stability. The 5 percent product is essentially iso-oncotic with plasma and can be used where blood volume expansion is indicated. The 25 percent solution has an albumin concentration about five times that of normal plasma; 100 ml of this is oncotically equivalent to 500 ml of plasma. With the 25 percent solution, a small-volume infusion may be used with little risk of circulatory overloading to treat hypoproteinemia or continued protein loss. Albumin is often used to treat extensive burns, pancreatitis, and, in selected patients, severe hypoalbuminemia.

Twenty-five percent albumin is a useful plasma volume expander in treatment of shock in patients who are not dehydrated. Its value in these patients depends on its oncotic effect, that is, a shift of fluid from extravascular spaces by means of high intravascular protein concentration. Thus, adequate hydration is essential when 25 percent albumin is employed to treat shock. In dehydration, there is little available extravascular fluid, so to be effective, the concentrated albumin must be administered with adequate amounts of supplemental fluid. In these cases, at least 500 ml of fluid such as saline or lactated Ringer's solution is required with each 100 ml of 25 percent albumin.

Albumin is said to be useful in erythroblastosis fetalis, since it binds bilirubin, and in so doing, should lessen the danger of kernicterus. Because of the small dose required, Albumin packaged in 25-ml vials can be used. Its effectiveness in this situation has not been impressive.

There has been much interest in the proper use of Albumin and Plasma Protein Fraction, caused, in part, by the rapidly increasing cost of medical care. Best estimates are that about 4 to 4.6 *million* liters of plasma were used in 1980 as starting material for the production of Albumin and Plasma Protein Fraction. The findings of a workshop on albumin use were summarized in two articles by Tullis [60]. He lists indications for appropriate or occasional use, uses requiring additional data, and uses that are unjustified (Table 8–11). Several studies have suggested that much Albumin and Plasma Protein Fraction are used inappropriately and thus contribute to the high cost of medical care without significant benefit to patients [61].

Table 8-11. Clinical Uses for Albumin Products*

Appropriate use
Shock
Burns
Adult respiratory distress syndrome
Pump prime for cardiopulmonary bypass
Hemolytic disease of the newborn
Plasma replacement in therapeutic plasmapheresis
Occasional use
Acute liver failure
Red cell resuspension medium
Ascites
Hypoproteinemia after surgery
Acute nephrosis
Renal dialysis
Use requiring additional data
Detoxification
Unjustified use
Undernutrition
Chronic nephrosis
Chronic cirrhosis

*Modified from J. L. Tullis. Albumin: 1. Background and use. 2. Guidelines for clinical use. *JAMA* 1977; 237:355–60 and 460–3. With permission.

Albumin is heat treated to inactivate viruses and can be given without risk of hepatitis or AIDS. Shelf life is from 2 to 5 years, depending on storage temperature and manufacturing process.

The gene for human albumin has been cloned, and a recombinant organism that produces albumin reported. There is no doubt that recombinant albumin can be produced, but many problems will have to be addressed before a recombinant product reaches the market [62]. Some of the problems are scientific, e.g., is the recombinant albumin truly identical with the natural product, and how will it function? Other problems are logistic, e.g., the estimated need for over 1.1×10^8 liters of culture and as much as 10 billion gallons of water per year to produce it [63]. Finally, there are economic considerations, since in Cohn fractionation, albumin, gamma globulin, and factor VIII are all harvested from the same starting plasma. A procedure that eliminates albumin as a revenue source would surely increase the cost of the other products. Recombinant albumin may be a reality, but its availability as a replacement product for the current product is doubtful.

IMMUNE GLOBULIN

Immune globulin, formerly known as gamma globulin or immune serum globulin, is the antibody-containing fraction of plasma [64]. The globulins can be separated from pooled plasma (fraction II of the Cohn process) and may be used prophylactically as replacement therapy in patients who have a deficiency of immunoglobulin, or therapeutically to treat a wide variety of conditions [65]. Immune globulin preparations are made for either intravenous or intramuscular use, but *the two are not interchangeable.* Specific immune globulins, such as Hepatitis B Immune Globulin and Rh Immune Globulin, are currently available in the United States only for intramuscular administration. Preparations of immune globulins for intramuscular use have generally been considered free from the risk of transmitting hepatitis B, even though they are prepared from large plasma pools prepared from many paid donations [66]. This has been ascribed partly to the presence of large amounts of anti-HBs in the product and partly to the small amount given by intramuscular injection. Recent widespread use of *intravenous* immune globulin in much larger doses has shown that it, unlike intramuscular IgG, may transmit non-A, non-B hepatitis [67].

Immune Globulin for Intramuscular Use

Immune globulin for intramuscular use is a 16.5 ± 1.5 percent solution of globulins containing $0.3\ M$ glycine as a preservative. It is tested to ensure that the FDA-required levels of antibodies for diphtheria, measles, and poliomyelitis are present and, although not specifically required to be present by regulation, almost always has adequate levels of antibodies against hepatitis A and B. Immune globulin is indicated for prophylaxis of hepatitis A and for the prevention or modification of measles. Since the introduction of the intravenous preparations, it is no longer used for replacement therapy in immunodeficient patients.

Immune Globulin for Intravenous Use

Several preparations of immune globulin for intravenous use are currently available. One contains 5 ± 1 percent protein stabilized with 10 ± 2 percent maltose and no preservatives. At least 90 percent of the protein is immunoglobulin. Another preparation is available as either a 3 or a 6 percent solution of protein of which 96 percent is immunoglobulin G. This is stabilized with 5 or 10 percent sucrose and also contains no preservatives. A third product is available as either a 2.5 or a 5.0 percent immunoglobulin solution.

These products are useful for maintenance therapy in immunodeficient patients and for patients with idiopathic thrombocytopenic purpura (ITP) [68]. In the latter condition, a dose of 0.4 gm/kg on 5 consecutive days is recommended, but lower doses may be adequate [69, 70]. In ITP, a beneficial effect is seen more frequently in children than in adults, but is often transient. Hence, it is most widely used in the management of acute situations and is of little, if any, value in long-term therapy. One disadvantage of intravenous gamma globulin is cost; a 5-day course for an adult costs approximately $6,000 in 1987.

Because of its effectiveness in ITP, intravenous gamma globulin has been tried in thrombocytopenic patients who are refractory to platelet transfusions. Although there have been occasional reports of success [71, 72], other evaluations have found it to be of no value [73]. We, too, have had little success and do not advise this extremely expensive therapy for refractory patients.

Immune Globulin Containing Specific Antibodies

Immune globulin products prepared from patients with high titers of particular antibodies, or from the serum of immunized animals, are useful in modifying the appropriate diseases. Some licensed immune globulin preparation used in the treatment, modification, or prevention of selected diseases are the following:

1. Rabies Immune Globulin
2. Lymphocyte Immune Globulin, Anti-Thymocyte Globulin
3. Pertussis Immune Globulin
4. $Rh_O(D)$ Immune Globulin
5. Tetanus Immune Globulin
6. Vaccinia Immune Globulin
7. Varicella-Zoster Immune Globulin
8. Hepatitis B Immune Globulin

Hepatitis B Immune Globulin is prepared from donors with high titers of anti-HBs and, when given to anti-HBs-negative persons exposed to hepatitis B, modifies the disease. Hepatitis B Immune Globulin is indicated in laboratory accidents where persons have been exposed to hepatitis B virus through cuts or needlesticks. The recommended dose in such cases is 0.06 ml per kilogram as soon as possible after exposure and within 24 hours if possible. At the same time, hepatitis B vaccination should be initiated. Both are also indicated in newborn infants whose mothers are HBsAg positive. The latest recommendations of the Immunization Practices Advisory Committee are published in the Morbidity and Mortality Weekly Report and should be followed [74].

Lymphocyte Immune Globulin, also known as anti-thymocyte globulin or ATG, is prepared from the serum of rabbits, goats, or horses immunized with cultured human lymphoblasts. It is used to enhance acceptance of allografted tissues in humans. Despite careful absorption of the product with human red cell stroma, various red cell–related antibodies remain, and patients who are treated with Lymphocyte Immune Globulin often have positive direct or indirect antiglobulin tests [75].

Rh Immune Globulin (RhIG) is prepared from donors with high titers of anti-Rh and is used to prevent Rh-negative persons from being immunized to Rh.

Rh-negative women, either during pregnancy or immediately after the delivery of an Rh-positive child, are candidates for RhIG therapy (see Chap. 9). RhIG can also be used in other individuals who are exposed to Rh-positive red cells and in whom it is appropriate to attempt to prevent Rh immunization. The most common circumstances in which such exposure occurs is when Rh-negative persons are transfused with Rh-positive platelets. While the platelets themselves do not have Rh antigens, almost all preparations of platelet concentrate contain some red cells and are, therefore, potentially immunogenic. Although the potential does exist, Rh immunization from platelet transfusion rarely occurs—probaby because most platelet recipients are immunosuppressed [76]. As a result, we do not advocate *routine* administration of RhIG to all Rh-negative persons who receive Rh-positive platelets, but suggest that each case be evaluated individually. In girls or in women of childbearing age or younger, even those who appear to be immunosuppressed, RhIG is appropriate. In the case of older women, men, or boys, RhIG is not usually necessary. The reasons to avoid a blanket recommendation for RhIG in all Rh-negative persons who receive Rh positive platelets are (1) cost, (2) waste of valuable material, and (3) possible confusion in subsequent serologic testing from the passively acquired anti-Rh.

Rh immunization has seldom been reported after the administration of Rh-positive fresh frozen plasma to an Rh-negative patient; the likelihood of immunization in such cases is so low that we do not advise RhIG.

A single dose of RhIG (approximately 300 micrograms) is adequate to prevent immunization after transfusion of 15 to 20 ml of Rh-positive red blood cells [77]. The material is taken up rapidly after intramuscular injection and can usually be detected circulating in plasma within 24 hours [78]. The half-disappearance time of intramuscular RhIG is about 21 to 24 days, the same as normal immunoglobulin [79].

RhIG has been used to attempt to prevent immunization after the administration of Rh-positive transfusions to Rh-negative recipients. Doses of 20 to 25 micrograms of RhIG per milliliter of Rh-positive red blood cells are suggested, but often require the intramuscular injection of large volumes of material. RhIG prepared for intravenous administration would be advantageous in such cases, but is not currently available in the United States.

DERIVATIVES AND COMPONENTS FOR THE TREATMENT
OF CLOTTING FACTOR DEFICIENCIES

At least 14 factors are involved in the coagulation of shed blood. Most are also needed for normal hemostasis in vivo, and a deficiency of any one (except factors IV and XII) may lead to hemorrhagic disease (Table 8–12). When this happens, treatment with plasma components or the specific factor itself may be required. The various deficiencies and the appropriate modes of replacement therapy are listed in Tables 8–12 and 8–13. Deficiencies of factors II, V, VII,

Table 8-12. Half-Life of Important Blood Coagulation Factors

Factor	Name	Estimated Half-Life		
		In vivo	In vitro, 4°C	In vitro, −20°C to −30°C
—	Platelets	4 days	24–48 hours**	—
I	Fibrinogen	3–6 days	Years	Years
II	Prothrombin	3 days	—	—
V	Labile factor, Proaccelerin	12–36 hours	10–14 days	6 months*
VII	Stable factor	1–7 hours	>21 days*	>6 months*
VIII	Anti-hemophilic factor	8–12 hours	7 days	>6 months*
IX	Plasma thromboplastin component	12–14 hours	>21 days	>6 months
X	Stuart-Prower factor	30–50 hours	—	—
XI	Plasma thromboplastin antecedent	48–77 hours	3–4 days	—
XIII	Fibrin-stabilizing factor	3–12 days	—	—
AT III	Antithrombin III	17–76 hours	>42 days	—

*These estimates, which are based on clinical studies, have not been confirmed by detailed laboratory studies.
**Can be stored five days or more at 20 to 24°C.

and X are listed together as prothrombin complex deficiencies because they are related, and because deficiencies of any or all of them are often manifested by prolonged prothrombin or partial thromboplastin times. These abnormalities are common in severe liver disease and, except for factor V, in patients taking warfarin.

Cryoprecipitate

When fresh frozen plasma is thawed in the cold, a white gelatinous precipitate forms. This material contains large quantities of factor VIII and fibrinogen, and can be harvested for the treatment of hemophilia. The method is adaptable to most blood banks, but careful attention to detail is important if optimum yields are to be obtained. Triple plastic containers allow the preparation of red blood cells, cryoprecipitate, and plasma from one blood donation, all in a closed system. Cryoprecipitate preparation, which can be done any time after the plasma has been completely frozen, begins by thawing the plasma at 4°C. This usually takes 12 to 14 hours, after which time the cryoprecipitate can be administered or, if not immediately needed, can be refrozen under conditions similar to those used for fresh frozen plasma.

Table 8–13. Components and Derivatives Used to Treat Coagulation Factor Deficiencies

Disease or Condition	Component	Derivative	Desired Therapeutic Goal or Factor Level	Usual Product of Choice
Hypofibrinogenemia	Cryoprecipitate		100 mg/dl	Cryoprecipitate
Prothrombin deficiency (II)	Fresh Frozen Plasma, Plasma	Factor IX Complex	10–40%	Fresh Frozen Plasma
Factor V deficiency	Fresh Frozen Plasma		10–25%	Fresh Frozen Plasma
Factor VII deficiency	Fresh Frozen Plasma, Plasma	Factor IX Complex	10–20%	Fresh Frozen Plasma
Factor VIII deficiency	Cryoprecipitate	Antihemophilic factor	30–50%	Antihemophilic Factor
Factor VIII deficiency with factor VIII antibodies		Anti-Inhibitor Coagulant Complex	Control bleeding	Anti-Inhibitor Coagulant Complex
Factor IX deficiency	Fresh Frozen Plasma, Liquid Plasma, Plasma	Factor IX Complex	30–50%	Factor IX Complex
Factor X deficiency	Fresh Frozen Plasma, Plasma	Factor IX Complex	15–20%	Fresh Frozen Plasma
Factor XI deficiency	Plasma, Liquid Plasma, Fresh Frozen Plasma		Control bleeding 30–50%* Factor XI level	Plasma or Fresh Frozen Plasma
Factor XIII deficiency†	Plasma, cryoprecipitate		5%	Plasma
Liver disease with bleeding or for surgery	Fresh Frozen Plasma		Control bleeding	Fresh Frozen Plasma
Warfarin overdose (acute)	Fresh Frozen Plasma		Control bleeding, normal prothrombin time	Fresh Frozen Plasma
DIC	Fresh Frozen Plasma, Cryoprecipitate‡		Control bleeding	Components usually ineffective unless DIC is reversed
von Willebrand's disease	Cryoprecipitate, Fresh Frozen Plasma		Normal bleeding time Factor VIII > 50%	Cryoprecipitate

*Individual response variable.
†Derivative concentrate available for experimental use.
‡Platelets may also be indicated.
DIC = disseminated intravascular coagulation.

When needed for transfusion, cryoprecipitate is thawed at 37°C and mixed. The material is infused through a transfusion set or injected with a syringe and a special infusion set containing a small filter. The factor VIII in cryoprecipitate is highly concentrated, and the bags must be emptied completely and the transfusion equipment washed out with saline to avoid losing significant amounts of factor VIII. Once the cryoprecipitate is thawed, the factor VIII activity is stable for about 24 hours, provided the material is stored at room temperature. Fibrinogen is stable for a much longer period.

Cryoprecipitate is also used as a source of fibrinogen, since each bag contains about 250 mg. Although fibrinogen can be prepared by Cohn fractionation, frequent contamination with hepatitis virus resulted in its removal from the market. When fibrinogen is required, we advise treatment with cryoprecipitate. If doses of 4 to 6 gm are indicated, it will be necessary to use as many as 16 to 24 bags of cryoprecipitate. The volume of this infusion is between 150 and 250 ml.

The factor VIII activity of cryoprecipitate per gram of protein is 12 to 60 times that present in fresh normal plasma. There is some protein loss in the conversion of fresh frozen plasma to cryoprecipitate, so the total amount of factor VIII in cryoprecipitate is about 50 to 70 percent of what was present in the original plasma. Anti-A and anti-B are present in cryoprecipitate, but are not concentrated. ABO-compatible cryoprecipitate is preferable, but ABO-incompatible material can be administered safely. Infectious diseases can be transmitted by cryoprecipitate.

Dosage schedules for factor VIII replacement are discussed on pages 322 through 323 and apply to both AHF concentrate and cryoprecipitate. Each bag of cryoprecipitate contains 80 to 100 units of factor VIII.

Cryoprecipitate is the therapy of choice for patients with von Willebrand's disease who are bleeding or being prepared for invasive procedures (see p. 326).

Cryoprecipitate has been reported to shorten the bleeding time and to control "major bleeding disorders" in patients with uremia [80]. These observations are unconfirmed, but have led many clinicians to use cryoprecipitate for such indications. The dose in adults is the content of 10 bags infused over 30 minutes.

Cryoprecipitate is also used as a source of *fibronectin,* the protein also known as *cold insoluble globulin.* Clinical interest in fibronectin stems from its role as an opsonic protein and the possibility that the reduced levels of fibronectin seen in some patients with surgical and traumatic shock, burns, malignancy, and similar illnesses may be deleterious [81]. There are reports that the administration of fibronectin in the form of cryoprecipitate had a beneficial effect in some patients. There is a large literature on this subject, well summarized by Snyder and Luban [82]. Occasional reports suggest benefit; others show no effect, but few of the studies have been controlled or randomized. We believe that current evidence is inadequate to justify the use of cryoprecipitate for its content of fibronectin in any but research settings.

Fibronectin is stable for up to 40 days at 1 to 6°C in whole blood and in unfrozen donor plasma and is well maintained in platelet concentrates stored for 3 to 5 days at room temperature [83]. In cryoprecipitate, the level of fibronectin is 4 mg/ml, an approximate tenfold increase over the levels of plasma.

Recently, cryoprecipitate has become popular with surgeons as a source of fibrinogen for the preparation of "fibrin glue." The combination of cryoprecipitate and topical thrombin produces a glue-like substance that is applied directly to bleeding sites. Excellent control of bleeding has been reported. The "glue" is prepared by mixing equal volumes of topical thrombin (1,000 units/ml) and cryoprecipitate; amounts of from 2 to 20 ml of final mixture have been used [84].

Antihemophilic Factor

Antihemophilic Factor, also known as Factor VIII Concentrate, is the derivative most often used for the treatment of patients with classic hemophilia. Replacement therapy is indicated for bleeding, for surgery, and at times, for prophylaxis. Usually, therapy is accomplished with a commercially prepared blood derivative, i.e., Antihemophilic Factor, although cryoprecipitate has some place in the management of factor VIII–deficient patients. As a rule, therapy is required to control major bleeding episodes, including hemorrhage into joints or muscles. The goal of treatment is to stop the bleeding; this usually requires enough AHF to raise the circulating level of factor VIII to about 30 percent of normal for surgery or major hemorrhage and to about 15 percent of normal for spontaneous bleeding into joints [85, 86].

A unit of factor VIII has been defined arbitrarily as the average amount of factor VIII in 1 ml of fresh, anticoagulated (1:9 dilution) plasma; all blood products for the treatment of hemophilia refer to this standard when describing the amount present. Levels in normal persons vary from 50 to 200 percent of an average or mean value; hence, a normal donor may have plasma levels of from 0.5 to 2 units per milliliter.

Antihemophilic factor is prepared commercially from large batches of fresh frozen plasma, about 75 percent of which is collected by plasmapheresis of paid donors. Because these concentrates have high factor VIII activity relative to their protein content, it is possible to administer sufficient factor VIII to control or prevent hemorrhage and to do this for long periods. AHF is used to treat joint or tissue hemorrhage after trauma, and to allow elective surgery. Prophylactic treatment is now widely prescribed, so that many hemophiliac patients lead more normal lives. The benefits from the widespread availability of antihemophilic concentrates have been so great that patients with hemophilia now reach adulthood and maturity.

The concentrates are supplied in lyophilized (freeze-dried) form, with the content in AHF units listed on each vial. Most concentrates contain between 200 and 400 units per vial and are intended to be diluted in 10 to 25 ml of diluent. Because of the high protein content, manufacturer's directions about mixing should be followed carefully to avoid foaming and failure of the concentrate to dissolve. Concentrates with higher specific activity, available at higher cost, are indicated when large doses over long periods are needed for surgery, severe trauma, or major hemorrhages. Hemolytic anemia due to anti-A in the concentrate has been a reported complication [87].

The increased use of large doses of factor VIII, particularly in the form of antihemophilic factor concentrate, has brought about a new awareness of the high frequency of liver disease in hemophiliacs [88]. The etiology is not clear, although the most reasonable possibility is increased exposure to hepatitis from multiple infusions of blood products, particularly those prepared from large donor pools. Because of the risk of contracting non-A, non-B hepatitis or AIDS from antihemophilic factor, all products currently on the market in the United States are heat treated. This treatment appears to inactivate HIV, but does not eliminate the risk of non-A, non-B hepatitis [89, 90]. (See Addenda.)

A second complication is the development of factor VIII inhibitors. These inhibitors are antibodies that react with and neutralize the infused factor VIII. As with hepatitis, their incidence seems at least partly related to increased exposure to factor VIII in the form of concentrate.

Patients with these antibodies are either "high responders" or "low responders," indicating that some patients make antibodies that are low in titer and others make antibodies that are present in high titer and difficult or impossible to neutralize. The management of patients with factor VIII antibodies, particularly the high responders, is difficult. When serious bleeding threatens or occurs, it can tax the resources of any blood bank. In the case of minor hemorrhage, replacement therapy should be withheld, since the infusion of factor VIII is almost inevitably followed by a rise in inhibitor titer. If treatment is essential, patients with relatively low titers of inhibitor (below 10 Bethesda units) can be given massive doses of antihemophilic factor in an attempt to neutralize the inhibitor. This is often possible in low responders but difficult or impossible in high responders, in whom a trial of activated factor IX concentrate, officially known as *Anti-Inhibitor Coagulant Complex,* may be warranted [91]. This concentrate is often effective because it contains activated coagulation factors that bypass the need for factor VIII itself. An anamnestic rise in inhibitor may be seen [92].

Antihemophilic factor from pigs has been used, both with and without plasmapheresis, to treat patients with factor VIII inhibitors [93]. Porcine AHF is highly immunogenic and can be used for only a short time before the patient develops antibodies against foreign proteins and has severe reactions. At times, however, porcine AHF may be lifesaving.

Factor IX Complex

Factor IX Complex is used to treat bleeding in patients who have hemophilia B, a hereditary deficiency of factor IX [94]. These patients have a clinical course and inheritance pattern that may be indistinguishable from those of classic hemophilia (factor VIII deficiency), hence, laboratory tests are needed to differentiate the two. The in vivo half-life of factor IX is about 18 to 36 hours, which means that treatment may have to be given two or three times a day if abnormal bleeding is to be controlled. The in vivo levels required to control hemorrhage are similar to those needed for the treatment of classic hemophilia. Factor IX is well preserved in ACD plasma at 4°C; almost all the original activity remains after 21 days of storage at this temperature. It is also stable at −20°C, and plasma frozen for 6 months loses only about 16 percent of its original factor IX activity [95]. Because of this, plasma up to 4 weeks old, fresh frozen plasma, and plasma from which the cryoprecipitate has been removed are all suitable therapeutic agents, but most patients who have abnormal bleeding or require surgery are treated with the Factor IX Complex available from several commercial sources. Antihemophilic Factor concentrates, intended for use in classic hemophilia, are devoid of factor IX activity and are of no value in patients with factor IX deficiency.

Techniques for the preparation of concentrated factor IX take advantage of the fact that factor IX can be adsorbed to and eluted from various chemicals such as tricalcium phosphate, barium sulfate, diethylaminoethyl (DEAE) cellulose, DEAE Sephadex, and aluminum hydroxide. When factor IX is prepared by such a process, the other vitamin K–dependent proteins, including factors II, VII, and X, are also concentrated. The factor IX content varies according to the manufacturing process. In addition to factors II, VII, IX, and X, some concentrates also contain measurable amounts of protein C (see p. 326). An experimental preparation of factor IX, essentially free from factors II, VII, and X, has been described, but products currently available all contain factors II, VII, IX, and X.

Because Factor IX Complex contains measurable amounts of factors II, VII, and X, it can be used to treat deficiencies of these coagulation proteins, and will reverse the effects of coumarin-type anticoagulants. Except for unusual circumstances, however, these conditions are better treated with coumarin antagonists such as vitamin K_1. Fresh frozen plasma can be used in emergency situations if rapid reversal of the coumarin effect is essential.

Hepatitis and disseminated intravascular coagulation are two serious and occasionally fatal complications of factor IX treatment [96, 97]. Because of the risk of these, Factor IX Complex should be used only for factor IX–deficient patients or when bleeding accompanies a *well-documented* deficiency of factor II, VII, or X. In the latter group, fresh frozen plasma is preferable if the patient can tolerate the amount required to control bleeding. Factor IX Complex is not

Von Willebrand's Disease

Von Willebrand's disease is characterized by a long bleeding time, deficient factor VIII, and an abnormality of platelet adhesiveness [99]. Both males and females are victims, and the disease appears to be inherited as an autosomal dominant. Treatment with fresh frozen plasma or with cryoprecipitate usually corrects the laboratory abnormalities and stops abnormal bleeding. Other concentrates of factor VIII are not effective and should not be used. Eight to ten bags of cryoprecipitate, given early in the course of bleeding, are reported to be an effective dose in an adult [100]. The deficiency of factor VIII is easier to correct than is the abnormal bleeding time, and infusions of fresh frozen plasma or cryoprecipitate will regularly raise the factor VIII level. The rise in the patient's factor VIII level is, in fact, greater than can be accounted for by the amount of factor VIII in the infused component (Fig. 8-3). This is because those components also contain a factor that stimulates the endogenous production of factor VIII.

Factor XI Deficiency

Deficiency of factor XI is, at times, associated with a bleeding tendency. The disease is inherited as an autosomal characteristic and is seen in male and female patients. Spontaneous bleeding is not a problem, and hemorrhage after surgery or dental extractions occurs only in major factor XI deficiency. Factor XI is labile during blood bank storage; half the original activity is lost after 3 or 4 days at 4°C, and transfused factor XI leaves the circulation with a half-life of approximately 40 to 80 hours [101]. Plasma or fresh frozen plasma is appropriate for transfusion therapy in this disease, one recommended dose being 10 to 20 ml per kilogram of body weight every 10 to 12 hours.

Deficiencies of Antithrombin III and Protein C

At least three proteins, antithrombin III, protein C, and protein S are potent anticoagulants required for the normal inhibition of intravascular clotting throughout the body. Deficiencies of any of these may be hereditary or acquired and can lead to intravascular thrombosis. Patients who have severe trauma and receive massive transfusion often have low levels of antithrombin III, but its clinical significance is unknown [102].

The role of replacement therapy in any of these deficiency states is not established. Antithrombin III is well preserved in stored whole blood, in fresh frozen plasma, and in cryoprecipitate-depleted plasma, so that stored and fresh frozen plasma are equally effective in the treatment of antithrombin III deficiency [103, 104]. A heat-treated concentrate of antithrombin III is under clinical investigation.

Table 8–14. Clinical Conditions Associated with Disseminated Intravascular Coagulation (DIC)

Acute DIC
    Amniotic fluid embolism
    Premature separation of placenta
    Sepsis
    Acute intravascular hemolytic event
    Fat embolism
    Snakebite with systemic absorption of venom
    Anaphylaxis
    Heat stroke
    Traumatic shock
    Massive brain injury

Chronic DIC
    Malignancy (adenocarcinomas)
    Eclampsia (possibly)
    Hepatic disease (rare)
    Intrauterine retention of dead fetus
    Infectious diseases
    Localized endothelial abnormalities
    Leukemia, especially promyelocytic

---

indicated for hemorrhage associated with severe liver disease or open-heart surgery.

OTHER HEMORRHAGIC CONDITIONS THAT ARE TREATED WITH BLOOD COMPONENTS

Disseminated Intravascular Coagulation

Disseminated intravascular coagulation (DIC) is a complex disorder that occurs when coagulation factors or platelets are consumed by widespread and uncontrolled clotting within the vascular system [98]. It is seen in many conditions including shock, major trauma, and sepsis (Table 8–14) and is generally controlled only after the initiating disease process is reversed. Physicians who treat such patients often prescribe large amounts of fresh frozen plasma and platelets in an attempt—usually futile—to reverse the bleeding tendency. Although there is little evidence that such aggressive therapy helps unless the underlying condition is corrected, it is difficult not to issue these components when there is active bleeding. In chronic DIC or in the absence of significant hemorrhage, component therapy given in an attempt to return abnormal laboratory values to normal is useless.

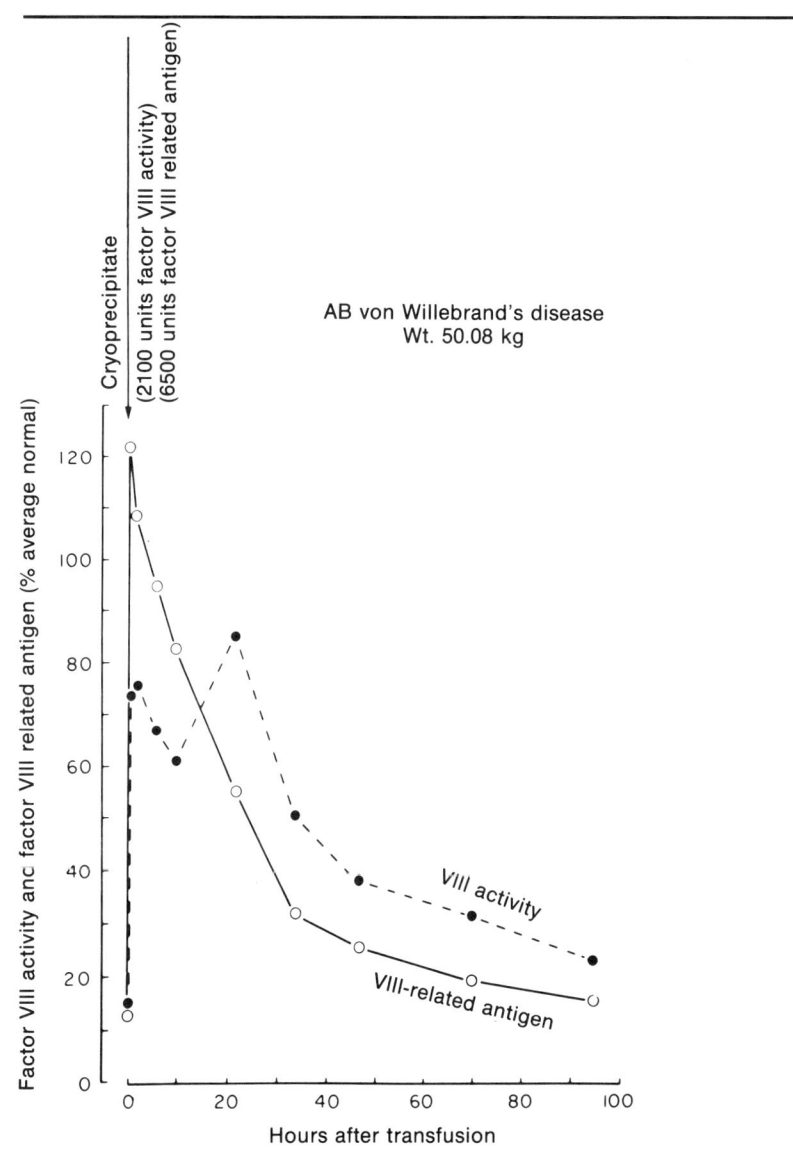

Figure 8–3
Transfusion response in a patient with von Willebrand's disease after treatment with cryoprecipitate. Note that the rise in factor VIII activity is greater and more persistent than expected from the administered dose of factor VIII. (From R. Biggs, D. R. Rizza (eds). *Human Blood Coagulation, Hemostasis and Thrombosis*. Oxford, England: Blackwell Sci, 1984. With permission.)

Platelets

Normal platelets are required for adequate hemostasis, and severe thrombocytopenia is almost always associated with a bleeding tendency.

The normal platelet count is between 150,000 and 300,000 per cubic millimeter. Abnormal bleeding almost always occurs in *severe* thrombocytopenia, and a correlation exists between the platelet count and the onset or severity of bleeding. There is, however, no absolute threshold or critical value of platelet count below which bleeding always occurs. When the platelet count is above 50,000 per cubic millimeter, bleeding is uncommon, and most patients can withstand a major stress such as surgery. Platelet levels between 10,000 and 50,000 per cubic millimeter are adequate to prevent spontaneous bleeding, but may not be sufficient in trauma or for surgery. Bleeding is usually evident in patients with platelet counts below 10,000 per cubic millimeter and, in most cases, is a serious threat.

The clinical correlation given above is approximate. It varies from patient to patient, or even from day to day in a single patient. Platelet counts, particularly in the low ranges, are relatively inaccurate and must be interpreted in this light. In addition, many factors besides the platelet count influence whether patients with thrombocytopenia will bleed abnormally. Some factors influencing bleeding in thrombocytopenic patients are the following:

1. Platelet count
    a. Below 10,000 per cubic millimeter: high risk
    b. 10,000 to 50,000 per cubic millimeter: moderate to low risk
    c. Above 50,000 per cubic millimeter: almost no risk
2. Age of circulating platelets: young platelets function better than old ones
3. Rapidity of onset of thrombocytopenia
4. Steroid therapy
5. Coagulation factor deficiencies
6. Medication such as aspirin

For example, it is common for patients with chronic idiopathic thrombocytopenic purpura, especially while being treated with adrenal steroids, to tolerate very low platelet counts without noteworthy bleeding. Conversely, hemorrhage from thrombocytopenia can be seen at far higher platelet counts in patients who have an abrupt onset of thrombocytopenia.

COLLECTION

Platelets can be obtained from a unit of whole blood collected into any of the currently licensed anticoagulant-preservative solutions. The platelets are harvested by centrifugation of the whole blood at a relatively low g force, removal of the platelet-rich plasma, and concentration of the platelets by a second centrifugation at a higher g force, followed by removal of most of the supernatant plasma. These platelets, often known as a unit of *random-donor platelets*, usually contain from 6 to 8 × 10^{10} platelets per bag, although federal regulations require only that ". . . 75 percent of the units tested contain not less than 5.5 × 10^{10} platelets." That value is an absolute minimum, and careful attention to details during collection and processing should produce a product with at least 6.5 × 10^{10} platelets per unit [105]. These platelets must be suspended in sufficient plasma—usually about 50 ml—to maintain a pH of 6.0 or greater throughout the storage period.

Platelets can also be collected by platelet apheresis procedures. Such preparations contain 3 to 6 × 10^{11} platelets in approximately 200 ml of plasma per bag.

STORAGE

Platelets that have been collected and processed in a closed system can be stored for 5 days. Early differences of opinion about optimal storage temperature have been resolved, and 20 to 24°C is the accepted storage temperature. While some transfusion services store platelets at "room temperature," this approach is adequate only if platelet temperature is maintained between 20 and 24°C. Temperatures below 20°C during platelet preparation and storage cause a striking increase in the number of large aggregates in the platelet concentrates.

The storage time of platelets has been extended beyond the original 3 days because newer plastic containers allow enhanced transfer of CO_2 from the container, and thus delay the fall in pH that is damaging to platelets [106]. The function of such stored platelets is adequate, but there is some evidence that these longer storage periods may be slightly deleterious [107].

Of greater concern, however, is the potential for bacterial growth during prolonged room-temperature storage. This was first noted with 3-day stored platelets. With the longer permissible storage period, it has surfaced as an even greater problem involving several deaths [108, 109]. Federal regulations, which formerly allowed 7 days of storage at 22 to 24°C, have now been modified to allow only 5 days of storage.

During storage, platelets must be subjected to constant, *gentle* agitation. The method of agitation is important in ensuring proper function, especially with longer storage times. Elliptical rotators may not be suitable for platelets stored in PL-732 plastic, and some flat-bed agitators may be less satisfactory than others for platelets in CLX plastic [110].

Platelets can be frozen for subsequent infusion, although protocols in current use are experimental and involve significant platelet loss. Frozen autologous platelets have been used in patients with leukemia who are undergoing intensive chemotherapy. Platelets harvested by platelet apheresis while the illness is in remission are stored frozen until needed later in the treatment. This approach seems to have promise for large cancer centers, but is of little practical use in average settings [111].

TRANSFUSION

Platelet transfusions are indicated in patients with severe thrombocytopenia and significant bleeding—for example, in leukemia and lymphoma, after cancer chemotherapy, or in bone marrow depression from drugs or irradiation. They may also be of value in *preventing* hemorrhage when given to some patients with extremely low platelet counts. They are seldom indicated for patients with idiopathic thrombocytopenic purpura, in whom circulating antibody usually destroys transfused platelets in a few minutes or hours. In these patients, even large transfusions are of little or no value. Splenectomy is often done in ITP, and preoperative transfusion with platelets has been advocated, but most patients with ITP can undergo splenectomy without platelet transfusions.

Several studies have addressed the specific platelet levels at which thrombocytopenic bleeding occurs. As far back as 1960, Raccuglia and Bethell showed a correlation between platelet count and hemorrhage [112]. In that study, most thrombocytopenic patients did not have clinical bleeding, and those who did usually had platelet counts below 20,000 per cubic millimeter. In patients with acute leukemia, visible bleeding is related to thrombocytopenia, and platelet levels above 10,000 per cubic millimeter are associated with a reduced risk of hemorrhage. There is an inverse relation between bleeding time and platelet count, and stool blood loss increases when the platelet count falls below 10,000 per cubic millimeter [113, 114]. While it is impossible to select an arbitrary level at which platelet transfusions are indicated, especially those given prophylactically, it seems reasonable to attempt to maintain platelet counts above 10,000 per cubic millimeter in patients with drug-induced marrow aplasia.

The dose of platelets required depends on the patient's size, and on the presence of splenomegaly, fever, sepsis, platelet antibodies, and other variables.

The response to platelet transfusions is best expressed in terms of the rise in platelet count per square meter of body surface area, in order to make the evaluation independent of blood volume and comparable from one individual to another. One useful guideline is to calculate a *corrected count increment* 1 to 2 hours after infusion using the following formula:

$$\text{Corrected count increment} = \frac{(\text{Postcount} - \text{Precount}) \times \text{Body surface area}}{\text{Number of platelets infused (in terms of } 10^{11})}$$

In this formula, the pre- and postcounts are in terms of platelets per cubic millimeter, the body surface area is in square meters (Figs. 8–4 and 8–5) and the number of platelets infused is in 10^{11} platelets. An example is shown in Table 8–15. Expected corrected count increments are between 10,000 and 20,000 per cubic millimeter 1 to 2 hours after infusion. Repeated poor responses suggest that the patient is in a refractory state.

Body Surface of Adults
Nomogram for determination of body surface from height and mass

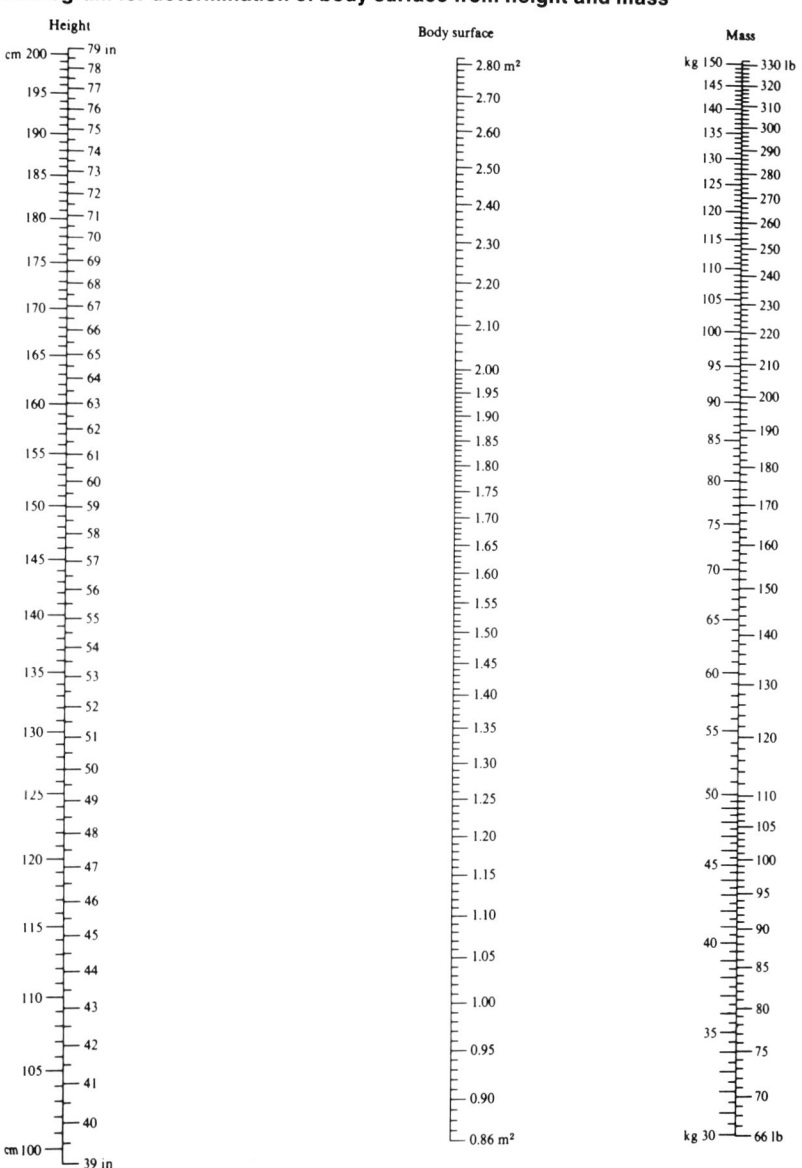

Height	Body surface	Mass
cm 200 – 79 in	2.80 m²	kg 150 – 330 lb
195 – 77, 78	2.70	145 – 320
190 – 75, 76	2.60	140 – 310
185 – 73, 74	2.50	135 – 300, 290
180 – 71, 72	2.40	130 – 280
175 – 69, 70	2.30	125 – 270, 260
170 – 67, 68	2.20	120 – 250
165 – 65, 66	2.10	115 – 240
160 – 63, 64	2.00, 1.95	110 – 230
155 – 61, 62	1.90, 1.85	105 – 220
150 – 59, 60	1.80, 1.75	100 – 210
145 – 57, 58	1.70, 1.65	95 – 200
140 – 55, 56	1.60, 1.55	90 – 190
135 – 53, 54	1.50, 1.45	85 – 180
130 – 51, 52	1.40, 1.35	80 – 170
125 – 49, 50	1.30, 1.25	75 – 160
120 – 47, 48	1.20, 1.15	70 – 150
115 – 45, 46	1.10, 1.05	65 – 140
110 – 43, 44	1.00	60 – 130
105 – 41, 42	0.95	55 – 120
	0.90	50 – 110, 105
cm 100 – 39 in	0.86 m²	45 – 100, 95
		40 – 90, 85
		35 – 80, 75
		kg 30 – 66 lb, 70

Figure 8–4
A line connecting the body weight (on the right) with the height (on the left) will intersect the central line at a point corresponding to the person's body surface area. (From *Geigy Scientific Tables*. With permission. Courtesy of Ciba-Geigy Limited, Basel, Switzerland.)

332 8. Blood Components, Fractions, and Derivatives

Body Surface of Children

Nomogram for determination of body surface from height and mass

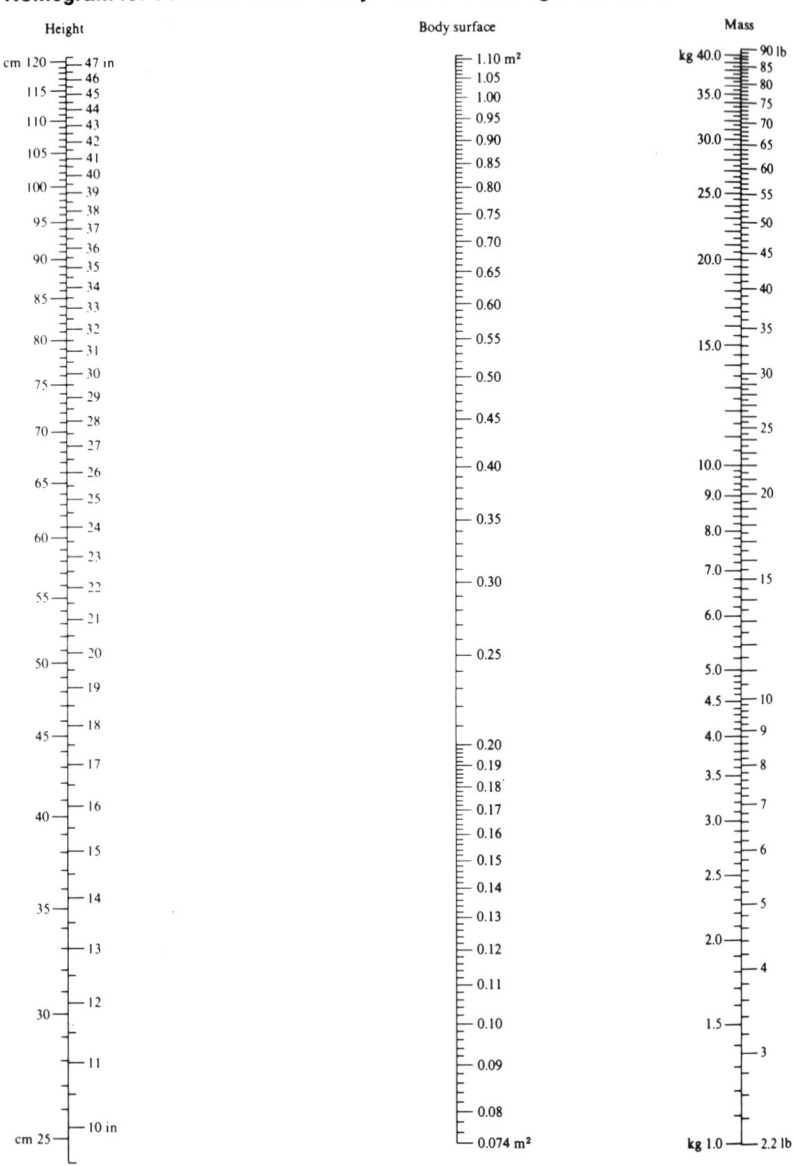

Height	Body surface	Mass

(Nomogram with three scales: Height from cm 25 (10 in) to cm 120 (47 in); Body surface from 0.074 m² to 1.10 m²; Mass from kg 1.0 (2.2 lb) to kg 40.0 (90 lb).)

Figure 8–5
Nomogram similar to that in Fig. 8–4, but for use with children. (From *Geigy Scientific Tables*. With permission. Courtesy of Ciba-Geigy Limited, Basel, Switzerland.)

Table 8–15. An Example of the Corrected Count Increment to Estimate Efficacy of a Platelet Transfusion

$$\text{CCI} = \frac{(\text{Postcount/mm}^3 - \text{Precount/mm}^3)\,(\text{Body surface area [m}^2\text{]})}{\text{Number of platelets infused (in terms of } 10^{11})}$$

$$\text{CCI} = \frac{(60{,}000 - 10{,}000)\,(1.7)}{3.6}$$

$$\text{CCI} = 23{,}600$$

In this example, a patient with a body surface area of 1.7 m² was given a platelet transfusion containing 3.6×10^{11} platelets. The platelet count rose from 10,000/mm³ to 60,000/mm³ after the transfusion. The corrected count increment is 23,600 per 10^{11} platelets per square meter of body surface area.

Another system for calculating the effectiveness of platelet transfusion is the *percent recovery* [115]. The formula is:

$$\text{Percent recovery} = \frac{(\text{Postcount} - \text{Precount}) \times \text{Blood volume}}{\text{Number of platelets transfused} \times \tfrac{2}{3}} \times 100$$

The factor of ⅔ accounts for splenic pooling of transfused platelets. Expected recoveries are above 60 percent at 1 hour, and above 40 percent at 24 hours.

A very rough estimate of the effectiveness of platelet transfusion can be made using the guideline that an average-size person should have a rise in platelet count of 5,000 to 10,000 per cubic millimeter for each unit transfused. Failure to show adequate responses is evidence of a refractory state, alloimmunization, or some other complicating factor such as sepsis.

Although platelets have ABO antigens, there is no conclusive evidence that these affect survival or function of platelets when they are transfused into ABO-incompatible recipients. ABO-compatible platelets are preferred, but there is no reason not to use incompatible ones. The use of Rh-positive platelets in Rh-negative recipients is discussed on page 318.

Each unit of platelet concentrate is suspended in about 50 ml of donor plasma, so the transfusion of 10 units is also a transfusion of about 500 ml of plasma. At times—for example, when group O donors are used for a group A recipient—the transfused anti-A may be sufficient to cause a positive antiglobulin test and hemolysis of the recipient's erythrocytes.

Platelet concentrates should be administered through a blood recipient set with a standard filter.

REFRACTORINESS

The failure to achieve satisfactory posttransfusion platelet increments or to control thrombocytopenic bleeding is a serious problem in the management of

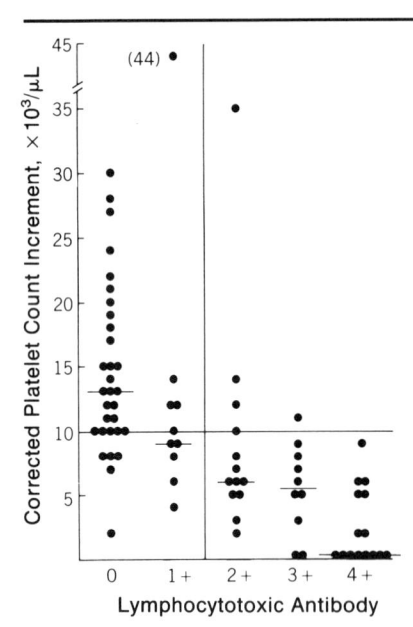

Figure 8-6
Increments in platelet count 1 hour after transfusion of random-donor platelets as a function of the presence of HLA antibodies in the recipient. The corrected increment plotted on the ordinate is equivalent to the rise in platelet count per square meter of body surface area for each 10^{11} of platelets transfused. (From P. A. Daly, C. A. Schiffer, J. Aisner, P. H. Wiernik, Platelet transfusion therapy: one-hour posttransfusion increments are valuable in predicting the need for HLA-matched preparations. *JAMA* 1980; 243:435–8. With permission.)

many patients with thrombocytopenia. This refractory state may be from fever, sepsis, splenomegaly, or DIC, or may be related to platelet alloimmunization.

Not all patients who receive multiple transfusions of platelets become immunized. In one series, only 46 percent of patients with acute leukemia became immunized within 6 months after intensive platelet support [116]. The incidence of alloimmunization is higher in patients with aplastic anemia, probably because they are not usually treated with immunosuppressive drugs. True alloimmunization is often difficult to detect clinically because of the numerous other factors that lead to poor recovery of transfused platelets. Platelet destruction caused by immunization can sometimes be differentiated by comparing the platelet counts 1 hour and 24 hours after transfusion. In immunized patients, neither the 1-hour nor the 24-hour counts show the expected rise, whereas in refractoriness from other causes, sepsis for example, the 1-hour count usually rises as expected, but shortened platelet survival leads to low counts again by 18 to 24 hours (Fig. 8-6) [117].

Table 8-16. Platelet Response after Transfusion from Donors Mismatched for HLA Antigens Within Cross-Reacting Groups (CREGs)*

Recipient Antigens or CREGs	Usual Transfusion Outcome with Platelet-Donor Antigens Specified	
	Good†	Poor†
A1 or 11	A 11 or 1	A3
A3		A1 or 11
A2	A28	
B5, 15, 17, 18, 21, 35	B16, 18, 15, 35 (variable)	B17, 21
B15, 17,		B5
B7, 22, 27, 40	B7, 22	B27
B12 or 21		B21 or 12
B8 or 14		B14 or 8
B18	B5	
BW6 or 4		BW4 or 6

*Data mostly from M. B. Dahlke, K. L. Weiss, Platelet transfusion from donors mismatched for crossreactive HLA antigens. *Transfusion* 1984; 24:299-302.
†Note that these outcomes are trends, rather than absolutes, in that all data on posttransfusion increments included substantial scatter.

If HLA-compatible platelets are available, either from a family member or from an HLA-matched donor, immunized patients often achieve good recovery and survival. Even with fully HLA-matched platelets, however, from 6 to 39 percent of platelet transfusions are unsuccessful, perhaps because of antibodies against platelet-specific antigens [115]. Good survival may be obtained even in the face of mismatching, provided the mismatch is for selected cross-reactive HLA antigens [118]. In view of the enormous number of HLA phenotypes, selection of matched platelets might seem impractical unless closely related donors are available. However, some phenotypes are relatively common, and furthermore, a good deal of cross-reactivity exists among HLA antigens. Within groups of cross-reacting antigens ("CREGs"), mutual immunogenicity is lower than would be the case between the antigens of different groups (see Chap. 3). In other words, the patient's immune system may not recognize cross-reacting antigens as foreign. By taking advantage of this phenomenon, alloimmunized recipients can achieve good platelet transfusion results from carefully selected donors without the need for an enormous panel of typed donors [118, 119]. See Table 8-16 for examples of good and poor transfusion results in various cross-reacting antigenic groups.

It is worth giving an example. A leukemic patient of HLA phenotype A1, 30/B8, 13 was severely refractory to unselected platelets. The patient had broadly reactive cytotoxic antibodies, but was able to achieve satisfactory platelet increments with one platelet apheresis concentrate a week for over a year, during which time most of his cytotoxic antibodies disappeared. This was done by selecting donors whose HLA antigens were cross-reactive with those of the patient, i.e., antigens A1-3-11-10, the whole Aw19 group, and B8-14-7-40-13, while avoiding A2, 28, and 9, as well as B17, 44, 21, and 27.

A somewhat peculiar observation, so far without explanation, is that patients negative for HLA A2 do not seem to become immunized to mismatched antigens as easily as those that do have the antigen [120]. Neither DR nor D series antigens seem to have any importance in transfusion therapy.

It is possible that using only small numbers of HLA-matched donors for transfusion support might prevent alloimmunization [121], but Schiffer and Slichter have concluded that ". . . patients with thrombocytopenia should receive pooled platelet concentrates from random donors as their initial source of platelet support," reserving single-donor HLA-matched donors for use ". . . only when refractoriness to random-donor platelets has been documented" [122]. Although it may be convenient to give single-donor (not necessarily HLA-matched), rather than random, platelets, there are few scientific data to support the frequent preference of clinicians for such products.

Removal of lymphocytes from platelet concentrates before transfusion has been reported to reduce the incidence of alloimmunization to HLA [123], but not everyone has found this to be effective [124]. If leukocytes are to be removed, either filtration or centrifugation is effective. Newer methods of platelet apheresis produce concentrates with minimal leukocyte contamination. Recently, ultraviolet irradiation of platelets has been reported to prevent transfusion-induced alloimmunization in dogs [125]. (See Addenda.)

Incompatibility of the HLA Bw4/Bw6 group of antigens has been shown to be related to poor response to platelets in some patients [126]. In this study of 21 patients who had become refractory to random-donor platelets, the mean recovery was significantly less for Bw4/Bw6 incompatible platelets. These observations have not been confirmed.

The use of intravenous IgG in patients who are refractory to platelet transfusions is discussed on page 317. The entire subject of platelet support for refractory patients is well reviewed by Menitove, and by Slichter [115, 127].

CROSSMATCHING

The relatively poor correlation between platelet refractoriness and demonstrable HLA antibodies has prompted investigations into platelet crossmatching. Many methods have been proposed, but all are cumbersome and poorly suited for routine use [128]. In some cases, the predictive value of such procedures is reported to be high, as is seen in Fig. 8–7 [129, 130].

ASPIRIN AND PLATELET TRANSFUSION

Aspirin ingestion leads to changes in platelet function, which in turn cause a prolonged bleeding time and a tendency to increased bleeding. Thus, to prevent

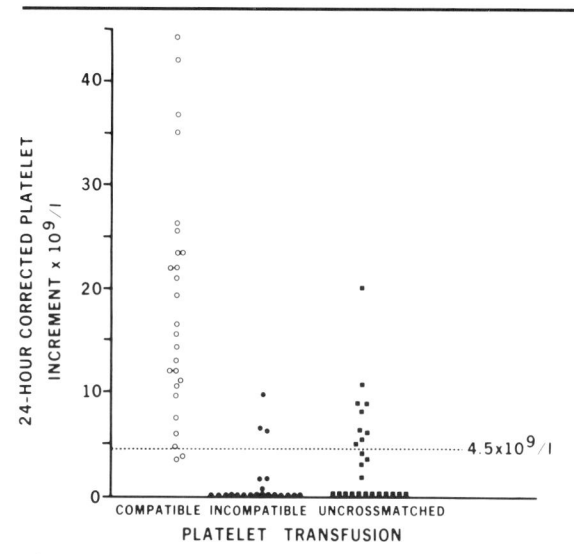

Figure 8–7
Twenty-four-hour-corrected platelet increments with transfusion of crossmatch-compatible, crossmatch-incompatible, and uncrossmatched random-donor platelets. (From J. Freedman, C. Hooi, M. B. Garvey, Prospective platelet crossmatching for selection of compatible random donors. *Br J Haematol* 1984; 56:9–18. With permission.)

abnormal bleeding at surgery, physicians may order platelet transfusions for patients who have taken aspirin. This should be restricted to urgent surgical procedures and then only after a prolonged bleeding time has actually been demonstrated. A single dose of platelets of 0.5 to 1 unit per 10 kilograms will be adequate, since aspirin-treated patients will regain normal function when as few as 20 percent of the circulating platelets have not been exposed to aspirin [131].

Because adequate function can be expected with so few normal platelets, there is no need to avoid preparing conventional platelets from donors who have ingested aspirin. For single-donor platelets, where the contribution on one donation may constitute more than 80 percent of the platelets available to the recipient after transfusion, aspirin ingestion within the 3 days before donation should preclude use of that donor.

Granulocytes (Neutrophils)

The increasingly intensive chemotherapeutic regimens used in the treatment of leukemia and cancer inevitably result in temporary bone marrow ablation and consequent pancytopenia. Transfusion support of the patient through this difficult period is critical. Treatment of anemia and thrombocytopenia with transfusions of red blood cells and platelets has been generally successful, and for the past 20 years or so, there have been attempts to treat or prevent infections due to neutropenia by transfusions of granulocytes. This has not been easy to accomplish because of the enormous turnover of neutrophils even in the normal state, the consequent difficulty in transfusing enough cells, and the very short survival of these cells in the circulation.

Clinical evaluation of granulocyte transfusion therapy has been singularly difficult, at least in part for the following reasons:

1. It is used only in desperately ill patients with complex disease processes.
2. Because of the above, it is always used in conjunction with other therapy, e.g., steroids, antibiotics, chemotherapeutic agents.
3. Even in reported studies, most transfusions have probably included less than the optimal number of granulocytes.
4. Cell collection methods differ as to quality, as well as quantity, of granulocytes.
5. Granulocytes probably function mostly outside the circulation, which means that posttransfusion increments are of little value in assessing the effects of transfusions.
6. The importance of immune compatibility is still uncertain.
7. Controlled studies have focused predominantly on gram-negative sepsis.
8. The number of patients studied in each controlled trial has been small, and there are too many uncontrolled variables between different institutions to allow direct comparisons or pooling of data.
9. During the time that experience has been gained with granulocyte transfusions, there have been simultaneous and overlapping changes and improvements in chemotherapy, antibiotic therapy, and general management of leukemia and cancer patients.

Despite these difficulties, most investigators have concluded that granulocyte transfusions are effective in appropriate clinical circumstances, that the tranfused cells do migrate to sites of infection, that they can kill bacteria, and that they favorably influence the clinical outcome [132]. The evidence is even stronger when all the studies are considered as a group, even though their results cannot be statistically pooled.

CRITERIA FOR GRANULOCYTE TRANSFUSION

The two basic criteria for granuloctye transfusion are neutropenia (peripheral blood neutrophil count below 500 per microliter) and infection. Counts approaching zero should be regarded even more seriously.

Since some patients with minimal granulocyte counts do not suffer infections, granulocyte transfusions are restricted to those with sepsis or a significant local infection (e.g., pneumonitis) not responding to a 2- or 3-day trial of appropriate antibiotic therapy [132]. If it seems likely that bone marrow function will return in a few days, granulocyte transfusions are probably not necessary. Giving granulocytes to patients who are moribund, or who are unlikely to regain marrow function, is useless, although a trial of 4 or 5 days of granulocyte transfusions may be reasonable. One or two transfusions are never clinically indicated.

Granulocyte transfusions may also be of benefit to newborns with sepsis [133]. In addition to sepsis, the criteria are severe neutropenia (as above), and a deficient marrow reserve of neutrophils. In such circumstances, a full adult dose of granulocytes (with the plasma removed to a bare minimum) may be lifesaving, and often does not need to be repeated. If the baby's marrow is packed with granulocyte precursors, transfusion will be ineffective. Exchange transfusion with freshly collected whole blood is another option, but one for which adequate data are not yet at hand [134]. It is doubtful that buffy coats from regular blood collections would provide enough neutrophils.

Because of the effectiveness of present-day antibiotic therapy and other infection-control measures, the use of granulocyte transfusions has decreased dramatically in the past 5 years.

The benefits of *prophylactic* granulocyte transfusions are equivocal at best [135]. The actual and potential hazards, however, are considerable, primarily relating to reactions and to alloimmunization [136]. The latter is important clinically, leading to decreased posttransfusion increments, impaired cell migration, diminished response to transfused platelets, and probably, shorter survival. With these considerations in mind, it is safe to say that general methods of preventing infections in neutropenic patients are probably more effective than granulocyte transfusions, and certainly safer.

DOSAGE

The normal daily turnover of neutrophils in *uninfected* people is about 10^{11}. Based partly on clinical experience and partly on old experiments with transfusions of cells from patients with chronic granulocytic leukemia, the general impression is that an adequate granulocyte transfusion should contain at least 10^{10} granulocytes. There is good evidence that larger doses are better [137, 138]. However, to obtain a minimum of 10^{10} cells per transfusion, the *mean* yield must be notably higher than that. We have found, for example, that with a mean yield of 1.3 to 1.4 × 10^{10} granulocytes, which is readily obtainable from normal donors without steroid premedication by continuous or intermittent centrifugation systems, about 25 percent of transfusions will have a granulocyte yield below 10^{10}, and may therefore be considered inadequate by the above standard.

The problem is that granulocyte yields are unpredictable and some donors have poor yields despite steroid stimulation and optimal techniques. Few investigators have given attention to this problem as it affects the transfused dose of cells. Therefore, to be sure of a *minimum* of 10^{10} granulocytes per transfusion, the *mean* leukapheresis yield probably needs to be at least 2×10^{10}, a figure not likely to be achieved by most cell separators without steroid premedication of the donors. The matter of dosage deserves more emphasis. With the cost, complexity, and risks (to both patient and donor) of granulocyte transfusions, every reasonable means should be taken to assure a maximal cell yield. If this cannot be done, granulocyte transfusions should probably not be given.

STORAGE

Granulocytes are generally stored in the same medium in which they were collected, i.e., citrated donor plasma containing hydroxyethyl starch. These cells tolerate storage poorly, and begin to lose their most highly integrative function, i.e., chemotaxis, even before 24 hours [139, 140]. Since chemotaxis is an essential cell function in the defense against infection, this sets a limit on storage, at least until some improvements in storage conditions are devised.

Storage seems to be better at room temperature than at 4°C, agitation is probably undesirable (in contrast with the needs of platelets), and freezing and thawing have not yet provided a usable product. Any granulocyte concentrate should be transfused as soon as possible, and should not be stored for more than a day.

COMPATIBILITY

Considerations regarding ABO and Rh are essentially the same as those discussed for platelet transfusions on page 333. One difference is that all granulocyte collections contain substantial numbers of red cells (15 to 50 ml or more of packed red cells). This means that red cell compatibility must be given some consideration. The red cells should be removed if they have an antigen that is incompatible with any potent antibody in the recipient's plasma (see Chap. 2).

The matter of HLA compatibility is more controversial in that some earlier work suggested a direct relationship between posttransfusion granulocyte recovery and HLA compatibility, as well as ABO compatibility [141]. The consensus nowadays is that there is little evidence to support HLA-matching for granulocyte transfusions to unimmunized patients. In the case of alloimmunized recipients, however, e.g., those who already exhibit refractoriness to platelet transfusions or who have cytotoxic antibodies, transfused unmatched granulocytes may not survive as well and can cause severe reactions in some patients [132]. Unfortunately, other than from platelet refractoriness and the occurrence of reactions, it is difficult to judge whether or not a patient is immunized.

REACTIONS AND COMPLICATIONS

In general, the same reactions and complications will occur as discussed for platelets and other components, because granulocyte transfusions involve not only granulocytes, but also platelets, mononuclear cells, red cells, and plasma, plus some anticoagulant and macromolecular agent. Symptomatic treatment or premedication is usually adequate (see Chap. 7). Mild febrile reactions are common and can usually be controlled by slowing the infusion rate. On the other hand, severe shaking chills and fever or respiratory distress leading to pulmonary edema probably indicate alloimmunization, and usually require the transfusion to be stopped.

One report found an increased incidence of lethal pulmonary reactions in patients receiving amphotericin B while receiving granulocyte transfusions [142]. Others found no such association [143]. The discrepancy is difficult to explain. Despite the findings in the former report, we do not think amphotericin B should be withheld from neutropenic patients receiving granulocyte transfusions if they have fungal infections, but it would be wise to observe them carefully and perhaps arrange for a few hours time interval between the drug and transfusion administration.

Pulmonary infiltrates are sometimes observed in patients receiving granulocyte transfusions. Diffuse infiltrates or those occurring a few days after the onset of a course of transfusions appear to represent an appropriate migration of granulocytes to a site of infection, and seem to have no ominous significance. On the other hand, localized infiltrates occurring 1 to 3 weeks after a series of transfusions was begun probably represent a resistant infection and a failure of transfusion therapy [144].

References

1. Mollison PL. Methods of determining the posttransfusion survival of stored red cells. *Transfusion* 1984; 24:93–6.
2. Peck CC. Evaluating the survival of stored red cells. *Transfusion* 1984; 24:97–9.
3. Moroff G, Sohmer PR, Button LN, and Members of the Ad Hoc Committee. Proposed standardization of methods for determining the 24-hour survival of stored red cells. *Transfusion* 1984; 24:109–14.
4. Hechtman HB, Grindlinger GA, Vegas AM, et al. Importance of oxygen transport in clinical medicine. *Crit Care Med* 1979; 7:419–23.
5. Miller LD, Oski FA, Diaco JF, et al. The affinity of hemoglobin for oxygen: Its control and in vivo significance. *Surgery* 1970; 68:187–95.
6. Woodson RD, Wranne B, Detter JC. Effect of increased blood oxygen affinity on work performance of rats. *J Clin Invest* 1973; 52:2717–24.
7. Collins JA, Stechenberg L. The effects of the concentration and function of hemoglobin on the survival of rats after hemorrhage. *Surgery* 1979; 85:412.
8. Broadie TA, Herman CM. Oxygen consumption from fresh versus 21-day-old ACD whole blood. *J Trauma* 1978; 18:381–6.
9. Beutler E, Wood L. The in vivo regeneration of red cell 2,3-diphosphoglyceric acid (DPG) after transfusion of stored blood. *J Lab Clin Med* 1969; 74:300–4.
10. Woodson RD. Physiological significance of oxygen dissociation curve shifts. *Crit Care Med* 1979; 7:368–73.
11. Valeri CR, Zaroulis CG. Rejuvenation and freezing of outdated stored human red cells. *N Engl J Med* 1972; 287:1307–13.

12. Valeri CR, Rorth M, Zaroulis CG, et al. Physiologic effects of transfusing red blood cells with high or low affinity for oxygen to passively hyperventilated, anemic baboon: systemic and cerebral oxygen extraction. *Ann Surg* 1975; 181: 106–13.
13. Dennis RC, Vito L, Weisel RD, et al. Improved myocardial performance following high 2-3 diphosphoglycerate red cell transfusions. *Surgery* 1975; 77:741–7.
14. Jalonen J, Rajamaki A, Laaksonen V, Inberg MV. The effects of elevated red blood cell 2,3-diphosphoglycerate concentration and metabolism during cardiopulmonary bypass. *J Thorac Cardiovasc Surg* 1980; 79:748–54.
15. Gibson JG, Murphy WP, Scheitlin WA, Rees SB. The influence of extracellular factors involved in the collection of blood in ACD on maintenance of red cell viability during refrigerated storage. *Am J Clin Pathol* 1956; 26:855–73.
16. Moroff G, Morse EE, Katz AJ, et al. Survival and biochemical characteristics of stored red cells preserved with citrate-phosphate-dextrose-adenine-one and two and prepared from whole blood maintained at 20 to 24°C for eight hours following phlebotomy. *Transfusion* 1984; 24:115–9.
17. Chapman RG. Effect of initial storage at room temperature on human red cell ATP, 2,3-DPG, and viability. *Transfusion* 1977; 17:147–50.
18. Robertson OH. Transfusion with preserved red blood cells. *Br Med J* 1918; 1:691.
19. Loutit JF, Mollison, PL, Young IM. Citric acid-sodium citrate-glucose mixtures for blood storage. *Q J Exp Physiol* 1943; 32:183.
20. Gibson JG II. A citrate-phosphate-dextrose solution for preservation of human blood. *Am J Clin Pathol* 1957; 28:569–78.
21. Simon ER, Chapman RG, Finch CA. Adenine in red cell preservation. *J Clin Invest* 1962; 41:351–9.
22. Falk JS, Lindglad TO, Westman BJM. Histopathological studies on kidneys from patients treated with large amounts of blood preserved with ACD-Adenine. *Transfusion* 1972; 12:376–81.
23. Högman CF, Hedlund K, Åkerblom O, Venge P. Red blood cell preservation in protein-poor media. I. Leukocyte enzymes as a cause of hemolysis. *Transfusion* 1978; 18:233–41.
24. Högman CF, Hedlund K, Sahleström Y. Red cell preservation in protein-poor media. III. Protection against hemolysis. *Vox Sang* 1981; 41:274–81.
25. Bailey DN, Bove JR. Chemical and hematological changes in stored CPD blood. *Transfusion* 1975; 15:244–9.
26. Simon GE, Bove JR. The potassium load from blood transfusion. *Postgrad Med* 1971; 49:61–4.
27. Moore GL, Peck CC, Sohmer PR, Zuck TF. Some properties of blood stored in anticoagulated CPDA-1 solution. A brief summary. *Transfusion* 1981; 21:135–7.
28. Polge C, Smith AU, Parkes AS. Revival of spermatozoa after vitrification and dehydration at low temperatures. *Nature* 1949; 164:666.
29. Meryman HT, Hornblower M. A method for freezing and washing red blood cells using a high glycerol concentration. *Transfusion* 1972; 12:145–56.
30. Mollison PL, Sloviter HA. Successful transfusion of previously frozen human red cells. *Lancet* 1951; 2:862.
31. Valeri CR, Szymanski IO, Runck AH. Therapeutic effectiveness of homologous erythrocyte transfusions following frozen storage at −80C for up to seven years. *Transfusion* 1970; 12:102–12.
32. Szymanski IO, Carrington EJ. Evaluation of a large-scale frozen blood program. *Transfusion* 1977; 17:431–7.
33. Carr JB, de Quesada AA, Shires DL. Decreased incidence of transfusion hepatitis

after exclusive transfusion with reconstituted frozen erythrocytes: studies in a dialysis unit. *Ann Intern Med* 1973; 78:693–5.
34. Alter HJ, Tabor E, Meryman HT, et al. Transmission of hepatitis B virus infection by transfusion of frozen-deglycerolized red blood cells. *N Engl J Med* 1978; 298:637–42.
35. Haugen RK. Hepatitis after the transfusion of frozen red cells and washed red cells. *N Engl J Med* 1979; 301:393–5.
36. Myhre BA, Nakasako YY, Schott R. Studies on 4C stored frozen-reconstituted red blood cells. I. Bacterial growth. *Transfusion* 1977; 17:454–9.
37. Kahn RH, McDonough B, Ellis FR, Pino B. The impact of converting to an all frozen blood system in a large regional blood center. *Transfusion* 1978; 18:304–11.
38. Chaplin H Jr. The proper use of frozen red blood cells for transfusion. *Blood* 1982; 59:1118–20.
39. Meryman HT, Hornblower M. The preparation of red cells depleted of leukocytes. Review and evaluation. *Transfusion* 1986; 26:101–6.
40. Perkins HA, Payne R, Ferguson J, Wood M. Nonhemolytic febrile transfusion reactions: quantitative effects of blood components with emphasis on isoantigenic incompatibility of leukocytes. *Vox Sang* 1966; 11:578–600.
41. Menitove JE, McElligott MC, Aster RH. Febrile transfusion reaction: what blood component should be given next. *Vox Sang* 1982; 42:318–21.
42. Eernisse JG, Brand A. Prevention of platelet refractoriness due to HLA antibodies by administration of leukocyte-poor blood components. *Exp Hematol* 1981; 9:77–83.
43. Fisher M, Chapman JR, Ting A, Morris PJ. Alloimmunisation to HLA antigens following transfusion with leucocyte-poor and purified platelet suspensions. *Vox Sang* 1985; 49:331–5.
44. Holohan TV, Terasaki PI, Deisseroth AB. Suppression of transfusion-related alloimmunization in intensively treated cancer patients. *Blood* 1981; 58:122–8.
45. Yap PL, Pryde AD, McClelland DBL. IgA content of frozen-thawed-washed red blood cells and blood products measured by radioimmunoassay. *Transfusion* 1982; 22:36–8.
46. Perkins HA, Senecal I, Howell E. Leukocyte contamination of red cells in leukocyte-poor and frozen-deglycerolized units. *Transfusion* 1973; 13:194–9.
47. Brady MT, Milam JD, Anderson DC, et al. Use of deglycerolized red blood cells to prevent posttransfusion infection with cytomegalovirus in neonates. *J Infect Dis* 1984; 150:334–9.
48. Braunstein AH, Oberman HA. Transfusion of plasma components. *Transfusion* 1984; 24:281–6.
49. NIH Consensus Conference. Fresh frozen plasma: indications and risks. *JAMA* 1985; 253:556–7.
50. Kakaiya RM, Morse EE, Panek S. Labile coagulation factors in thawed fresh frozen plasma prepared by two methods. *Vox Sang* 1984; 46:44–6.
51. Luff RD, Kessler CM, Bell WR. Microwave technology for the rapid thawing of frozen blood components. *Am J Clin Pathol* 1985; 83:59–64.
52. Rock G, Tackaberry ES, Dunn JG, Kashyap S. Rapid controlled thawing of fresh-frozen plasma in a modified microwave oven. *Transfusion* 1984; 24:60–5.
53. Milam JD, Buzzurro CJ, Austin SF, Stansberry SW. Stability of factors V and VIII in thawed fresh frozen plasma units. *Transfusion* 1980; 20:546–8.
54. Martin DJ, Lucas CE, Ledgerwood AM, et al. Fresh frozen plasma supplement to massive red blood cell transfusion. *Ann Surg* 1985; 202:505–11.

55. Mannucci PM, Federici AB, Sirchia G. Hemostasis testing during massive blood replacement: a study of 172 cases. *Vox Sang* 1982; 42:113–23.
56. Counts RB, Haisch C, Simon TL, et al. Hemostasis in massively transfused trauma patients. *Ann Surg* 1979; 109:91–9.
57. Reed RL, Ciavarella D, Heimbach DM, et al. Prophylactic platelet administration during massive transfusion: a prospective, randomized, double-blind clinical study. *Ann Surg* 1986; 203:40–8.
58. Nilsson L, Hedner IM, Nilsson IM, Robertson B. Shelf-life of bank blood and stored plasma with special reference to coagulation factors. *Transfusion* 1983; 23:377–81.
59. Finlayson JS. Albumin products. *Semin Thromb Hemost* 1980; 6:85–120.
60. Tullis JL. Albumin: 1. Background and use. 2. Guidelines for clinical use. *JAMA* 1977; 237:355–60; 460–3.
61. Alexander MR. Therapeutic use of albumin. *JAMA* 1979; 241:2527–9.
62. Kahn RA, Allen RW, Baldassare J. Alternate sources and substitutes for blood components. *Blood* 1985; 66:1–12.
63. Drees TC, Downing M, Hildebrandt C. Biotechnology, here today or tomorrow. *Plasma Quart* 1983; 5:120–1.
64. Finlayson JS. Immune globulins. *Semin Thromb Hemost* 1979; 6:44–74.
65. Stiehm ER. Standard and special human immune serum globulins as therapeutic agents. *Pediatrics* 1979; 63:301–19.
66. Gerety RJ, Aronson DL. Plasma derivatives and viral hepatitis. *Transfusion* 1982; 22:347–51.
67. Lever AML, Webster ADB, Brown D, Thomas HC. Non-A, non-B hepatitis occurring in agammaglobulinemic patients after intravenous immunoglobulin. *Lancet* 1984; 2:1062–4.
68. Bussel JB, Hilgartner MW. The use and mechanism of action of intravenous immunoglobulin in the treatment of immune haematologic disease. *Br J Haematol* 1984; 56:1–7.
69. Imbach P, d'Apuzzo V, Hirt A, et al. High-dose intravenous gammaglobulin for idiopathic thrombocytopenic purpura in childhood. *Lancet* 1981; 1:1228–30.
70. Emilia G, Sacchi S, Torelli G, et al. Low-dose intravenous pepsin-treated gammaglobulin for idiopathic thrombocytopenic purpura in adults. *Br J Haematol* 1984; 58:761–64.
71. Junghans RP, Ahn YS. High-dose intravenous gamma globulin to suppress alloimmune destruction of donor platelets. *Am J Med* 1984; 64:204–8.
72. Baumann MA, Menitove JE, Aster RH, Anderson T. Urgent treatment of idiopathic thrombocytopenic purpura with single-dose gammaglobulin infusion followed by platelet transfusion. *Ann Intern Med* 1986; 104:808–9.
73. Schiffer CA, Hogge DE, Aisner J, et al. High-dose intravenous gammaglobulin in alloimmunized platelet transfusion recipients. *Blood* 1984; 64:937–40.
74. Recommendations for protection against viral hepatitis. *MMWR* 1985; 34:313–35.
75. Ballas SK, Draper EK, Dignam CM. Pre-transfusion testing problems caused by anti-lymphocyte globulin and their solutions. *Transfusion* 1985; 25:254–6.
76. Lichtiger B, Surgeon J, Rhorer S. Rh-incompatible platelet transfusion therapy in cancer patients. *Vox Sang* 1983; 45:139–43.
77. Mollison PL. *Blood Transfusion in Clinical Medicine*, 7th ed. Oxford, England: Blackwell Sci, 1983; 383–5.
78. Smith GN, Griffiths B, Mollison D, Mollison PL. Uptake of IgG after intramuscular and subcutaneous injection. *Lancet* 1972; 1:1208–12.
79. Eklund J, Hermann M, Kjellman H, Pohja P. Turnover rate of anti-D IgG injected during pregnancy. *Br Med J* 1982; 284:854–5.

80. Janson PA, Jubelier SJ, Weinstein MJ, Deykin D. Treatment of the bleeding tendency in uremia with cryoprecipitate. *N Engl J Med* 1980; 303:1318-22.
81. Saba TM, Dillon B, Lanser ME. Fibronectin and phagocytic host defense: relationship to nutritional support. *J Parent Ent Nutr* 1983; 7:62.
82. Snyder EL, Luban NLC. Fibronectin: applications to clinical medicine. *CRC Crit Rev Clin Lab Sci* 1986; 23:15-34.
83. Snyder EL, Ferri PM, Mosher DF. Fibronectin in liquid and frozen stored blood components. *Transfusion* 1984; 24:53-6.
84. Lupinetti FM, Stoney WS, Alford WC Jr, et al. Cryoprecipitate-topical thrombin glue. Initial experience in patients undergoing cardiac operations. *J Thorac Cardiovasc Surg* 1985; 90:502-5.
85. Kitchens CS. Surgery in hemophilia and related disorders. A prospective study of 100 consecutive procedures. *Medicine (Baltimore)* 1986; 65:34-45.
86. Aledort LM. *Current Management in the Treatment of Hemophilia: A Physician's Manual.* New York: National Hemophilia Foundation, 1986.
87. Rosati LA, Barnes B, Oberman HA, Penner JA. Hemolytic anemia due to anti-A in concentrated antihemophilic factor preparations. *Transfusion* 1970; 10:139-41.
88. Hilgartner MW, Giardina P. Liver dysfunction in patients with hemophilia A, B and von Willebrand's disease. *Transfusion* 1977; 17:495-9.
89. Petricciani JC, McDougal JS, Evatt BL. Case for concluding that heat-treated licensed antihemophilic factor is free from HTLV-III. *Lancet* 1985; 2:890-1.
90. Gomperts ED. Procedures for the inactivation of viruses in clotting factor concentrate. *Am J Hematol* 1986; 23:295-305.
91. Lusher JM, Shapiro SS, Palascak JE, et al. Efficacy of prothrombin-complex concentrates in hemophiliacs with antibodies to factor VIII. A multicenter therapeutic trial. *N Engl J Med* 1980; 303:421-5.
92. Laurian Y, Girma JP, Lambert T, et al. Incidence of immune responses following 102 infusions of Autoplex in 18 hemophilic patients with antibody to factor VIII. *Blood* 1984; 63:457-62.
93. Kernoff PBA, Thomas ND, Lilley PA, et al. Clinical experience with polyelectrolyte-fractionated porcine factor VIII concentrate in the treatment for hemophiliacs with antibodies to factor VIII. *Blood* 1984; 63:31-41.
94. Aronson DL. Factor IX complex. *Semin Thromb Hemost* 1979; 6:28-43.
95. Aggeler PM. Physiological basis for transfusion therapy in hemorrhagic disorders: a critical review. *Transfusion* 1961; 1:71-86.
96. Gerety RJ, Aronson DL. Plasma derivatives and viral hepatitis. *Transfusion* 1982; 22:347-51.
97. Cederbaum A, Blatt P, Roberts H. Intravascular coagulation with use of human prothrombin complex concentrates. *Ann Intern Med* 1976; 84:683-7.
98. Ratnoff OD. Disseminated intravascular coagulation. In: Ratnoff OD, Forbes CD (eds). *Disorders of Hemostasis.* Orlando: Grune, 1984; 289-319.
99. Bloom AL. The von Willebrand syndrome. *Semin Hematol* 1980; 17:215-27.
100. Perkins HA. Correction of the hemostatic defects in von Willebrand's disease. *Blood* 1967; 30:375-80.
101. Horowitz HI, Fujimoto MM. Survival of factor XI in vitro and in vivo. *Transfusion* 1965; 5:538-42.
102. Seyfer AE, Seaber AV, Dombrose FA, Urbaniak JR. Coagulation changes in elective surgery and trauma. *Ann Surg* 1981; 193:210-3.
103. Mintz PD, Blatt PM, Kuhns WJ, Roberts HR. Antithrombin III in fresh frozen plasma, cryoprecipitate, and cryoprecipitate-depleted plasma. *Transfusion* 1979; 19:597-8.

104. Inkster M, Sherman LA, Ahmed P, et al. Preservation of antithrombin III activity in stored whole blood. *Transfusion* 1984; 24:57–9.
105. Slichter SJ, Harker LA. Preparation and storage of platelet concentrates. I. Factors influencing the harvest of viable platelets from whole blood. *Br J Haematol* 1976; 34:395–402.
106. Murphy S, Kahn RA, Holme S, et al. Improved storage of platelets for transfusion in a new container. *Blood* 1982; 60:194–200.
107. Lazarus HM, Herzig RH, Warm SE, Fishman DJ. Transfusion experience with platelet concentrates stored for 24 to 72 hours at 22°C. *Transfusion* 1982; 22:39–43.
108. Heal JM, Singal S, Sardisco E, Mayer T. Bacterial proliferation in platelet concentrates. *Transfusion* 1986; 26:388–90.
109. Braine HG, Kickler TS, Charache P, et al. Bacterial sepsis secondary to platelet transfusion: an adverse effect of extended storage at room temperature. *Transfusion* 1986; 26:391–3.
110. Snyder EL, Pope C, Ferri PM, et al. The effect of mode of agitation and type of plastic bag on storage characteristics and in vivo kinetics of platelet concentrates. *Transfusion* 1986; 26:125–30.
111. Schiffer CA, Aisner J, Wiernik P. Frozen autologous platelet transfusions for patients with leukemia. *N Engl J Med* 1978; 299:7–12.
112. Raccuglia G, Bethell FH. Platelet transfusions and administration of platelet derivatives in man. I. Evaluation of laboratory technics used for prognostic purposes. *Am J Clin Pathol* 1960; 34:495–504.
113. Harker LA, Slichter SJ. The bleeding time as a screening test for evaluating platelet function. *N Engl J Med* 1972; 287:155–9.
114. Slichter SJ, Harker LA. Thrombocytopenia: mechanisms and management of defects in platelet production. *Clin Haematol* 1978; 7:523–39.
115. Menitove JE. Platelet transfusion for alloimmunized patients. *Clin Oncol* 1983; 2:587–609.
116. Dutcher JP, Schiffer CA, Aisner J, Wiernik PH. Long-term follow-up of patients with leukemia receiving platelet transfusions: identification of a large group of patients who do not become alloimmunized. *Blood* 1981; 57:395–8.
117. Daly PA, Schiffer CA, Aisner J, Wiernik PH. Platelet transfusion therapy: one-hour posttransfusion increments are valuable in predicting the need for HLA-matched preparations. *JAMA* 1980; 243:435–8.
118. Duquesnoy RJ, Filip DJ, Rodey GE, et al. Successful transfusion of platelets "mismatched" for HLA antigens to alloimmunized thrombocytopenic patients. *Am J Hematol* 1977; 2:219–26.
119. Dahlke MB, Weiss KL. Platelet transfusion from donors mismatched for cross-reactive HLA antigens. *Transfusion* 1984; 24:299–302.
120. Duquesnoy RJ, Filip DJ, Aster RH. Influence of HLA-A2 on the effectiveness of platelet transfusions in alloimmunized thrombocytopenic patients. *Blood* 1977; 50:407–12.
121. Gmur J, von Felten A, Osterwalder B, et al. Delayed alloimmunization using random single donor platelet transfusions: a prospective study in thrombocytopenic patients with acute leukemia. *Blood* 1983; 62:473–9.
122. Schiffer CA, Slichter SJ. Platelet transfusions from single donors. *N Engl J Med* 1982; 307:245–8.
123. Murphy MF, Metcalfe P, Thomas H, et al. Use of leucocyte-poor blood components and HLA-matched-platelet donors to prevent HLA alloimmunization. *Br J Haematol* 1986; 62:529–34.
124. Schiffer CA, Dutcher JP, Aisner J, et al. A randomized trial of leucocyte-depleted

platelet transfusion to modify alloimmunization in patients with leukemia. *Blood* 1983; 52:815–20.
125. Deeg HJ, Aprile J, Graham TC, et al. Ultraviolet irradiation of blood prevents transfusion-induced sensitization and marrow graft rejection. *Blood* 1986; 67: 537–9.
126. McElligott MC, Menitove JE, Dequesnoy RJ, et al. Effect of HLA BW4/BW6 compatibility on platelet transfusion responses of refractory thrombocytopenic patients. *Blood* 1982; 59:971–5.
127. Slichter SJ. Controversies in platelet transfusion therapy. *Annu Rev Med* 1980; 31:509–640.
128. Kakaiya RM, Gudino MD, Miller WV, et al. Four crossmatch methods to select platelet donors. *Transfusion* 1984; 24:35–41.
129. Kickler TS, Braine H, Ness PM. The predictive value of crossmatching platelet transfusion for alloimmunized patients. *Transfusion* 1985; 25:385–9.
130. Freedman J, Hooi C, Garvey MB. Prospective platelet crossmatching for selection of compatible random donors. *Br J Haematol* 1984; 56:9–18.
131. Stuart MJ, Murphy S, Oski FA, et al. Platelet function in recipients of platelets from donors ingesting aspirin. *N Engl J Med* 1972; 287:1105–9.
132. Higby DJ, Burnett D. Granulocyte transfusions: current status. *Blood* 1980; 55:2–8.
133. Christensen RD, Anstall H, Rothstein G. Neutrophil transfusion in septic neutropenic neonates. *Transfusion* 1982; 22:151–3.
134. Christensen RD, Anstall H, Rothstein G. Use of whole blood exchange transfusion to supply neutrophils to septic, neutropenic neonates. *Transfusion* 1982; 22:504–6.
135. Strauss RG, Connett JE, Gale RP, et al. A controlled trial of prophylactic granulocyte transfusions during initial induction chemotherapy for acute myelogenous leukemia. *N Engl J Med* 1981; 305:597–603.
136. Schiffer CA, Aisner J, Daly PA, et al. Alloimmunization following prophylactic granulocyte transfusion. *Blood* 1979; 54:766–74.
137. Vogler WR, Winton EF. A controlled study of the efficacy of granulocyte transfusions in patients with neutropenia. *Am J Med* 1977; 63:548–55.
138. Aisner J, Schiffer CA, Wiernick PH. Granulocyte transfusions: evaluation of factors influencing results and a comparison of filtration and intermittent centrifugation leukapheresis. *Br J Haematol* 1978; 38:121–9.
139. Glasser L. Effect of storage on normal neutrophils collected by discontinuous-flow centrifugation leukapheresis. *Blood* 1977; 50:1145–50.
140. Steigbigel RT, Baum J, MacPherson JL, Nusbacher J. Granulocyte bactericidal capacity and chemotaxis as affected by continuous flow centrifugation and filtration leukapheresis, steroid administration, and storage. *Blood* 1978; 52:197–209.
141. Graw RG, Goldstein I, Eyre H, Terasaki P. Histocompatibility testing for leukocyte transfusions. *Lancet* 1970; 2:77–8.
142. Wright DG, Robichaud KJ, Pizzo PA, Deisseroth AB. Lethal pulmonary reactions associated with the combined use of amphotericin B and leukocyte transfusions. *N Engl J Med* 1981; 304:1185–9.
143. Dana BW, Durie BGM, White RF, Huestis DW. Concomitant administration of granulocyte transfusions and amphotericin B in neutropenic patients: lack of significant pulmonary toxicity. *Blood* 1981; 57:90–4.
144. Dana BW, Durie BGM, White RF, et al. The significance of pulmonary infiltrates developing in patients receiving granulocyte transfusions. *Br J Haematol* 1983; 53:437–43.

9. Hemolytic Disease of the Newborn

Unlike the chapter on this topic in our previous editions, this one covers only those aspects of hemolytic disease of the newborn (erythroblastosis fetalis) that directly involve the blood bank. Other aspects can be found in texts on obstetrics, pediatrics, and clinical pathology.

Maternal Alloimmunization

A mother can be immunized to any fetal blood group antigen she does not herself possess, and the resulting antibody, if it is of the IgG type, can cross the placenta and cause disease in a fetus that has the corresponding antigen. Thus, erythroblastosis can occur in the fetuses of Rh-positive mothers and can also be caused by incompatibility in other blood group systems, including the ABO system. Maternal antibodies to platelet and white cell antigens can also affect the corresponding cells in the fetus, causing, for example, neonatal thrombocytopenia or leukopenia. The controlling factors are the likelihood of presence of antigen in the fetus and its absence in the mother, its immunogenicity, the mother's capacity for making antibodies, and the ability of the antibody to reach the fetus.

The antigens usually concerned in alloimmunization of pregnancy are those of the ABO and Rh-Hr systems, with occasional cases involving other blood groups—Kell, Duffy, Kidd, MNSs, and others [1]. Once maternal immunization has taken place, erythroblastosis can be expected if the fetus possesses the antigen and if the antibody is of the type that can cross the placenta (IgG). Discovery of "new" blood group antigens and antibodies has often hinged on such occurrences. Most blood group antigens are clearly detectable at early stages of fetal development, and Rh antibodies transferred from the mother have been detected in fetal serum and body fluids at 2 or 3 months of gestation.

For immunization to take place during pregnancy, fetal red cells entering the maternal circulation must apparently remain there long enough to stimulate the mother's antibody-producing mechanisms. For example, ABO incompatibility protects to some extent from Rh hemolytic disease, and probably from other less-common maternofetal incompatibilities as well, such as K and c. Experimentally, volunteers produce Rh antibody less readily when injected with ABO-incompatible Rh-positive blood [2, 3]. Maternal anti-A or anti-B possibly destroys ABO-incompatible fetal Rh-positive red cells before they can stimulate Rh antibody production. This protection, of course, depends on the fetus's ABO group rather than the father's. However, in about 20 percent of families with erythroblastotic babies, the mother becomes immunized despite ABO incompatibility.

Passage of Fetal Red Cells into the Mother

Since Rh antigens are not present in body tissues other than red blood cells, these cells must cross the placental barrier to immunize the Rh-negative mother. The likelihood of Rh immunization is increased in women who have received a relatively large influx of fetal cells, just as it is in women who have had actual transfusions of Rh-positive blood. Immunization seems to take place largely in response to a major incursion of fetal cells, such as 1 to 5 ml, which may occur particularly at the time of delivery.

Even before Rh immunosuppressive therapy, less than 10 percent of Rh-negative mothers with Rh-positive husbands became immunized during the first pregnancy. Many Rh-positive fathers are, of course, heterozygous and thus have an even chance of fathering Rh-negative offspring. Since smaller fetal leakages of Rh-positive blood appear to be less immunizing than larger ones, placental permeability to fetal red cells must be important. It has also been noted that about 30 percent of Rh-negative subjects are "nonresponders," that is, they fail to become immunized even to repeated injections of Rh-positive red cells [4]. As would be expected, the more Rh-positive pregnancies, the more likely a mother is to become immunized. The likelihood, however, seems greatest with the second pregnancy, perhaps simply because women who get through two Rh-positive pregnancies without producing Rh antibody are not so prone to immunization.

Once a person begins to form Rh antibody, it usually remains detectable in the serum almost indefinitely, although the titer may decrease without further stimulation. This perseverance applies to the IgG type. IgM Rh agglutinins often disappear rapidly and do not reappear even with repeated antigenic exposure.

Rh Immune Globulin

Passive immunization with Rh immune globulin (RhIG) is very effective in the prevention of primary Rh immunization. The exact mechanism by which RhIG brings about immunosuppression is not yet clear, but it is probably not the same as the way in which ABO incompatibility protects against Rh immunization. ABO incompatibility probably results in hemolysis and phagocytosis of red cells in the liver, where the immunogenicity of the cell fragments is minimal. Experimentally, volunteers are less likely to produce Rh antibody in response to Rh-positive red cells if the cells are coated with Rh antibody before injection [2, 3]. Passively given Rh antibody may act by blocking surface antigenic determinants on the red cells, with resultant suppression of antibody response by host lymphocytes [5]. The development of the concept of Rh immunosuppression is described in vivid and personal terms by Zimmerman [6].

Application of this work to the prevention of immunization in pregnancy has largely been based on the premise that the big influx of fetal red cells into the mother takes place at the time of delivery. A single dose of 100 to 300 μgm of RhIG after delivery prevents immunization by 5 to 15 ml, respectively, of fetal red cells, an ample margin for most deliveries. The standard dose in North America is 300 μgm for full-term deliveries. Smaller doses are used in European countries. This procedure is 95 percent effective. Failures are for the most part due to immunization *during* pregnancy, less often due to a prior immunization in which antibody was too weak to detect, or occasionally to a fetal blood leakage in excess of 15 ml of red cells [7].

Larger-than-usual fetomaternal hemorrhage can be detected at delivery by using the Kleihauer technique [8], or by observing an apparent D^u type among mothers previously typed as D-negative, or by a rosetting technique [9]. Once the extent of the fetal cell influx has been estimated in milliliters of red cells, the dosage of RhIG can be increased as needed [10].

Immunization *during* pregnancy can be effectively prevented by giving a suitable dose of RhIG at 28 weeks of gestation. If the baby turns out to be Rh-positive, a second dose of the same magnitude is given within 3 days of delivery [11]. This has been found to reduce the failure rate of RhIG from 1.8 to 0.07 percent, without causing any fetal damage.

Standard procedure in North America is to give RhIG intramuscularly within 72 hours of delivery to all unimmunized Rh-negative mothers who have given birth to an Rh-positive baby. A lower dose may be used for those who have undergone a first trimester abortion [12]. The use of RhIG in this way has resulted in a sharp drop in the number of immunized mothers [13].

The D^u Mother

Controversy continues as to whether RhIG should be administered to mothers of type D^u. The reasons for this are the following:

1. An occasional type D^u person has produced anti-D [14].
2. If a mother were to become immunized, the obstetrician might be held liable for failure to give RhIG.
3. The injection of RhIG is generally harmless ("when in doubt, treat").

Others, however, counter with these arguments:

1. In addition to type D^u, an occasional phenotypically D-positive person has also been able to make anti-D. Both situations are exceedingly rare [15], and nobody seriously suggests that RhIG be given to all Rh-positive mothers.
2. There is little scientific evidence that RhIG prevents Rh immunization in a type D^u person [16].

3. There seems to be no logical reason why RhIG should be effective in this setting [14, 17]. In fact, most of the RhIG will be directly adsorbed onto the mother's own red cells.
4. As a matter of therapeutic principle, a treatment not positively indicated is contraindicated.

One could also argue that standards of practice do not require the use of RhIG in D^u mothers, nor is the recommendation to do so given by the manufacturers. Unfortunately, the recommendation was published in an official obstetrical bulletin, thus in effect, creating a standard [18]. This has more recently been abrogated [19, 20]. The weight of opinion seems now to be that RhIG is not indicated in mothers of type D^u, unless there is doubt as to the true Rh type [19, 20]. In this regard, it is especially important to be sure that what appears to be a D^u mother is not, in fact, a D-negative mother showing the effects of a large fetomaternal hemorrhage.

At least part of this problem seems to be semantic. For a long time, many blood banks reported the D^u phenotype as "Rh-negative, D^u-positive," a confusing designation. Since D^u antigen is a variant of D and is itself potentially (if weakly) immunizing, it makes more sense and is certainly less confusing to report the phenotype as "Rh-positive, type D^u," or "Rh-positive (D^u)."

Effects of Antibody on the Fetus

Maternal Rh antibodies cause excessive breakdown of fetal red cells, presumably from the earliest stages at which erythrocytic antigens appear. Those fetuses that fail to compensate adequately by increased production of red cells may die in the uterus, usually in a massively edematous state known as *hydrops fetalis*. This condition seems to be the result of proliferation of hematopoietic cells in the hepatic sinusoids, hepatomegaly, portal hypertension, and hypoproteinemia, rather than of fetal heart failure, as was once thought [21, 22]. Babies born alive can usually be saved with adequate and rapid treatment. This is one valid indication for transfusion of uncrossmatched red blood cells in the delivery room. Since the likelihood of a favorable outcome roughly parallels the baby's hemoglobin level, severe anemia is a bad prognostic sign.

Despite excessive red cell destruction, bilirubin does not accumulate to any great extent in intrauterine life. It may be that this metabolite is cleared in some way through the placenta to the mother's circulation. Bilirubin *in the adult* is partly eliminated by being conjugated in the liver to a glucuronide form, predominantly by the enzyme glucuronyl transferase. It seems that a certain amount of *un*conjugated bilirubin needs to accumulate in the newborn to activate this enzyme, which may explain why it appears to be deficient in the neonatal liver [23, 24]. Unconjugated bilirubin is toxic to the brain of the newborn baby, and permanent brain damage (*kernicterus,* or bilirubin encephalopathy) may result if jaundice is permitted to progress unchecked. This condition has about 70 percent mortality. Children who survive may suffer a form of cerebral palsy.

Prenatal Diagnosis

The history of prior pregnancies is crucial in Rh disease. If there have been no previous pregnancies and no transfusions, the likelihood of serious erythroblastosis in the current fetus is slight. If there have been previous pregnancies but no neonatal jaundice, the probability of involvement in the current pregnancy is greater, but still low. If previous babies have had hemolytic disease, the present fetus (if Rh-positive) will be affected, probably at least as severely as the last one. If the last baby was stillborn because of erythroblastosis, the chances are about two out of three that the present one will be stillborn if the pregnancy is allowed to go to term.

The foregoing are generalizations, and exceptions to them must be expected. They apply to Rh hemolytic disease, but not to that caused by ABO incompatibility. Although it is true that the trend is to more severe involvement of successive Rh-positive fetuses, the course of erythroblastosis is not definitely predictable, and unexpectedly mild cases occur. Even a history of one or more stillbirths does not always mean that the next baby will be stillborn.

BLOOD TYPING

In each pregnancy, at the time of her first visit to the obstetrician, every patient should have a blood sample drawn for ABO and Rh typing (if this is not already known) and a test for unexpected blood group antibodies. It is also important to test apparently Rh-negative mothers for D^u. This is not because women of type D^u are likely to make Rh antibody, but for future reference at the time of delivery. At that time, a positive D^u result in a woman previously noted to be D^u-negative most likely represents leakage of a larger than usual amount of the baby's Rh-positive blood. This would require quantitation to determine the dose of RhIG needed to prevent immunization of the mother.

ANTIBODY DETECTION TESTS

A test for unexpected antibodies should be done even if the patient is Rh-positive. Although blood group immunization is infrequent in Rh-positive people, it may be an unexpected cause of erythroblastosis. In addition, some people have had transfusions and do not know about it. Any transfusion may be immunizing, and pregnancy with a fetus possessing the corresponding antigen may result in erythroblastosis. Finally, if the mother herself requires transfusions, prior knowledge of an antibody will save a great deal of hurried laboratory work and prevent delay in providing compatible blood.

Early in the course of a woman's prenatal visits to the physician, if she is Rh-negative or has an unexpected antibody that could cause fetal hemolytic disease, it is advisable to obtain a blood sample from the husband for ABO and Rh or other relevant typing. Do not rely on old records from some unknown laboratory.

If the mother is Rh-negative, it is helpful to know whether the father is Rh-positive and, if so, whether he is homozygous or heterozygous (see Chap. 3). If the father is Rh-negative, the likelihood of erythroblastosis is much less. When there is reasonable doubt as to the identity of the father, remember that test results from the male partner may be seriously misleading and should not deter one from routine antibody screening.

Unimmunized Rh-negative mothers with Rh-negative husbands require no additional serologic testing unless there is some particular reason to look further. Repeated stillbirths, or a previous baby with jaundice, justify additional tests with more sensitive methods or investigation for possible ABO hemolytic disease. When no antibody can be detected but a strong suspicion of erythroblastosis exists, the mother's serum can be tested against the father's red cells, provided they are ABO-compatible. This procedure can reveal immunization to a low-incidence antigen possessed by the father, hence possibly also by the fetus, but not present in the usual reagent red blood cells used for antibody detection.

An Rh-negative mother with an Rh-positive husband and no antibodies is unlikely to encounter serious difficulty due to Rh incompatibility in the current pregnancy, although this can occur. As a precaution in such cases, it is wise to test for antibody once again about a month before the due date, to detect any antibody that may have developed and reached significant strength. This would not be done if Rh immune globulin had been administered during pregnancy.

ANTIBODY IDENTIFICATION

Once an unexpected antibody is detected, the antibody specificity must be determined. Some, like the Lewis antibodies or cold anti-P_1, do not cause erythroblastosis. Others, like those of the Kell and Duffy systems [1], may be important *if* the father has the corresponding antigen. If there is doubt as to the antibody identity, blood samples should be submitted for identification to a laboratory capable of providing this service.

OTHER ANTIBODIES

In the case of an IgG antibody other than anti-D, the father should be tested to determine whether he has the corresponding antigen and, if possible, whether he is homozygous or heterozygous for the gene that produces that factor. If the father does not have the antigen concerned, then the antibody is of no significance as a cause of hemolytic disease. In any event, the patient should be notified of the presence of a blood group antibody and warned of its possible significance in transfusion. This information should be provided in comprehensible written form to the patient's physician as well as to the medical record.

Antibody Titration

When the usual Rh antibody has been identified, a titration should be done. Titers are an indication of the degree of immunization of the mother, even though the value itself may bear little relation to the severity of the disease affecting the fetus. A few generalities may help put this into better perspective:

1. The initial appearance of anti-D almost always means that the fetus is Rh-positive.
2. The pregnancy during which anti-D first appears is not often seriously affected by erythroblastosis.
3. Low titers of antibody (less than 8) are seldom associated with serious fetal disease.
4. A rising antibody titer usually means that the fetus is Rh-positive and thus potentially affected.
5. Even with an Rh-positive fetus, many immunized women maintain a fixed antibody titer. This does not necessarily mean that the fetus is Rh-negative or that it is not seriously affected.

As titers increase, the numbers get bigger and the difference from one dilution to the next looks correspondingly more impressive. Thus the difference between a titer of 2 and one of 8 does not look like much, while a step from 64 to 256 seems a very great change indeed. In reality, both represent only a two-tube difference, which is the borderline of significance. More strictly quantitative hemagglutination techniques or automatic methods have little application to clinical testing.

Since the advent of diagnostic amniocentesis (see below) and fetal blood sampling, the value of serial antibody titrations has decreased. The important things are the *detection* of antibody in sufficient strength to be clinically significant, and its *identification*.

The titration technique should be one suitable for the detection of IgG-type antibodies. Titers obtained by these techniques will give results that roughly parallel each other, although some variation must be expected. Since small differences of techniques can make large differences in titers, the titers obtained in one laboratory should not be directly compared with those of another.

Amniocentesis

Antibody titers do not answer the following questions: (1) whether a pregnancy should be allowed to go to term, thus risking stillbirth if the fetus is seriously involved; (2) whether the fetus should be delivered early by induction or cesarean section, thus risking unnecessary prematurity if the fetus is not seriously affected; or (3) whether the fetus is a candidate for intrauterine transfusion.

The only widely available method to determine the effect of maternal antibody on the fetus is to examine the amniotic fluid and measure the bilirubinoid

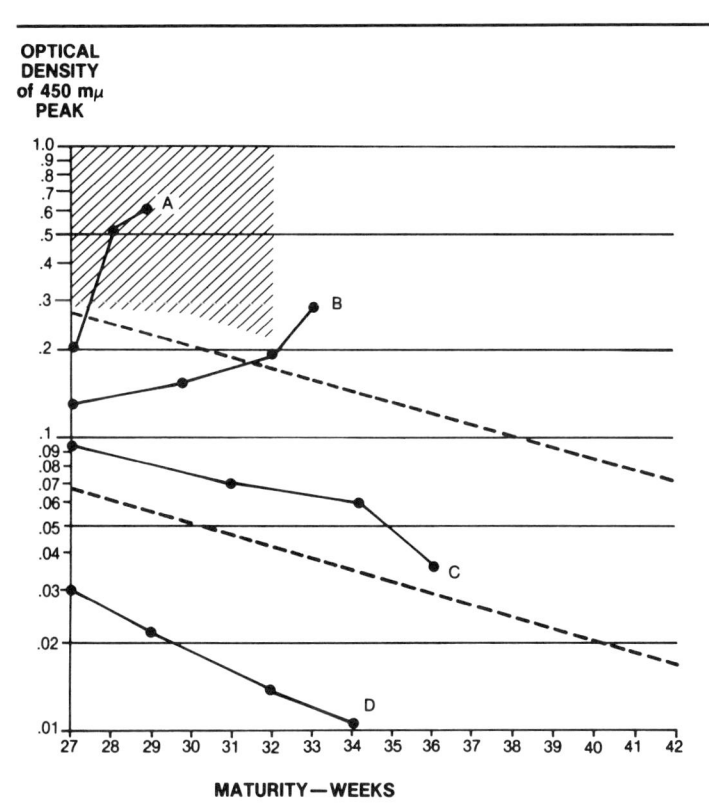

Figure 9–1
Chart of amniotic fluid optical density (at 450 nm) related to fetal gestational age, based in part on Liley's data [34]. The dashed lines separate three zones: the top zone indicates severe fetal hemolytic disease; the middle one, moderate involvement; and the bottom, mild disease or an unaffected fetus. The shaded zone indicates where intrauterine transfusion is usually necessary. The solid lines show readings on individual patients in the following circumstances: (A) intrauterine fetal death, (B) severe hemolytic disease with survival, (C) mild hemolytic disease, (D) Rh-negative fetus.

pigments by a change in optical density at 450 nm. Procedural and other details can be found in the literature on obstetrics [25, 26]. The data so obtained must be correlated with the history and ultrasound findings to serve as a guide to appropriate clinical action. Examples are shown in Fig. 9–1. If, for example, the father is heterozygous, optical density readings consistently in the low zone probably indicate an Rh-negative fetus or one that is only mildly affected. The pregnancy in such a case could be allowed to proceed to term, thus avoiding the hazards of unnecessary prematurity.

Amniotic fluid optical-density difference (*delta OD*) readings in the intermediate zone are difficult to judge and will probably require serial determinations before a confident evaluation is possible. The trend of the delta OD readings should be downward; therefore, successive specimens maintaining the same delta OD indicate increasing severity of disease. Severe disease or stillbirth in a previous pregnancy should serve as a warning that there is an increased chance of stillbirth in the present fetus. At this stage, intrauterine transfusion is an option. If the obstetrician estimates that fetal pulmonary maturity will permit preterm delivery, the fetus will have to withstand the dangers of prematurity, delivery, and the effects of erythroblastosis, including the probability of exchange transfusion. The situation calls for the utmost in clinical judgement and careful coordination between the obstetrician, the neonatologist, and the laboratory.

ULTRASOUND IMAGING

The use of ultrasound imaging has had many beneficial effects [27]. It obviates fluoroscopy or other X-ray techniques with their potentially harmful effects on the fetus. In addition, it permits detection and evaluation of edema, pericardial effusion, or other evidences of fetal hydrops. Finally, it enables the placing of needles for direct fetal intravascular transfusion or intrauterine peritoneal transfusion [28].

Testing of the Newborn

ABO AND RH TYPING

Blood grouping, Rh typing, and a direct antiglobulin test are done on the blood of all babies born to Rh-negative mothers or to those with a history of erythroblastosis in previous infants. The Rh typing is occasionally misleading when the patient's Rh antibodies are of the "blocking" type. Such antibodies may occupy all the antigenic sites of a baby's Rh-positive red cells, preventing agglutination by Rh antiserums, especially those reactive in saline, and thereby giving a false-negative result. The opposite may also occur, with heavily coated red cells reacting indiscriminately with high-protein antiserums, resulting in a positive reading regardless of Rh status. Blocking is not a common event, but when it does occur, the laboratory staff must be alert to the apparent inconsistency of a positive direct antiglobulin test on the "Rh-negative" baby's red cells and the presence of an antibody in the baby's and mother's serum. A further refinement in such cases is to elute antibody from the baby's cells (see Chap. 5) and determine its specificity. The same eluate can then also be used to crossmatch donor blood for exchange transfusion.

If elution is carefully done, it sometimes frees enough binding sites so that the same cells from which the eluate was prepared can be correctly typed as Rh-positive. However, any typing done on cells that have been treated by an elution procedure needs to be interpreted with great caution.

DIRECT ANTIGLOBULIN TEST

When Rh antibody is present in significant amounts in an Rh-positive baby's serum, the direct antiglobulin (Coombs) test is almost always positive, indicating antibody coating the baby's red cells. The test therefore shows hemolytic disease but gives no indication whether exchange transfusion is likely to be needed. In mild cases, or in ABO erythroblastosis, the direct antiglobulin test is often only weakly positive or even negative.

Babies who have received intrauterine transfusions may have a negative or weakly positive direct antiglobulin test at birth and may appear to be Rh-negative because of substitution of Rh-negative donor blood for the baby's own blood. The results obtained will depend on the amount of donor blood given, the time that has passed since the transfusion, and the baby's own rate of blood cell replacement. Such findings must not be taken to indicate that exchange transfusion is not needed, or that the baby is really Rh-negative.

HEMOGLOBIN LEVEL

The primary danger of hemolytic disease in fetal life is hydrops fetalis. Liveborn babies, on the other hand, are at particular hazard of anemia and heart failure in the immediate neonatal period, that is, the first day or two. The key test at the time of birth is, therefore, the umbilical cord blood hemoglobin level. A level below 15 gm/dl indicates anemia, and less than 12 gm/dl constitutes severe anemia.

OTHER TESTS

Once the baby is a few hours old, the dangers of jaundice predominate, and management hinges mostly on serial bilirubin determinations. The rate of rise of serum bilirubin is important and must be correlated with the actual bilirubin level and with the baby's gestational age. In general, a rise of more than 0.5 mg/dl per hour indicate severe disease. Kernicterus rarely occurs in uncomplicated erythroblastosis in term infants unless the unconjugated serum bilirubin exceeds 20 mg/dl. Although many authorities warn against the too-ready use of such a "magic number," it still represents a useful guideline. It must be correlated, however, with the rate of rise and with other clinical factors, particularly the baby's state of maturity.

Other clinical and laboratory factors of importance are discussed in the literature on pediatrics [29, 30].

Removal of Rh Antibody by Plasmapheresis

A number of attempts have been made to remove the Rh antibody by plasmapheresis, first by older manual methods and then with greater enthusiasm when machines for plasmapheresis became available (see Chap. 10). The results have not been impressive so far, probably no better than those obtainable using intrauterine transfusion and early delivery [5, 31]. The removal of enormous amounts of plasma (35 to 150 or more liters in a pregnancy) may cause some reduction in antibody titer, but the effect on fetal survival is at best debatable [29]. It is possible that the procedure is self-defeating by affecting feedback mechanisms that control more antibody formation. The proceedings of a meeting held on this topic in England may be consulted by the interested reader [32]. Controlled studies are needed and these have not been done [33].

Intrauterine Transfusion

A bold venture, pioneered by Liley in 1963, attacks the problem of early intrauterine death [34]. Noting that red cells injected into the peritoneal cavity of a fetus are absorbed into its circulation, Liley succeeded in transfusing compatible Rh-negative erythrocytes into the fetal abdominal cavity by means of transabdominal puncture of the mother. Red cells are absorbed from the fetal abdomen via the subdiaphragmatic lymphatics.

The mortality and success rates in terms of live births are difficult to assess for intrauterine transfusion, largely because of widely differing criteria for the procedure, as well as technical differences in various centers [35, 36]. Furthermore, with the incidence of Rh hemolytic disease diminishing because of the use of Rh immune globulin, fewer intrauterine transfusions are being done.

The general principle is to keep the fetus alive until it is feasible to deliver it with a reasonable chance of survival, that is, to reserve intrauterine transfusion to fetuses who would otherwise die of hydrops before 30 to 32 weeks of gestation. Even some fetuses with evidence of fetal hydrops have been saved by intrauterine transfusion. After 30 weeks, the same criteria probably better serve to indicate a need for early delivery.

Other routes of fetal transfusion have been developed, particularly to treat fetuses that are already hydropic. In England, Rodeck and co-workers reported reversal of hydrops by direct intravascular transfusion of fetuses under fetoscopy [37]. More recently, Grannum and his associates at Yale have carried out intrauterine *exchange* transfusions by using ultrasound imaging to insert a needle into the umbilical vein [38]. Clearly, the technique is extremely demanding, and not one that is likely to become routine in the community hospital [28].

Blood Selection

Concentrated red cells (hematocrit 85 to 90 percent) compatible with the mother's serum are prepared from Rh-negative blood that has preferably been less than 3 days in storage. The quantity to transfuse ranges from 40 ml at 24 weeks, to 100 to 120 ml at 32 weeks [25]. Overtransfusion can interfere with fetal circulation and may be fatal [35, 39]. Several transfusions may be needed at 2- to 4-week intervals.

Although the mother's washed red cells would be perfectly suitable, and probably preferable, fresh type O, Rh-negative red blood cells are used in most centers. One may avoid the complications of the presence of anti-A and anti-B and reduce the risk of graft-versus-host disease by washing the red cells before transfusion or by using reconstituted frozen red cells. Either expedient probably also lowers the likelihood of transmission of donor-borne viruses. In addition to either of these measures, the blood should probably also be irradiated to eliminate the possibility of graft-versus-host reaction [40]. Irradiation does not harm the red cells (see Chap. 6, p. 235).

The literature on obstetrics may be consulted for technical details of intrauterine transfusion [25, 39].

Exchange Transfusion

There are two aims in the treatment of erythroblastosis of the newborn, and their importance relative to each other depends on the stage of the disease. The first is the correction of anemia, with or without attendant heart failure, and the second is the reduction of hyperbilirubinemia to prevent brain damage. Anemia is usually the prime consideration in severely diseased infants immediately after delivery; the second becomes more important after the first day.

The only effective way of accomplishing both aims is the removal of the baby's own blood and its replacement by donor blood (exchange transfusion). Allen and Diamond's 1957 account of this procedure is a classic and still worth reading for background [41].

Special Considerations

Exchange with a full unit of donor whole blood achieves nearly 90 percent replacement of the average-sized baby's blood, which is generally considered adequate. The use of about 160 to 180 ml of donor whole blood per kilogram of the baby's body weight has been recommended as a maximum [29]. Since a unit of blood as usually collected consists of 450 ml of donor blood plus anticoagulant, it is within this range. This quantity is also referred to as a *two-volume exchange,* since it is about twice the average-sized newborn's blood volume.

Maternal Blood

Although few obstetricians seem to want to use it, maternal blood is ideal in many respects for exchange transfusion [36]. Its red cells are always compatible with respect to the antibody causing erythroblastosis. For exchange transfusion, it is best to remove the mother's plasma as completely as possible, preferably by washing the cells with isotonic saline solution and resuspending them in AB plasma. There is another way of accomplishing the same thing in blood banks with access to the necessary facilities. First, one or two units of blood are taken from the mother during pregnancy, with precautions to avoid significant clinical anemia. The red cells are then frozen for eventual transfusion to either baby or mother. After reconstitution, the red cells are free of plasma. They should be resuspended in antibody-free compatible plasma for exchange transfusion.

Blood Group
Since the antibody that causes erythroblastosis is formed by the mother, it stands to reason that its titer is at least as high in the mother's serum as in the baby's. For this reason, the usual practice has been to select blood for transfusion to the baby on the basis of compatibility with the mother's serum. A crossmatch using the baby's serum as well is then superfluous. When the mother's serum is not immediately available, as when erythroblastotic babies born elsewhere are sent to a hospital without the mother, serum from the baby may, of course, be used for crossmatch to avoid delaying an urgently needed transfusion. If time permits, an eluate from the baby's cells may be prepared and used instead of, or in addition to, the baby's serum.

ABO. Blood of the baby's own group is preferable if it is compatible with the mother's serum. When this is not possible, authorities differ as to the best policy to follow. One must choose between blood of the baby's own group (although it may be incompatible with the mother's serum) and O blood, which would be compatible with the baby's and mother's serums, but has the disadvantage of plasma incompatibility with the baby's red cells. Table 9–1 gives a guide to blood selection. Group O blood does have the further advantage that it can be prepared before delivery, without knowledge of the baby's blood group, and is being increasingly used for exchange transfusions and for other transfusions in the neonatal period. Group O red cells can, of course, be resuspended in AB plasma for exchange transfusions.

RH TYPE. In Rh erythroblastosis, Rh-negative blood must be used to obtain the best results with the fewest exchanges. When hemolytic disease is known or suspected to be due to factors other than D, the blood selected must lack the antigen or antigens concerned and should be serologically compatible. In case of difficulty in finding suitable blood, remember that a transfusion with incompatible blood is better than allowing a needed exchange to await the unraveling of an immunohematologic problem. Incompatible blood will not cause reactions in infants, and will help the baby, although multiple exchanges may be necessary to lessen hyperbilirubinemia.

In the case of exchange transfusion for conditions other than hemolytic disease, the mother's antibody or blood type is less important. Blood may then be selected according to the baby's blood type and crossmatched with the baby's serum.

Table 9–1. Selection of Blood by ABO Group for Exchange Transfusion to Babies with Rh Hemolytic Disease*

Baby's ABO Group	Mother's ABO Group			
	O	A	B	AB
O	O	O	O	
A	A or O	A	A or O	A or O
B	B or O	B or O	B	B or O
AB		AB or A	AB or B	AB or A or B

*In all cases, the blood will be Rh-negative. Type O red blood cells with AB plasma added can be used effectively for almost any case.

Blood Storage

Blood used for exchange transfusion should be reasonably fresh, a requirement for which there is no generally accepted definition. The idea is to provide red cells that have suffered as little damage from storage as possible, thus permitting good survival in the baby and contributing the least possible to the baby's accumulation of bilirubin. Another advantage of fresh blood is that it has a relatively low plasma potassium level, an important consideration in avoiding the possible hazard of potassium toxicity. Since there is little detectable difference in the viability of red cells within the first week after collection, and little potassium accumulation, it has been traditional to limit donor blood to less than 5 days of storage. In very sick babies, particularly prematures, the blood selected should always be *as fresh as possible,* provided that difficulties in finding fresh blood do not delay the exchange. Removal of a portion of the plasma decreases the amount of potassium and citrate transfused.

Another consideration is the capability of the red cells to transport and release oxygen [42]. Except in newborns who already have a demonstrated problem with tissue oxygenation, this seldom seems to be a significant concern. With currently used anticoagulants (i.e., CPDA-1), 2,3-DPG is well maintained for at least a week after the collection of donor blood.

Heparinized blood was at one time preferred in some centers, particularly for acidotic or hypocalcemic babies [29], but its short dating period means that donors must be ready and waiting to be drawn for the exchange transfusion. Such an approach is no longer clinically justifiable. In addition, heparin has some potentially undesirable metabolic effects [43, 44], and heparinized blood is no longer available.

Temperature

Since exchange transfusion with cold blood may be dangerous to a very sick baby, the blood should be warmed in some way. This should be done with great care, because prolonged or excessive warming has deleterious effects on stored blood. Rather than warming the whole container of blood, which would mean that some of the blood would be kept warm for a considerable period, it is better to warm the blood on its way from container to baby. This can be accomplished by passing the delivery tubing through a warming device. Special heat exchangers are available from a number of manufacturers.

ABO Hemolytic Disease

Erythroblastosis caused by maternofetal incompatibility in the ABO system is more common than that caused by Rh incompatibility, but is also subtler, usually milder, and consequently more difficult to diagnose [45–47]. This may cause unnecessary delay in instituting therapy. ABO erythroblastosis is caused by antibodies that are normally present in the plasma of people who have not necessarily been exposed to any obvious antigenic stimulus. Thus, it is as likely to strike the first pregnancy as a later one, and there is not necessarily any progression in severity from one pregnancy to the next. Because the incompatibility causing ABO erythroblastosis tends to protect against Rh disease, the two do not often coincide.

Although ABO hemolytic disease may be associated with high titers of maternal anti-A or anti-B, the titers as such are of little value in assessing the likelihood or severity of fetal disease. Therefore, prenatal efforts to detect cases in which the incompatibility might give rise to trouble are of no value. There are several reasons for this. First, although about 20 percent of babies are incompatible with their mothers, maternal anti-A and anti-B do not enter the fetus as easily as Rh antibodies. Second, A and B substances are present not only on the fetal red cells like the Rh factor, but also in other body tissues and (in secretors) in the body fluids. Thus, Allen and Diamond likened the fetus to a sponge that soaks up maternal anti-A and anti-B and absorbs or neutralizes the antibodies before they can have much effect on the red blood cells [41]. Stillbirth or severe erythroblastosis is seldom caused by ABO incompatibility.

Antibody Characteristics

There is a correlation between the qualitative nature of the maternal anti-A and anti-B and the occurrence of erythroblastosis. When the maternal antibody is of the IgG type, it can reach the fetus and cause disease. Such antibody occurs predominantly in people of group O, less often in those of groups A and B, and it involves primarily the anti-A component. It follows, then, that ABO erythroblastosis involves principally the babies of group O mothers with group A husbands. The disease obviously does not occur if the father is group O, or if the mother is group AB, or if the fetus is group O.

Although rises in titer of anti-A and anti-B may take place after the birth of ABO-incompatible babies, there is no evidence that increased titers have any effect on the likelihood of disease. The reason for the occurrence of IgG forms of these antibodies is not well understood. Pregnancy may sometimes play a role, but more often the presence of IgG antibodies may be due to other exposures to A and B substances, such as may take place in medical immunization procedures.

Routine laboratory testing cannot determine directly whether a father is homozygous or heterozygous with respect to A or B (that is, *AA* or *AO*; *BB* or *BO*), but this can sometimes be deduced from family studies. If any one of his children or either of his parents is group O, he is heterozygous. The absence of group O parents or offspring proves nothing. Since the heterozygous man may father group O babies, the likelihood of ABO erythroblastosis in his offspring is less.

DIAGNOSIS

The diagnosis of ABO hemolytic disease is primarily a matter of recognizing the problem in the newborn rather than in the prenatal stage. The condition usually presents as unexpected jaundice on the third or fourth day of life, sometimes even later.

Serologic Studies

Unexpected blood group antibodies are not detected in the serum of mother or baby, since the reagent red cells used in the test are group O. The presence of IgG-type anti-A or anti-B in the mother's serum is no help, since this type of antibody is common, especially in group O people. The first clue may well be that the mother of a jaundiced baby is group O and the baby, group A. The demonstration of any anti-A or anti-B in a baby's serum, incompatible with its own red cells, is an important point. Such an incompatible antibody may be presumed to be the cause of excessive destruction of the infant's red cells, even though fixation of the antibody to the cells may not be demonstrable.

The *direct antiglobulin test* is often weak or negative, apparently because the number of antibody molecules fixed to the red cells is at the lower limits of sensitivity of this test [48]. When the test is positive, and sometimes even when it is negative, it is often possible to elute antibody from the baby's red cells by the usual methods (heat elution works well, see Chap. 5). The resulting eluate is then tested against A, B, and O red cells to demonstrate the expected pattern of reactivity. Distinction of the A_1 and A_2 phenotypes is not clear in newborns, but the group A babies that are affected eventually turn out to be type A_1, probably because A_1 red cells have more A receptors.

Table 9–2 illustrates the serologic findings in a case of ABO hemolytic disease.

Jaundice

The jaundice resulting from ABO incompatibility usually occurs later and develops more slowly than in Rh erythroblastosis, although it still occurs at a

Table 9–2. Blood Grouping Results in a Typical Case of ABO Erythroblastosis

	Known Serums, Anti-			Known Red Cells			Direct Antiglobulin Test
	A	B	A,B	A	B	O	
Mother	0	0	0	+*	+	0	0
Baby	+	0	+	+	Weak	0	+
Eluate from baby's cells				+	0	0	

*Hemolysis.
Note that the mother has hemolytic anti-A and that anti-A was eluted from the baby's red cells. Incompatible maternal anti-A as well as some anti-B are present in the baby's serum, an important diagnostic point.

notably faster rate than physiologic jaundice. Its great danger to the newborn lies in its insidiousness and in the fact that the direct antiglobulin test is often negative, which may result in the jaundice being lightly regarded. The nursery staff must be trained to recognize the onset of jaundice, to be alert to it, and to notify the physician promptly when it is noticed. Once the existence of ABO hemolytic disease is recognized, or indeed, in any case of severe jaundice even when the cause is not clear, the need for exchange transfusion will be based on clinical and laboratory evaluation of the hyperbilirubinemia.

EXCHANGE TRANSFUSION

In ABO erythroblastosis, type O blood or red blood cells must be used for any exchange transfusion. If whole blood is used, it should probably lack hemolytic anti-A and anti-B, although data to support this recommendation are lacking. Other considerations regarding the decision for exchange transfusion and its performance are essentially the same as for hemolytic disease of other causes.

References
1. Weinstein L. Irregular antibodies causing hemolytic disease of the newborn: a continuing problem. *Clin Obstet Gynaecol* 1982; 25:321–32.
2. Stern K, Davidsohn I, Masaitis L. Experimental studies on Rh immunization. *Am J Clin Pathol* 1956; 26:833–43.
3. Stern K, Goodman HS, Berger M. Experimental isoimmunization to hemoantigens in man. *J Immunol* 1961; 87:189–98.
4. Mollison PL. Clinical aspects of Rh immunization. *Am J Clin Pathol* 1973; 60:287–301.
5. Bowman JM. Suppression of Rh isoimmunization. A review. *Obstet Gynecol* 1978; 52:385–93.
6. Zimmerman DR. Rh. *The Intimate History of a Disease and Its Conquest.* New York: Macmillan, 1973.
7. Davey MG. Epidemiology of failures of Rh immune globulin asnd ABO protection.

In: Ortho Research Institute of Medical Sciences. Proceedings of Symposium on Rh Antibody Mediated Immunosuppression. Raritan, NJ: Ortho Diagnostics, 1976; 109–13.
8. Mollison PL. *Blood Transfusion in Clinical Medicine,* 7th ed. Oxford, England: Blackwell Sci, 1983; 792–4.
9. Sebring ES, Polesky HF. Detection of fetal maternal hemorrhage in Rh immune globulin candidates. *Transfusion* 1982; 22:468–71.
10. Lee CL. Estimation of fetal red cells in mother. *N Engl J Med* 1976; 295:1080 (letter).
11. Bowman JM, Chown B, Lewis M, Pollock JM. Rh immunization during pregnancy: antenatal prophylaxis. *Can Med Assoc J* 1978; 118:623–7.
12. Keith L, Bozorgi N. Small-dose anti-Rh therapy after first trimester abortion. *Int J Gynaecol Obstet* 1977; 15:1–3.
13. Berger GS, Keith L. Utilization of Rh prophylaxis. *Clin Obstet Gynaecol* 1982; 25:267–75.
14. Lacey PA, Caskey CR, Werner DJ, Moulds JJ. Fatal hemolytic disease of a newborn due to anti-D in an Rh-positive Du variant mother. *Transfusion* 1983; 23:91–4.
15. White CA, Stedman CM, Frank S. Anti-D antibodies in D- and Du-positive women: a cause of hemolytic disease of the newborn. *Am J Obstet Gynecol* 1983; 145:1069–75.
16. Schneider J. German trials. In: Ortho Research Institute of Medical Sciences. Proceedings of Symposium on Rh Antibody Mediated Immunosuppression. Ortho Diagnostics, 1976; 63–6.
17. Mollison PL. *Blood Transfusion in Clinical Medicine,* 7th ed. Oxford, England: Blackwell Sci, 1983; 398–9.
18. American College of Obstetricians and Gynecologists. The selective use of Rho(D) immune globulin (RhIG). Technical Bulletin No. 61, 1981.
19. Konugres AA, Polesky HF, Walker RH. Rh immune globulin and the Rh-positive, Du variant, mother. *Transfusion* 1982; 22:76–7.
20. American College of Obstetricians and Gynecologists. Management of isoimmunization of pregnancy. Technical Bulletin No. 90, 1986.
21. James LS. Shock in relation to hydrops. *Ann Ostet Ginecol Med Perinat* 1971; 92:599–601.
22. Phibbs RH, Johnson P, Tooley WH. Cardiorespiratory status of erythroblastotic infants: II. Blood volume, hematocrit, and serum albumin concentration in relation to hydrops fetalis. *Pediatrics* 1974; 53:13–23.
23. Porter EG, Waters WJ. A rapid micromethod for measuring the reserve albumin binding capacity in serum from infants with hyperbilirubinemia. *J Lab Clin Med* 1966; 67:660–8.
24. Thaler MM. Perinatal bilirubin metabolism. *Adv Pediatr* 1972; 19; 215–35.
25. Queenan JT. *Modern Management of the Rh Problem,* 2nd ed. Hagerstown, MD: Harper & Row, 1977.
26. Queenan JT. Current management of the Rh-sensitized patient. *Clin Obstet Gynaecol* 1982; 25:293–301.
27. Frigoletto FD, Greene MF, Benacerraf BR, et al. Ultrasonographic fetal surveillance in the management of the isoimmunized pregnancy. *N Engl J Med* 1986; 315:430–2.
28. Queenan JT. Erythroblastosis fetalis: closing the circle. *N Engl J Med* 1986; 314:1448–9.
29. Oski FH, Naiman JL. *Hematologic Problems in the Newborn.* 3rd ed. Philadelphia: Saunders, 1982; 283–346.

30. Klaus MH, Fanaroff AA. *Care of the High-Risk Neonate*, 3rd ed. Philadelphia: Saunders, 1986.
31. Peddle LJ. The antenatal management of the Rh sensitized woman. *Clin Perinatol* 1984; 11:251–66.
32. Entwhistle CC, Bowell PJ (organizers). Symposium proceedings, Oxford, England. *Plasma Ther Transf Technol* 1984; 5:5–109.
33. Klein HG, Balow JE, Dau PC, et al. Clinical applications of therapeutic apheresis. Report of the Clinical Applications Committee, American Society for Apheresis. *J Clin Apheresis* 1986; 3:77–8.
34. Liley AW. Intrauterine transfusion of the fetus in haemolytic disease. *Br Med J* 1963; 2:1107–9.
35. Crosby WM, Brobmann GF, Chang ACK. Intrauterine transfusion and fetal death. *Am J Obstet Gynecol* 1970; 108:135–8.
36. Hamilton EG. Intrauterine transfusion. Safeguard or peril? *Obstet Gynecol* 1977; 50:255–60.
37. Rodeck CH, Kemp JR, Holman CA, et al. Direct intravascular fetal blood transfusion by fetoscopy in severe rhesus isoimmunization. *Lancet* 1981; 1:625–7.
38. Grannum PA, Copel JA, Plaxe SC, et al. In utero exchange transfusion by direct intravascular injection in severe erythroblastosis fetalis. *N Engl J Med* 1986; 314:1431–4.
39. Bowman JM. The management of Rh-isoimmunization. *Obstet Gynecol* 1978; 52:1–16.
40. Parkman R, Mosier D, Umansky I, et al. Graft-versus-host disease after intrauterine and exchange transfusions for hemolytic disease of the newborn. *N Engl J Med* 1974; 290:359–63.
41. Allen FH Jr, Diamond LK. Erythroblastosis fetalis. Boston: Little, Brown, 1957.
42. Delivoria-Papadopoulos M, Morrow G, Oski F. Exchange transfusion in the newborn infant with fresh and "old" blood: the role of storage on 2,3-diphosphoglycerate, hemoglobin-oxygen affinity, and oxygen release. *J Pediatr* 1971; 79:898–903.
43. Odell GB, Poland RL, Ostrea EM. Neonatal hyperbilirubinemia. In: Klaus MH, Fanaroff AA (eds). *Care of the High-Risk Neonate*. Philadelphia: Saunders, 1973.
44. Schiff D, Aranda JV, Chan G, et al. Metabolic effects of exchange transfusion. I. Effect of citrated and of heparinized blood on glucose, non-esterified fatty acids, 2-(4-hydroxybenzeneazo) benzoic acid binding, and insulin. *J Pediatr* 1971; 78:603–9.
45. Gold ER, Butler NR. *ABO Haemolytic Disease of the Newborn*. Bristol, England: John Wright, 1972.
46. Peevy KJ, Wiseman HJ. ABO hemolytic disease of the newborn: evaluation of management and identification of racial and antigenic factors. *Pediatrics* 1978; 61:475–8.
47. Dufour DR, Monoghan WP. ABO hemolytic disease of the newborn. A retrospective analysis of 254 cases. *Am J Clin Pathol* 1980; 73:369–73.
48. Romano EL, Hughes-Jones NC, Mollison PL. Direct antiglobulin reaction in ABO-haemolytic disease of the newborn. *Br Med J* 1973; 1:524–6.

10. Therapeutic Hemapheresis

We have already described hemapheresis for the collection of blood components, such as platelets or leukocytes (see Chap. 1). These procedures involve an extracorporeal system, usually centrifugal, by means of which certain blood components are separated and retained, while others, e.g., red cells and plasma, are returned to the donor. *Therapeutic* hemapheresis is the application of this principle to the separation and removal of a harmful blood constituent from a patient. Such a procedure is usually applied to the removal of a deleterious plasma component (therapeutic plasmapheresis or plasma exchange), although it may also be used to remove excessive numbers of platelets or leukocytes (therapeutic cytapheresis, or cytoreduction), or even for red cell exchange.

Our reason for discussing these blood manipulations in a book on transfusion is that they require the use of blood cell separators, many of which are operated in blood banks. These procedures are therefore within the field of blood bank activity, and are a relatively new and certainly interesting part of it.

Plasma Exchange

Plasma exchange, the commonest form of therapeutic hemapheresis, is a procedure in which plasma is extracted from a patient's whole blood, usually by passing the blood continuously or in batches through a blood cell separator. As the plasma is removed, an approximately equal amount of replacement solution is substituted, usually 5 percent albumin solution or normal plasma, and the patient's red cells are returned more or less continuously along with the replacement solution. The procedure is thus a form of extracorporeal blood modification or manipulation. Since its greatest clinical application is in immune disorders, it may be considered a form of immunologic modulation or even "immunosurgery."

Although the first removal, washing, and return of the blood of a human (uremic) patient was reported in France as early as 1909 [1], the widespread clinical application of plasma exchange had to await the advent of mechanical blood cell separators, which made such procedures reasonably safe and expeditious.

METHODS

Blood cell separators were described in detail in our third edition, and more briefly earlier in this book (see Chap. 1). Plasma exchange can be carried out with almost any blood cell separator. *Intermittent-flow* systems require the separation of plasma from successive batches of the patient's blood, with such batches, or cycles, being repeated as often as needed to remove a desired quantity of plasma. For example, if 250 ml of plasma is obtained per cycle, then

Table 10–1. Factors Important in Membrane Plasma Separation

Membrane structure and porosity
Blood flow rate and pressure
Transmembrane pressure
Geometry of flow pathway
Area of blood-to-membrane exposure
Biocompatibility of membrane material
Sterilizability
Cost

10 cycles will remove 2,500 ml, although not all of that quantity would be the patient's plasma, because of dilution by incoming replacement fluid. Intermittent-flow systems are relatively slow and cause large fluctuations in the extracorporeal volume of blood as well as in the patient's blood volume. This creates additional risks for some patients. An advantage of intermittent flow is that it can be carried out with a single venipuncture.

Continuous-flow systems are generally more convenient for plasma exchange, involve a smaller extracorporeal volume of the patient's blood, and because of continuous separation, do not occasion as much fluctuation in the blood volume. They have the disadvantage of generally requiring two venipunctures, one for outflow, the other for return of blood.

Membrane plasma separation devices are continuous-flow systems in which the blood passes by a membrane of varying geometry through which the plasma perfuses, leaving the blood cells to be returned to the patient along with replacement fluid [2]. Membrane technology has been used primarily in the field of hemodialysis for the removal of non-protein-bound solutes from blood. More recently, it has been applied increasingly to plasma exchange for removing protein-bound pathogenic substances. To achieve this, the membrane must be of such porosity to permit the passage of plasma protein molecules while barring the blood cells. Many variables affect the operating efficiency of such systems (Table 10–1).

The geometric configuration of such devices is of two major types. The first is that of blood flowing between flat sheets of membrane (a "sandwich" arrangement); the second, that of passage through multiple, capillary-like membranous tubules (hollow-fiber type). In both, the hydrodynamic force of blood flow parallel to the membrane surfaces creates a transmembrane filtration pressure leading to plasma flow at right angles through the membrane. Mathematical formulas have been derived to express the relationship, but in practice, the plasma flow is affected by many variables, such as the tendency of blood cells and protein molecules to pile up against a membrane [2, 3].

Membranes must be porous enough to allow molecules as large as immune

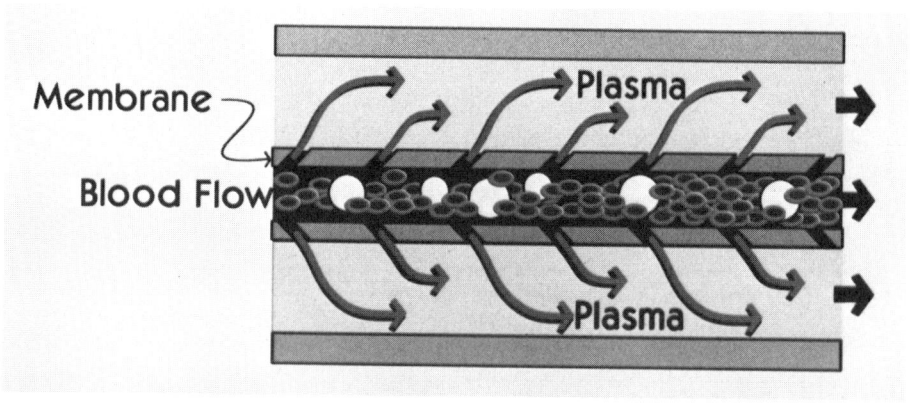

Figure 10-1
Diagrammatic representation of the separation of plasma from whole blood by means of a membrane. Hydrostatic forces cause a flow of liquid (plasma) through the pores of the membrane. The pores are large enough to allow passage of protein molecules, but too small to let blood cells through. The principle applies equally to a "sandwich" membrane configuration or to multiple hollow fibers.

complexes to pass through, while retaining all the blood cells. Maximum pore sizes of 0.2 to 0.6 micrometer (10^{-6}M) are usually satisfactory. If clogging occurs, the efficiency of filtration will decrease as blood flow continues (see Fig. 10-1). Such membranes must, of course, be biocompatible. There should be little or no adverse effects on blood cells exposed to the membrane, no toxic effects, no harmful substances leached from the plastic, and minimal complement activation [4].

Some devices include two stages of filtration, the first to separate plasma from blood cells, the second to separate large molecules, such as globulins or immune complexes, from the plasma. This is referred to as *cascade filtration* [5]. Cascade systems may even include several successive stages with progressively finer molecular sieving, but these are not yet available for routine clinical use. Other techniques pass the separated plasma through a cryoprecipitation chamber that separates cryoglobulins or immune complexes. Both of these modifications enable the patient to receive back his own modified plasma and avoid the expensive and relatively more risky use of albumin or homologous plasma.

Quantitative Considerations

When plasma is removed, any pathogenic component is removed with it. Although such a component cannot be totally eliminated, the extent of its removal is roughly proportional to the amount of plasma exchanged. Making certain

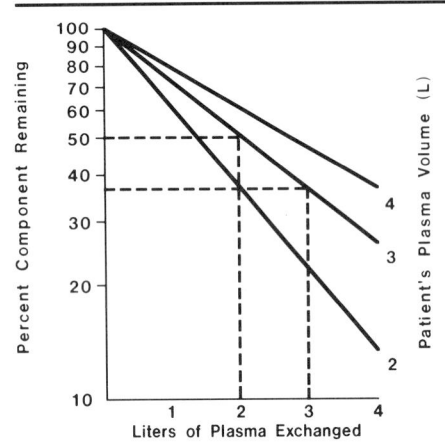

Figure 10-2
Curves relating the removal of a plasma component to the amount of plasma exchanged in patients with different plasma volumes. Plotted from a formula in reference 6. (From D. W. Huestis, Therapeutic plasmapheresis. In: J. D. Cash, *Progress in Transfusion Medicine*, Vol. 1. Edinburgh: Churchill, 1986; 78–94. With permission.)

assumptions that may not be entirely valid (such as considering the abnormal substance to be entirely intravascular), this relationship can be calculated mathematically [6], or expressed as a series of curves relating the volume of plasma exchanged to the patient's plasma volume and the amount of the substance remaining (Fig. 10–2).

Using the example of an IgM protein, which is found largely in the vascular compartment, such calculations show that an exchange of one plasma volume removes about 60 to 65 percent of that protein. Alternatively, and somewhat more easily, exchange of 40 ml of plasma per kilogram of body weight achieves approximately the same effect and is a more widely used guideline. By either measurement, an exchange of *one plasma volume* per session is adequate for most patients. Of course, one may do larger or smaller exchanges, depending on clinical needs. Very large plasma exchanges reach a point of diminishing efficiency, are expensive in time and materials, and increase the risk of complications.

As might be expected, plasma exchange is relatively effective in the removal of IgM proteins or immune complexes, since these are largely intravascular. Furthermore, the removal of circulating immune complexes sometimes seems to take place faster than would be predicted mathematically, apparently because even partial removal diminishes their inhibitory effects on suppressor T lymphocytes [7], which may then be able to cut down the production of IgM globulins. This may explain the occasional clinical remission apparently

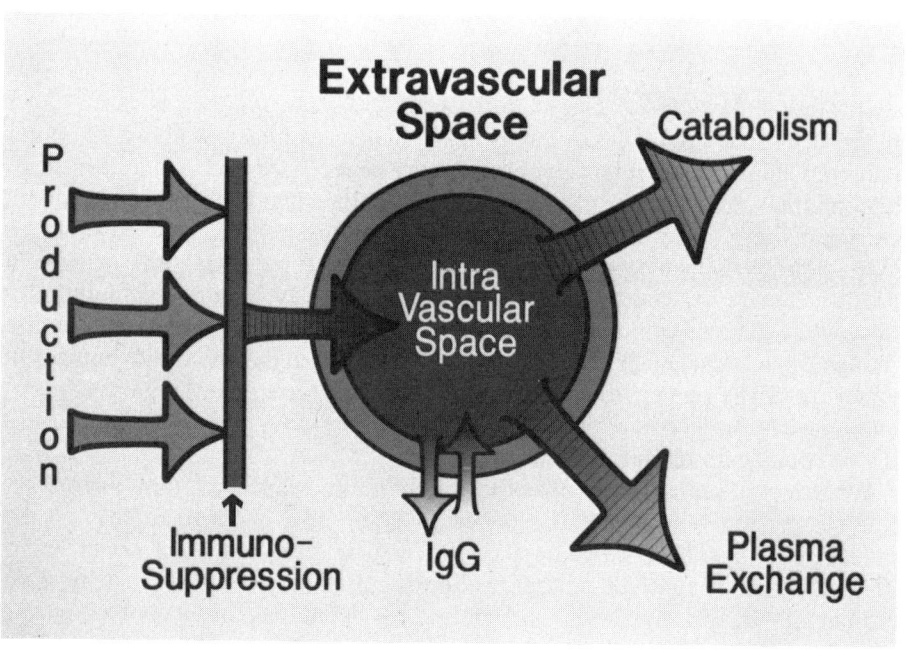

Figure 10-3
A diagram illustrating some of the complex interrelationships between the production, diffusion, and catabolism of a pathogenic plasma constituent, including the added effect of intervention by plasma exchange.

brought about by one or two plasma exchanges of a quantity that would seem to be inadequate to produce such an effect.

On the other hand, a plasma constituent such as IgG, which diffuses readily between the intravascular and extravascular compartments, will obviously not be removed as efficiently by plasma exchange. Larger or more frequent exchanges are needed. Similarly, if the substance to be removed is replaced rapidly and continuously by the body, very frequent exchanges may be necessary. In some cases, adequate reduction seems to be nearly impossible, perhaps because of some kind of compensatory rebound in production. The complex interrelationships are illustrated in Fig. 10-3.

Concurrent Immunosuppression

The efficiency of plasma exchange in removing deleterious plasma substances such as antibodies or immune complexes is enhanced by the concurrent application of immunosuppressive or cytotoxic therapy to inhibit antibody formation. In fact, these two forms of therapy are combined in most diseases treated by plasma exchange. The combination has the further advantage of permitting generally lower doses of immunosuppressive agents, thus reducing the risk of side effects.

Replacement Media

In small plasma exchanges, such as half a plasma volume, or about 20 ml per kilogram at infrequent intervals, plasma may be replaced with a simple electrolyte solution, usually isotonic saline. On the other hand, in large or frequent exchanges, e.g., one or more plasma volumes, the plasma must be replaced with some protein. No consensus exists as to the type or quantity of protein needed. Some physicians have used almost exclusively 5 percent albumin solution, while others have used plasma protein fraction or normal plasma. At first thought, plasma seems more physiologic. However, it has the disadvantages of exposure of the patient to disease transmission, citrate and allergic reactions, and possibly other complications. Albumin and plasma protein fraction cause fewer complications but are more costly.

What sort of replacement does the patient really need as a temporary substitute for plasma? Clearly, it is not necessary in most cases to replace all the plasma protein that has been removed. In fact, replacement of about half 5 percent albumin and half isotonic saline seems to be well tolerated by most patients [8, 9]. When insufficient protein is replaced, the patient soon manifests symptoms of hypovolemia even during a single exchange. This is rapidly correctable by the infusion of additional protein. Hypoproteinemia and hemodilution will also be demonstrable on laboratory testing.

During an exchange, the patient's fluid balance must be maintained by the continuous substitution of fluid in quantities approximately equal to that of the plasma lost. This is more difficult in intermittent-flow systems than in continuous-flow systems. Specific electrolyte deficiencies may need correction in some patients. Coagulation factors are unquestionably depleted during plasma exchange, but only very rarely does this seem to be a problem clinically. In the case of a large series of exchanges in immunodepressed patients, one should consider supplementing or following replacements with an intravenous infusion of immune serum globulin [10]. It is also important to remember that blood levels of any medications being given to the patient will be reduced by plasma exchange; supplementation during or after the procedure may be necessary.

Diseases Treated by Plasma Exchange

THE PATIENT

The physician whose blood bank has one or more blood cell separators will surely be asked, sooner or later, to use them for plasma exchange, unless another hospital service already has responsibility for such procedures. The blood bank staff in these circumstances must exercise an appropriate degree of caution in carrying out manipulative extracorporeal procedures on sick people, which are not the same as procedures for collecting blood components from healthy donors.

The decision to do one or more plasma exchanges must be shared between the blood bank physician, who has the responsibility for the exchange itself, and the clinical physician. There should be a definite rationale, based on established clinical indications (see below), otherwise, the procedure is experimental. Informed consent is essential. Some thought should also be given to the cost, since plasma exchanges are time-consuming and expensive. The clinical physician should also be acquainted with the known risks of plasma exchanges, particularly in cases involving critically ill, small, or elderly patients and those with poor vascular access or with circulatory problems.

RATIONAL BASIS FOR PLASMA EXCHANGE

Two fundamental criteria must be met for the rational application of plasma exchange to any disease state: first, there must be some known pathogenic substance in the plasma; second, it must be possible to remove this substance more rapidly and effectively than it can be renewed in the body. This means that plasma exchange resembles dialysis, the difference being that plasma exchange can remove protein-bound toxic substances, which dialysis cannot. Even when the above criteria are met, and when it can be shown that exchange reduces the quantity of a circulating pathogenic factor, clinical improvement does not necessarily follow; and to make the picture more confusing, some patients improve after plasma exchange despite the absence of demonstrable changes in the plasma, and some improve after sham procedures in controlled studies. The possibility of a placebo effect, or of some nonspecific effect of the procedure itself, must always be considered. The basic mechanisms by which plasma exchange influences disease processes are given in Table 10–2.

In a few conditions, particularly thrombotic thrombocytopenic purpura [11], the disease appears to be related to a missing plasma factor, which is supplied by the substitution of normal plasma in plasma exchange. In such a case, the exchange permits infusion of large enough quantities of plasma without volume overload.

Since plasma exchange is almost always combined with other forms of therapy, e.g., immunosuppression, and since the removal of immune components is never totally effective at a single session, a series of exchanges is usually applied to patients with appropriate diseases that are not responding to conventional therapy. The number and extent of treatments must be individualized for each person and disease. A single exchange is thus a rare exception. Also, because it is a complex and expensive supplemental therapy, plasma exchange is not often used as chronic maintenance treatment.

Although thousands of articles have been written about the application of plasma exchange to numerous conditions [12], most such publications are of uncontrolled studies of only a few patients. Because it is easy to publish appar-

Table 10–2. Possible Mechanisms for the Effects of Plasma Exchange on Disease

Removal of
  Antibodies (auto- or allo-)
  Immune complexes
  Toxins (protein-bound)
  Paraproteins

Provision of deficient plasma factors

Other possible effects
  Alteration of antigen-to-antibody ratio
  Alteration of mediators of inflammation or immunity
  Improved clearance of immune complexes
  Placebo

ently successful results but difficult either to arouse interest in negative findings or to persuade journals to accept them, a false impression exists of the efficacy of plasma exchange in some diseases. Only within the past few years have the results of prospective controlled studies begun to appear [13, 14].

The following discussion is by no means complete, but includes a number of conditions in which plasma exchange appears to have some definite benefit and others in which its effectiveness is debatable.

Diseases in Which Plasma Exchange Is Generally Effective

Hyperviscosity Syndrome

Excessive quantities of abnormal proteins in the plasma, usually associated with Waldenström's macroglobulinemia, may cause hyperviscosity. Treatment of this syndrome was one of the first, and remains one of the most effective, applications of plasma exchange [15]. Most patients do not require exchanges unless they manifest central nervous system symptoms or some other severe complication. In our experience, most of them need only one or two immediate exchanges while definitive chemotherapy is established, and thereafter, from time to time if the response to chemotherapy is inadequate. The amount of plasma to be removed depends on the degree of hyperviscosity and the severity of clinical symptoms. It is generally inadvisable to include any protein in the replacement fluid, particularly in relatively small procedures.

Cryoglobulinemia

Plasma exchange can effectively remove cryoglobulins on a short-term basis, and even on a long-term basis when the response to other therapy is inadequate. In this case, it may be possible to avoid the use of costly and potentially hazardous replacement media, such as albumin or normal plasma, by returning the patient's own plasma after cryoprecipitation [16, 17] (see p. 380).

Myasthenia Gravis

Autoantibody to the acetylcholine receptors at the neuromuscular junction plays a role in the pathogenesis of myasthenia gravis, although clinical severity is not necessarily related to the presence of the antibody or its titer. Nevertheless, a reduction in antibody titer after plasma exchange is usually correlated with clinical improvement, often dramatic [18, 19]. The efficacy of plasma exchange has been challenged on the grounds that the series of patients studied have been largely uncontrolled, and that virtually all of them also received immunosuppressive therapy [13]. However, many of these patients have shown striking improvement on plasma exchange after increasing dosage of immunosuppression and even thymectomy failed, and have then relapsed on withdrawal of plasma exchanges. The consensus is that plasma exchange is effective in combination with immunosuppressive drug therapy in appropriately selected patients for the short-term control of severe symptoms and before and after thymectomy [20, 21]. Occasional patients that do not readily tolerate therapeutic doses of immunosuppressive or cytotoxic agents seem to respond well to chronic courses of plasma exchange.

Goodpasture's Syndrome

Autoantibody to glomerular basement membrane characterizes Goodpasture's syndrome, the clinical manifestations of which are rapidly progressive glomerulonephritis and pulmonary hemorrhages. Plasma exchange lowers the plasma antibody level, and in combination with immunosuppressive therapy, usually controls the lung hemorrhages and often improves renal function, particularly in patients who are not anuric [22]. However, the correlation of clinical status with antibody level is by no means absolute, and plasma exchange plus immunosuppression has not been compared with immunosuppression alone. Nonetheless, the use of a course of plasma exchange in patients who are not responding to aggressive conventional therapy is considered an important option, even an emergency, by many specialists treating such patients. For reasons that are not clear, there have been occasional long remissions following such treatment.

Thrombotic Thrombocytopenic Purpura

We know little about the pathogenesis of thrombotic thrombocytopenic purpura, a severe and usually fatal disease, which seems to be related to a deficiency of some as-yet-unidentified plasma factor, possibly related to prostacyclin [23]. Anti-platelet drugs, plasma transfusions, and exchange transfusions have all been tried and reported to be effective in some patients [11, 24, 25]. Despite the lack of controlled trials (one is under way in Canada, comparing plasma exchange and plasma transfusions), the widespread application of plasma exchange along with other forms of therapy in this disease seems to have produced a marked decrease in mortality. Replacement with normal plasma (usually fresh frozen) is more effective than that with albumin, and is probably essential. The exchanges may thus be simply a means of increasing the level of the deficient plasma factor. Prolonged remissions have followed successful therapy. Of course, isolation and purification of the deficient factor at some future time may make plasma exchange unnecessary in this disease.

On the basis of fewer clinical data, it appears that the related conditions hemolytic-uremic syndrome and microangiopathic hemolytic anemia respond to the same type of exchange described above. (See Addenda.)

Guillain-Barré Syndrome

The Guillain-Barré syndrome, especially in its acute form, is prone to spontaneous remission, like multiple sclerosis. For this reason, even apparently dramatic responses must be regarded with suspicion. One controlled trial in England concluded that plasma exchange brought about a slight but insignificant improvement in this disease [26]. However, that paper must be interpreted with some caution. The study was set up to detect a marked effect, as pointed out by the authors. Their "slight improvement" included a lower death rate, a smaller number of patients on the respirator for less total days, and fewer patients showing clinical deterioration in the exchanged group. In fact, similar findings were seen in a much larger, multi-institutional, controlled trial of plasma exchange in the United States and Canada [27]. Based on these two studies, it is clear that plasma exchange does not produce dramatic effects in Guillain-Barré syndrome, but that it does bring about improvement in appropriate cases, and may even be the only form of active therapy that has any effect at all. The recommendations are that it be restricted to seriously ill patients, and that it be instituted early in the course of the disease [20, 27].

Another controlled study has been reported in which plasma exchange produced more marked improvement when normal plasma was used as the replacement medium, compared to when albumin was used [28]. If confirmed, this may be an important finding.

Other Conditions

High-titer factor VIII inhibitor can be temporarily reduced by exchanges, e.g., in preparing a hemophiliac patient for surgery, or in the treatment of a severe hemorrhage [29]. Plasma exchange has also been reported to bring about some remissions in cases of *posttransfusion purpura* [30]. Finally, the technique may be a useful adjunct to dietary treatment in reducing blood levels of phytanic acid in *Refsum's disease,* a rare, inherited metabolic condition [31].

Table 10-3 lists some of the diseases in which plasma exchange seems to be effective in appropriately selected cases.

Table 10-3. Diseases in Which Plasma Exchange Seems to be Effective*

Hyperviscosity syndrome
Myasthenia gravis
Goodpasture's syndrome
Thrombotic thrombocytopenic purpura
Cryoglobulinemia
Hemophilia with inhibitor
Guillain-Barré syndrome
Posttransfusion purpura
Refsum's disease

*Effective is defined as producing significant improvement that is better than transitory, even though, in many cases, controlled studies are lacking.

DISEASES IN WHICH THE EFFICACY OF PLASMA EXCHANGE IS LESS CERTAIN

Systemic Lupus Erythematosus and Fulminant Crescentic Nephritis

Systemic lupus erythematosus and fulminant crescentic nephritis are generally associated with the presence of immune complexes in the blood and tissues, and plasma exchange can effectively reduce the levels of such complexes [32].

Significant improvement occurs in about half the patients exchanged, who have usually been treated with immunosuppression as well. The only controlled study was in mild cases of a type that should not ordinarily require plasma exchange. Not surprisingly, it showed no difference between the plasma exchange and the control groups [33]. However, in severe active lupus, plasma exchange does appear to be useful when the patient has reached the limits of tolerance of immunosuppressive therapy without adequate response. Under those circumstances, plasma exchange may bring about a temporary or even a long-lasting remission, or may permit lower doses of immunosuppression [7]. Unfortunately, controlled studies are lacking, and correlation of clinical status with blood immune complex levels is uncertain.

Rheumatoid Arthritis

It has been said that rheumatoid arthritis may be considered an extravascular immune-complex disease [34]. If it is so, the pathogenic immune complexes may be inaccessible to plasma exchange, which may explain the uncertain results obtained in various clinical trials.

Initial enthusiasm for plasma exchange, based on uncontrolled observations, gave way to greater caution as controlled studies were undertaken. One carefully controlled, double-blind crossover study led to conclusions that plasma exchange produced improvements in laboratory values, but did not bring about clinical benefit in chronic disease [35]. On the other hand, one may conclude from various reports that plasma exchange has a moderately beneficial effect in severe complications of rheumatoid arthritis, such as vasculitis with circulating immune complexes. In other active phases of the disease, it is difficult to distinguish a true therapeutic effect from that of a placebo. Various American professional societies, as well as governmental bodies, recommend that plasma exchange should be limited to clinical study protocols except in severe life-threatening complications [36]. Certainly, more research is needed.

Lymphocytapheresis and lymphoplasmapheresis have also been investigated in rheumatoid arthritis. The first involves removing lymphocytes; the second, lymphocytes and plasma. Both are in a sense intensifications of plasma exchange, and remove mainly T lymphocytes, since these predominate in the peripheral blood. T lymphocytes are also found in large numbers in rheumatoid synovial tissue, where they seem to contribute to the inflammatory process, so it seems reasonable to test the effects of T-lymphocyte reduction on the progress of the disease. Two studies using sham procedures on the control patients showed significant improvements in the treated groups [37, 38], but the effects tended to be only transitory.

Unlike most other diseases treated by plasma exchange, rheumatoid arthritis affects millions of patients worldwide. Because of the immense potential cost of this form of treatment, the conflicting results of clinical trials, and the strong placebo effect, wider application of apheresis procedures in this disease should await the results of more extensive studies. The answer to the hitherto conflicting results may lie in patient selection, the criteria for which are not yet established.

Multiple Sclerosis

Few areas of scientific enquiry seem to have spawned more inadequate studies and unwarranted recommendations than that of multiple sclerosis, and the history of this disorder is one of a long and continued series of false claims of cure [39]. This is an area in which cures and reputations evaporate.

Although its pathogenesis is uncertain, multiple sclerosis seems to be an autoimmune process in the white matter of the central nervous system, perhaps mediated by activated T lymphocytes [40]. Theoretically, lymphoplasmapheresis and lymphocytapheresis could affect the progress of the disease by reducing circulating T cells with and without hypothetical antibodies, while plasma exchange could reduce antibodies. In practice, plasma exchange produced an apparent transitory improvement in uncontrolled trials, but had no effect in a controlled setting [41]. Depletion of lymphocytes has produced some changes in laboratory measurements [42], and some clinical improvement in uncontrolled trials [43, 44]. Others have found any improvement transitory and confined to a small proportion of patients. As in the case of rheumatoid arthritis, or perhaps even more so, any therapeutic intervention in this disease has a strong placebo effect [45]. At this time, the best conclusion is probably to consider any form of hemapheresis experimental rather than a therapeutic alternative in multiple sclerosis [20].

Rh Hemolytic Disease of the Newborn

As a result of immunoprophylaxis with Rh immune globulin, Rh immunization in Rh-negative women has decreased markedly. For women who are already immunized, the possible usefulness of plasma exchange to reduce the quantity of circulating antibody must be contrasted with the efficacy of established methods of treating the affected fetuses in a diminishing number of Rh-negative pregnancies. In the United States, there has been relatively little interest in plasma exchange in this setting, in contrast to its much greater use in the United Kingdom and other parts of Europe [46].

Removal of plasma may significantly lower Rh antibody titers in some patients. However, the extent to which this affects fetal survival is debatable, and the trials have so far been uncontrolled. What may be particularly important is that pregnant mothers are not given immunosuppressive or cytotoxic therapy, whereas this therapy is used in most other conditions treated by plasma exchange. Perhaps because of the absence of immunosuppression, antibody rebound is seen in at least some patients. The interested reader should consult the proceedings of a symposium held on this topic in Oxford, England, in July, 1983 [47].

Other Conditions

Plasma exchange can effectively remove a patient's anti-A and anti-B before ABO-incompatible *bone marrow transplantation* [48], thus preventing hemolysis of incompatible donor red cells in the transplant. Immunoadsorption (see below), or some system for removing red cells from the transplanted marrow, may turn out to be better systems for this purpose.

Both plasma exchange and lymphocytapheresis have been used to treat *renal transplant rejection* associated with humoral antibodies [49], but the results appear to be equivocal.

In some cases of life-threatening *cold-antibody hemolytic anemia* unresponsive to other measures, plasma exchange has been reported to bring about remissions. In cold antibody disease, extraordinary measures must sometimes be taken to prevent the effects of cool ambient temperatures on the blood, e.g., the use of one or more blood warmers, or even carrying out the procedure in a warm room.

Plasma exchange can reduce the levels of cholesterol and low-density lipoproteins in *familial hypercholesterolemia* [50], but here too, the effects of the procedure on the atherosclerosis that is a consequence of the disease are as yet uncertain, and a specific immunoadsorption procedure might be better in the long run.

Table 10-4. Diseases in Which Plasma Exchange is of Debatable Efficacy*

Systemic lupus erythematosus
Fulminant crescentic nephritis
Rheumatoid arthritis
Multiple sclerosis
Rh hemolytic disease of the newborn
ABO-incompatible bone marrow transplantation
Renal transplant rejection
Hypercholesterolemia (familial)
Cold-antibody hemolytic anemia

*A partial listing of conditions in which plasma exchange has produced equivocal results, or slight transitory improvement, or where convincing controlled studies are lacking.

Experience with *idiopathic thrombocytopenic purpura* is limited, but the results suggest useful effects in some patients [51].

Table 10–4 lists diseases in which plasma exchange is of doubtful efficacy.

Extracorporeal Adsorption and Related Techniques

The removal of whole plasma and its substitution or partial substitution by albumin or some similar product depletes many useful nonpathogenic proteins. In fact, the proportion may be as much as 100 gm of useful protein with each gram of pathogenic material [52]. Furthermore, albumin, the usual replacement medium, is expensive and its availability is dependent on commercial blood donation sources. More selective methods of extracting pathogenic substances from blood or plasma are highly desirable from the pathophysiologic, as well as economic, points of view. Developmental work in this field represents an interesting merging and crossfertilization of hemapheresis and dialysis technologies.

A number of possibilities exist. For example, a simple off-line system can be used for the removal of cryoglobulins and some immune complexes, whereby whole plasma is first removed from the patient by any process, substituting, for example, albumin. The plasma may then be subjected to a cryogelation or cryoprecipitating procedure, the cold-insoluble material removed, and the modified plasma returned to the patient at the next plasma exchange [16]. The efficacy of such a procedure is subject to many variables, e.g., the ability of the cryoglobulin to gel or precipitate at the selected temperature. Moreover, any off-line processing technique is cumbersome, requiring the capability to collect, treat, store, and separate large volumes of plasma.

On-Line Cryogelation

Systems are available now for the removal of cryoglobulins and immune complexes by cooling and aggregation at 4° C followed by micropore filtration at a pore size of about 0.1 micron [53]. As might be expected, clogging of the micropore filter can be a problem. In addition, losses of noncryoglobulins (classic cryoprecipitate, fibrinogen complexes, and entrapped gels) have continued to be a problem. Cryogelation has been applied predominantly to rheumatoid arthritis, but the studies have been neither controlled nor compared with conventional plasmapheresis [54].

IMMUNOADSORPTION

The principle of immunoadsorption is that of binding an antibody (usually covalently) to an inert solid matrix, then passing separated plasma through a column of such material so that the bound antibody (the *sorbent*) removes its corresponding antigen from the plasma. A wide variety of matrices can be used to hold sorbents of various sorts. This technique has the capability of exquisite specificity, i.e., of removing a pathogenic substance and nothing else [52]. In addition to strictly immunologic sorbents, various biochemical and biophysical reactions can be used in the same setting, sometimes with great efficacy. Staphylococcal protein A used as a sorbent, for example, has affinity for IgG classes 1, 2, and 4, and has been used particularly in experimental cancer therapy in an attempt to bolster immune defences against malignancy by releasing "blocked" tumoricidal antibodies [55]. The approach is interesting and perhaps hopeful.

The whole field of immunoadsorption technology holds a great deal of promise and is exciting much current interest. It seems certain that a wide variety of sorbents will be developed for various clinical purposes. Table 10–5 lists some of the important current clinical applications and investigations.

Some important considerations with immunoadsorption are those of stability of columns, adsorptive capacity, cost, possible elution of either matrix or sorbent into the patient's circulation, ability to recycle and resterilize (for reuse with the same patient), and selection of optimal flow geometry.

A special challenge is that of possible compatibility of immunoadsorbent materials with whole blood rather than plasma, which would have the enormous advantage that the preliminary separation of plasma from blood cells would be unnecessary. Some preliminary tests appear hopeful [56], but thrombocytopenia has been a problem.

OTHER SYSTEMS

Various types of electrophoretic or electrodialytic techniques of plasma protein separation have been tried on a small scale [57, 58], as have enzymatic systems. None of these seems yet to have reached a clinical stage, and they remain as speculative possibilities for the future. Recently, an experimental form of extracorporeal photo-activation of a chemotherapeutic agent has been applied to the treatment of cutaneous T-cell lymphoma [59]; this novel modification of hemapheresis appears promising.

Table 10-5. Some Plasma Immunoadsorption Systems

Sorbent	Matrix	Substance Removed	Clinical Disorder
Anti-LDL	Sepharose	LDL (cholesterol)	Hypercholesterolemia
Charcoal	Glass beads	Bile acids	Cholestatic pruritus
A and B substances	Silica	Anti-A, -B	Marrow transplant
DNA	Charcoal-collodion	ANA, immune complexes	Lupus
Protein A	Charcoal-collodion	Cancer "blocking agents," immune complexes	Cancer, Kaposi sarcoma
Tryptophane-PV alcohol resin		AChR antibody	Myasthenia gravis

LDL = low-density lipoprotein; ANA = antinuclear antibody; AChR = acetylcholine receptor; PV = polyvinyl.

Therapeutic Cytapheresis

Removal of blood cells, as opposed to plasma, is carried out, for the most part, to correct extraordinarily high cell counts in various leukemias, predominantly in chronic granulocytic leukemia. In the latter condition, cytapheresis has been used to control the less-florid phases of the disease for long periods, although it is now apparent that better control can be achieved at less cost by appropriate chemotherapy. At one time, such collected granulocytes were used for transfusions to infected leukopenic patients, the procedure from which normal granulocyte transfusions evolved [60]. With the general decrease in the use of granulocyte transfusions nowadays, this procedure is rarely done.

At present, most therapeutic cytapheresis is for the immediate reduction of severe thrombocytosis or leukocytosis in acute or chronic leukemia, when there is a risk of hemorrhage, thrombosis, or pulmonary or cerebral leukostasis [61]. It is thus a stopgap treatment to lower the body's tumor burden while definitive chemotherapy is being instituted. The general guidelines are given in Table 10-6.

In thrombocytosis, platelet apheresis is particularly efficient, probably because platelets are not replaced as fast as leukocytes. Two or three procedures usually suffice to reduce platelet counts to levels that are considered safe, although there is some evidence that counts below 2 million per microliter may present no particular risk [62]. Therapeutic leukapheresis, on the other hand, does not reduce leukocyte counts as quickly, but is capable of removing kilo-

Table 10-6. Indications for Cytoreduction Procedures

Leukapheresis	
WBC count × 1,000/mm^3	< 100: Seldom necessary
	100–200: Occasionally necessary
	> 200: Often urgent (except in chronic lymphocytic leukemia)*
Clinical indication	Evidence of vascular insufficiency (leukostasis), especially pulmonary or cerebral
Platelet apheresis	
Platelet count/mm^3	> 1,500,000: In presence of spleen (but not in reactive thrombocytosis)
Clinical indication	Thrombosis or hemorrhage

*Particularly when there is a high proportion of blasts.

grams of buffy coat in a few procedures, and is often very effective in relieving symptoms of leukostasis and in reducing spleen size. In contrast to granulocytes, removal of lymphocytes does not seem to have much effect on chronic lymphocytic leukemia.

Therapeutic erythrocytapheresis is a procedure in which the cell separator is used to remove defective red cells and substitute healthy ones [63]. It has been used predominantly in patients with sickle cell anemia during pregnancy or before surgical procedures.

In acute leukemia, leukapheresis can be used to reduce tumor burden and also to collect stem cells for experimental immunotherapy, and in cancer to collect autologous lymphocytes for immune modification [64]. (See Addenda.)

Complications of Therapeutic Hemapheresis

The complications that occur in plasma exchange and therapeutic cytapheresis are much the same, except that cytapheresis does not involve the use of a replacement fluid and is usually done only a few times in succession. Most of this discussion will center on plasma exchange.

Plasma exchange is often thought to be a benign procedure with little or no risk. It is in part this attitude that has led to trials of hemapheresis in many diseases where there is little or no scientific rationale for the application of this kind of procedure. The false impression of safety may be based on the knowledge that hemapheresis procedures are readily tolerated by healthy blood donors and therefore should be equally well tolerated by patients. This is not so. Although plasma exchange is *relatively* safe, there are many minor, and a few major, risks [65, 66].

Vascular Damage

Plasma exchange generally requires two excellent vein access sites, and the patients who require these procedures have often already had considerable vein damage as a consequence of intensive hospital treatment. Therefore, radical approaches may be needed if a series of exchanges is to be possible. Artificial shunts or arteriovenous fistulas may be necessary. These require the intervention of a vascular surgeon, and carry their own intrinsic risks as well, e.g., perforation, thrombosis, infection, and sepsis.

Procedural Reactions

Volume Effects

All cell separators involve the temporary sequestration of a certain quantity of blood outside the body, which can cause hypovolemia, hypotension, and vasovagal responses. These are undoubtedly aggravated by psychological factors. Such reactions resemble those encountered in regular blood donation, and can usually be controlled by the operator without too much difficulty by the infusion of extra fluid.

Fluid input in excess of outflow can cause hypervolemia, and this can be a problem with some patients, particularly when the blood outflow is stopped near the end of a procedure. It pays to observe the patient's vital signs closely during any apheresis procedure.

Replacement Media

At least partial protein replacement is important in large exchanges, and inadequate protein input can cause hypoproteinemia and hypotension. Infusion of additional protein corrects this quickly. In repeated exchanges, the patient's serum protein and immunoglobulin levels should be checked regularly, and corrective therapy instituted if necessary.

Unless it is specifically indicated, normal plasma should not be used as the replacement medium. It tends to cause allergic and idiosyncratic reactions, citrate toxicity, exposure to viral diseases such as hepatitis and AIDS, and problems referable to its anti-A and anti-B content and possibly to antileukocyte or other less-well-understood antibodies.

Citrate Effects

Citrate reactions result from a reduction in serum ionized calcium and are characterized by increased neuromuscular excitability, e.g., circumoral paresthesias, a tremorous feeling in the chest, chills, and occasionally even overt tetany [67]. Such reactions can be severe, particularly if the patient hyperventilates as well. Citrate reactions can be controlled by slowing the blood flow rate or decreasing the proportion of citrate to blood [68]. Heparin can be used as partial replacement of citrate in the anticoagulant in the case of patients who may be particularly sensitive to citrate. Supplementation with an infusion of ionized calcium [69] should seldom be necessary.

DELAYED COMPLICATIONS

Hemorrhage or Thrombosis
Any replacement medium other than normal plasma will deplete all clotting factors, an effect that can be readily measured [70–73]. Despite this, hemorrhagic or thrombotic complications are rare and more likely to be related to the patient's underlying disease.

Infections
Like clotting factors, immunoglobulins too are depleted, and many of the patients are immunosuppressed [72]. Complicating infections have been observed in patients with renal disease [74]. The prophylactic administration of immune serum globulin has been recommended [10], but is probably not necessary in most cases. If immunoglobulin levels fall significantly during a series of exchanges (e.g., IgG to 200 mg/dl or less), corrective infusion of intravenous immunoglobulin should be considered.

Table 10–7. Complications of Plasma Exchange

Vascular Complications	Shunts, Fistulas	Catheters
Hemorrhage, hematoma Sclerosis of veins Thrombosis, embolism	Surgical procedure Thrombosis Infection Circulatory interference	Perforation Infection
Procedural Complications	Citrate Effects	Volume Changes
Vasovagal reaction Chilling Hemolysis, mechanical Allergy, anaphylaxis Acute pulmonary edema Hypoproteinemia	Tremors, paresthesia Tetany Cardiac arrhythmia, arrest	Hypovolemia Hypervolemia, overload
Delayed Complications	Infections	
Clotting factor depletion Thrombocytopenia Hemorrhage Hypoproteinemia DIC, thrombosis	Bacterial (sepsis) Viral hepatitis	

Hepatitis has been reported, as might be expected, following the use of plasma as replacement. Theoretically, any disease transmissible by plasma could be acquired by a patient in these circumstances, but to our knowledge no cases have been reported.

Table 10-7 summarizes the major complications associated with therapeutic hemapheresis.

Mortality

We have estimated a case fatality rate of about 3 per 10,000 therapeutic procedures, most of these being related to the occurrence of acute pulmonary edema (adult respiratory distress syndrome) or acute cardiac arrhythmia occurring during or immediately after the procedure [66]. Almost all such deaths seem to be associated with the use of plasma as the replacement medium, but the precise pathogenesis of them remains uncertain. Considering that plasma exchange is applied to seriously ill patients with disorders that are not responding to aggressive conventional therapy, such a mortality does not seem excessive. Nevertheless, physicians electing to use this form of treatment should be aware of its limitations in the various disease states as well as its incurrence of morbidity and mortality.

References

1. Fleig C. L'autotransfusion de globules lavés comme procédé de lavage du sang dans les toxhémies. *Bull Mens Acad Sci Let Montpellier* 1909; 1:4–9.
2. Stromberg RR, Hardwick RA, Friedman LI. Membrane filtration technology in plasma exchange. In: MacPherson JL, Kasprisin DO (eds). *Therapeutic Hemapheresis*, Vol. I. Boca Raton, FL: CRC, 1985; 135–47.
3. Chmiel H. The effects of pressure, flow conditions, and surface composition on the filtration properties of plasma separation modules. *Plasma Ther Transfus Technol* 1983; 4:387–96.
4. Wegmuller E, Kazatchkine MD, Nydegger UE. Complement activation during extracorporeal blood bypass. *Plasma Ther Transfus Technol* 1983; 4:361–71.
5. Gregory MC, Shettigar UR, Kolff WJ. Theoretical value of cascade plasmapheresis. *Plasma Ther Transfus Technol* 1984; 5:517–29.
6. Calabrese LH, Clough JD, Krakauer RS, Hoeltge GA. Plasmapheresis therapy of immunologic disease. *Cleve Clin Q* 1980; 47:53–72.
7. Jones JV, Clough JD, Klineberg JR, Davis P. The role of therapeutic plasmapheresis in the rheumatic diseases. *J Lab Clin Med* 1981; 97:589–98.
8. McLeod BC, Sassetti RJ, Stefoski D, Davis FA. Partial plasma protein replacement in therapeutic plasma exchange. *J Clin Apheresis* 1983; 1:115–8.
9. Lasky LC, Finnerty EP, Genis L, Polesky HF. Protein and colloid osmotic pressure changes with albumin and/or saline replacement during plasma exchange. *Transfusion* 1984; 24:256–9.
10. Dau PC. Immune globulin intravenous replacement after plasma exchange. *J Clin Apheresis* 1983; 1:104–8.
11. Taft EG. Thrombotic thrombocytopenic purpura and dose of plasma exchange. *Blood* 1979; 54:842–9.

12. American National Red Cross. Therapeutic Hemapheresis Bibliography, 3rd ed. Washington, DC: American National Red Cross, 1984.
13. Shumak KH, Rock G. Therapeutic plasma exchange. *N Engl J Med* 1984; 310:762–71.
14. Rock G, Pineda AA. Controlled trials—necessity and progress. In: MacPherson JL, Kasprisin DO (eds). *Therapeutic Hemapheresis*, Vol. II. Boca Raton, FL: CRC, 1985.
15. Schwab PJ, Fahey JL. Treatment of Waldenström's macroglobulinemia by plasmapheresis. *N Engl J Med* 1960; 263:574–9.
16. McLeod BC, Sassetti RJ. Plasmapheresis with return of cryoglobulin-depleted autologous plasma (cryoglobulinpheresis) in cryoglobulinemia. *Blood* 1980; 55:866–70.
17. Malchesky PS, Asanuma Y, Zawicki I, et al. On-line separation of macromolecules by membrane filtration with cryogelation. In: Sieberth HG (ed). *Plasma Exchange*. Stuttgart: Schattauer, 1980; 133–9.
18. Dau PC, Lindstrom JM, Cassel CK, et al. Plasmapheresis and immunosuppressive drug therapy in myasthenia gravis. *N Engl J Med* 1977; 297:1134–40.
19. Kornfeld P, Ambinder PE, Mittag T, et al. Plasmapheresis in refractory generalized myasthenia gravis. *Arch Neurol* 1981; 38:478–81.
20. Consensus Conference. The utility of plasmapheresis for neurological disorders. *JAMA* 1986; 256:1333–7.
21. Newsom-Davis J, Wilson SG, Vincent A, Ward CD. Long-term effects of repeated plasma exchange in myasthenia gravis. *Lancet* 1979; 1:464–8.
22. Lockwood CM, Rees AJ, Pearson TA, et al. Immunosuppression and plasma exchange in the treatment of Goodpasture's syndrome. *Lancet* 1976; 1:711–5.
23. Remuzzi G, Misiani R, Marchesi D, et al. Haemolytic-uraemic syndrome: deficiency of plasma factor(s) regulating prostacyclin activity? *Lancet* 1978; 2:871–2.
24. Bukowski RM, King JW, Hewlett JS. Plasmapheresis in the therapy of thrombotic thrombocytopenic purpura. *Blood* 1977; 50:413–7.
25. Sennett ML, Conrad ME. Treatment of thrombotic thrombocytopenic purpura. Plasmapheresis, plasma transfusion, and vincristine. *Arch Intern Med* 1986; 146:266–7.
26. Greenwood RJ, Newsom-Davis J, Hughes RAC, et al. Controlled trial of plasma exchange in acute inflammatory polyneuropathy. *Lancet* 1984; 1:877–9.
27. The Guillain-Barré Syndrome Study Group. Plasmapheresis and acute Guillain-Barré syndrome. *Neurology* 1985; 35:1096–104.
28. Shumak KH, Humphrey JG, Chiu JY, et al. Toronto General Hospital controlled trial data plasma exchange therapy in Guillain-Barré syndrome. *J Clin Apheresis* 1985; 2:326–31.
29. Slocombe GN, Newland AC, Colvin MP, Colvin BT. The role of intensive plasma exchange in the prevention and management of haemorrhage in patients with inhibitors to factor VIII. *Br J Haematol* 1981; 47:577–85.
30. Slichter SJ. Post-transfusion purpura: response to steroids and association with red blood cell and lymphocytotoxic antibodies. *Br J Haematol* 1982; 50:599–605.
31. Gibberd FB, Billimoria JD, Page NG, Retsas S. Heredopathia atactica polyneuritiformis (Refsum's disease) treated by diet and plasma exchange. *Lancet* 1979; 1:575–8.
32. Lockwood CM, Peters DK. Plasma exchange in glomerulonephritis and related vasculitides. *Ann Rev Med* 1980; 31:167–9.
33. Wei N, Klippel JH, Huston DP, et al. Randomised trial of plasma exchange in mild systemic lupus erythematosus. *Lancet* 1983; 1:17–22.

34. Zvaifler NJ. The immunopathology of joint inflammation in rheumatoid arthritis. *Adv Immunol* 1973; 13:265–336.
35. Dwosh IL, Giles AR, Ford PM, et al. Plasmapheresis therapy in rheumatoid arthritis. *N Engl J Med* 1983; 308:1124–9.
36. Office of Technology Assessment, U.S. Congress. The safety, efficacy, and cost effectiveness of therapeutic apheresis. Washington DC: U.S. Government Printing Office, 1983; 37–8.
37. Karsh J, Wright DG, Klippel JH, et al. Lymphocyte depletion by continuous flow centrifugation in rheumatoid arthritis: clinical effects. *Arthritis Rheum* 1979; 22:1055–9.
38. Wallace D, Goldfinger D. Lowe C, et al. A double-blind, controlled study of lymphocytapheresis versus sham apheresis in rheumatoid arthritis. *N Engl J Med* 1982; 306:1406–10.
39. Masland J, cited by McFarlin DE. Treatment of multiple sclerosis. *N Engl J Med* 1983; 308:215–7.
40. Merrill JE, Kutsanai S, Mohlstrom C, et al. Proliferation of astroglia and oligodendroglia in response to human T-cell derived factors. *Science* 1984; 224:1428–30.
41. Hauser SL, Dawson DM, Lehrich JR, et al. Intensive immunosuppression in progressive multiple sclerosis. A randomized, three-arm study of high dose intravenous cyclophosphamide, plasma exchange and ACTH. *N Engl J Med* 1983; 308:173–80.
42. Kateley JR, Morehouse R, Berlinsky P, et al. Influence of lymphatic depletion by leukocytapheresis on lymphocyte populations and interferon production in patients with multiple sclerosis. *Plasma Ther Transfus Technol* 1983; 4:5–10.
43. Giordano GF, Masland W, Ketchel SJ, et al. An investigation of lymphocytapheresis in multiple sclerosis. *Plasma Ther Transfus Technol* 1982; 3:417–22.
44. Giordano GF. Role of lymphocytapheresis in immune-mediated diseases: consequences of lymphocyte depletion. In: MacPherson JL, Kasprisin DO (eds). *Therapeutic Hemapheresis,* Vol. II, Boca Raton, FL: CRC, 1985.
45. National Multiple Sclerosis Society. *Therapeutic Claims in Multiple Sclerosis.* New York: NMSS, 1982.
46. Robinson EAE, Tovey LAD. Intensive plasma exchange in the management of severe Rh disease. *Br J Haematol* 1980; 45:621–31.
47. Entwhistle CC, Bowell PJ (organizers). Symposium Proceedings, Oxford, England. *Plasma Ther Transfus Technol* 1984; 5:5–109.
48. Bensinger WI. Plasma exchange and immunoadsorption for removal of antibodies prior to ABO-incompatible bone marrow transplantation. *Artif Organs* 1981; 5:254–8.
49. Cardella CJ. Does plasma exchange have a role in renal transplant rejection? *Plasma Ther Transfus Technol* 1982; 3:153–6.
50. Thompson GR. Plasma exchange for hypercholesterolemia. *Lancet* 1981; 1:1246–8.
51. Blanchette VS, Hogan VA, McCombie NE, et al. Intensive plasma exchange therapy to patients with idiopathic thrombocytopenic purpura. *Transfusion* 1984; 24:388–94.
52. Lysaght MJ, Samtleben W, Schmidt B, Gurland HJ. Closed-loop plasmapheresis. In: MacPherson JL, Kasprisin DO (eds). *Therapeutic Hemapheresis,* Vol. I. Boca Raton, FL: CRC, 1985; 149–68.
53. Abe Y, Smith JW, Malchesky PS, Nose Y. Cryofiltration: development and current status. *Plasma Ther Transfus Technol* 1983; 4:405–14.
54. Horiuchi T, Malchesky PS, Smith JW, Nose Y. Selective removal of mac-

romolecules by cryofiltration. In: Pineda AA (ed). *Selective Plasma Component Removal.* Mount Kisko, NY: Futura Pub, 1984: 169–209.
55. Terman DS. Immunoadsorbents in autoimmune and neoplastic diseases. *Plasma Ther Transfus Technol* 1983; 4:415–33.
56. Nilsson IM, Freiburghaus C, Sundquist SB, Sandberg H. Removal of specific antibodies from whole blood in a continuous extracorporeal system. *Plasma Ther Transfus Technol* 1984; 5:127–34.
57. Bing DH. Chemical precipitation and removal of IgG and immune complexes. In: Pineda AA (ed). *Selective Plasma Component Removal.* Mount Kisko, NY: Futura Pub, 1984; 139–68.
58. Bier M, Cuddeback RM, Kopwillem A. Preparative plasma protein fractionation by isotachophoresis in sephadex columns. *J Chromatogr* 1977; 132:437–50.
59. Edelson R, Berger C, Gasparro F, et al. Treatment of cutaneous T-cell lymphoma by extracorporeal photochemotherapy. Preliminary results. *N Engl J Med* 1987; 316:297–303.
60. Morse EE, Freireich EJ, Carbone PP, et al. The transfusion of leukocytes from donors with chronic myelocytic leukemia to patients with leukopenia. *Transfusion* 1966; 6:183–92.
61. Hester J. Therapeutic cytapheresis. In: MacPherson JL, Kasprisin DO (eds). *Therapeutic Hemapheresis,* Vol. II. Boca Raton, FL: CRC, 1985; 143–53.
62. Buss DH, Stuart JJ, Lipscomb GE. The incidence of thrombotic and hemorrhagic disorders in association with extreme thrombocytosis: an analysis of 129 cases. *Am J Hematol* 1985; 20:365–72.
63. Kleinman SH, Hurvitz CG, Goldfinger D. Use of erythrocytapheresis in the treatment of patients with sickle cell anemia. *J Clin Apheresis* 1984; 2:170–6.
64. Rosenberg SA, Lotze MT, Muul LM, et al. Observations on the systemic administration of autologous lymphokine-activated killer cells and recombinant interleukin-2 to patients with metastatic cancer. *N Engl J Med* 1985; 313:1485–92.
65. Editorial. Hazards of apheresis. *Lancet* 1982; 2:1025–6.
66. Huestis DW. Mortality in therapeutic haemapheresis. *Lancet* 1983; 1:1043.
67. Watson DK, Penny AF, Marshall RW, Robinson EAE. Citrate induced hypocalcaemia during cell separation. *Br J Haematol* 1980; 44:503–7.
68. Hester JP, McCullough J, Mishler JM, Szymanski IO. Dosage regimens for citrate anticoagulants. *J Clin Apheresis* 1983; 1:149–57.
69. Buskard NA, Vargheze Z, Willis MR. Correction of hypocalcaemic symptoms during plasma exchange. *Lancet* 1976; 2:344–5.
70. Flaum MA, Cuneo RA, Appelbaum FR, et al. The hemostatic imbalance of plasma-exchange transfusions. *Blood* 1979; 54:694–702.
71. Keller AJ, Chirnside A, Urbaniak SJ. Coagulation abnormalities produced by plasma exchange on the cell separator with special reference to fibrinogen and platelets. *Br J Haematol* 1979; 42:593–603.
72. Orlin JB, Berkman EM. Partial plasma exchange using albumin replacement: removal and recovery of normal plasma constituents. *Blood* 1980; 56:1055–9.
73. Chirnside A, Urbaniak SJ, Prowse CV, Keller AJ. Coagulation abnormalities following intensive plasma exchange on the cell separator. II. Effects on factors I, II, V, VII, IX, X, and antithrombin III. *Br J Haematol* 1981; 48:627–34.
74. Wing EJ, Bruns FJ, Fraley DS, et al. Infectious complications with plasmapheresis in rapidly progressive glomerulonephritis. *JAMA* 1980; 244:2423–6.

Addenda

Chapter 4. Testing of Donor Blood

Page 161. A prospective study by McEvoy et al. (*Br Med J* 1987;1:1595–7) of 150 health-care workers in Britain who had been accidentally exposed to blood or body fluids containing human immunodeficiency virus (HIV), found the risk of occupational infection to be very low. A similar study in the United States by Gerberding et al. (*J Inf Dis* 1987;156:1–8) concluded that health-care workers are at minimal risk for HIV, cytomegalovirus, and hepatitis B virus transmission from occupational exposure to patients with AIDS or AIDS-related complex, even when intensively exposed for long periods of time. Both groups of investigators, however, stressed the need for safe procedures by health-care workers at all times. The Centers for Disease Control have issued new recommendations for the prevention of HIV transmission in health-care settings (*MMWR* 1987;36 suppl 2S:1S–18S). This document does not specifically address the precautions appropriate in the donor room environment, but implies that they are the same as in any other health-care situation. While we agree that sensible precautions are appropriate in handling blood and other body fluids at any time, we believe there is an important distinction between patients and healthy blood donors.

Chapter 6. Red Blood Cell Transfusion

Page 214. One important cause of anemia in hospitalized patients is blood loss as a result of sampling for laboratory tests. (B. R. Smoller and M. S. Kruskall, *N Engl J Med* 1986;314:1233–5.)

Page 226. Autologous transfusion has become of major importance as a result of widespread concern about transfusion-associated AIDS. Patients fear the disease and physicians fear, in addition, their own medicolegal exposure. The procedure is applicable to children (A. J. Silvergleid, *JAMA* 1987;257:3403–4), cardiac surgery candidates (T. R. Love, et al., *Ann Thorac Surg* 1987;43:508–12), pregnant women (M. S. Kruskall, S. Leonard, H. Klapholz, *Obstet Gynecol* 1987;70:938–41) and the elderly (J. Pindyck, *JAMA* 1987;257:1186–8) but appears to be underutilized (P. T. C. Y. Toy, *N Engl J Med* 1987;316:517–20). A major unsettled question is whether autologous donation units that meet federal and AABB standards, if not used by the autologous donor, can be transfused to others. The FDA Advisory Panel has voted against such "crossing over," but many blood bankers do not support this position because they believe that the units in question are safe and that discarding them is wasteful (M. A. Popovsky, *Transfusion* 1987;27:544). The issue is in doubt.

Chapter 7. Complications of Transfusion
Page 276. As of December 21, 1987, the number of transfusion-associated AIDS cases was as follows: 1,121 adults, 96 children, in addition to 484 hemophiliac adults and 40 hemophiliac children (J. Allen, personal communication, December 1987).

Page 280. 1. As of November 1987, 11 blood recipients in the United States are known to have become HIV-seropositive following transfusion of blood components from antibody-negative donors (American Association of Blood Banks. *Blood Bank Week,* 1987;4[44]:1).
2. Despite persistent efforts to educate the public to the contrary, a more recent poll showed that 29 percent still cling to a belief that the AIDS virus can be acquired by donating blood (Gallup Poll, *The Washington Post,* December 1, 1987).

Page 281. These findings were reported in more detail by Bove et al. (*Transfusion* 1987;27:201–2). Their statement that look-back was about half finished has been challenged by Busch, Samson, and Perkins (*Transfusion* 1987;27:503–4), who pointed out that most high-risk donors have self-deferred, so that blood banks are unaware of their antibody status and prior donations. The latter authors have evidence that substantially more cases will be found by a more aggressive approach involving active identification of AIDS patients who have donated blood and of donors implicated in transfusion-transmitted HIV infections. This is perfectly valid, but goes beyond the scope of look-back as originally set up.
The probability exists of even more testing of donor blood, specifically for the human T-cell lymphotropic virus, type I (HTLV-I). The American Association of Blood Banks, American National Red Cross, and Council of Community Blood Centers have issued a joint statement, the essence of which is that HTLV-I is a virus that should be excluded from blood transfusion as soon as a reliable and confirmable test is available (November 20, 1987). The grounds are that HTLV-I is associated with diseases in which at least seropositivity is transmissible by blood, that it has a long latent period, can cause serious disease in animal models, and that the technology is available. Counter arguments are that the benefits of such testing are unknown, since transfusion-associated disease has not been reported, that the test is unlicensed and its specificity uncertain, and that nobody would know what to tell a seropositive donor. (See S. G. Sandler and J. R. Bove. HTLV-I and blood transfusion. *Transfusion* [editorial] in press.) In the present climate of ever-increasing testing of donor blood, we would not be surprised to see HTLV-I testing adopted. The philosophy and rationale behind attempts to achieve a "zero-risk" blood supply are well discussed by Zuck (*Transfusion* [editorial] 1987;27:447–8).

Page 282. In November 1987, the American Association of Blood Banks and the FDA recommended that blood banks permanently disqualify as donors those persons that have received human pituitary-derived growth hormone. This is because of the possibility that Creutzfeldt-Jakob disease (a rare, fatal, neurologic disorder) may be spread by transfusion. The disqualification does not apply to recipients of *recombinant* growth hormone, which has been available commercially since 1985. A fact sheet is available from the FDA.

Chapter 8. Blood Components, Fractions, and Derivatives

Page 323. The very high incidence of HIV infection in patients treated with antihemophilic factor concentrates has led to the introduction of new and safer products. Most materials are now heat-treated to reduce infectivity. There is evidence that heating in solution ("pasteurization") produces a safer product than heating after the material has been lyophilized (dry heat). Two new procedures, solvent-detergent treatment and purification by adsorption to and elution from a column coated with antibodies to the von Willebrand factor are also used, and may produce even safer products. Factor VIII prepared by recombinant technology is in clinical trials. The subject is well reviewed by Roberts and Macik (H. R. Roberts and B. G. Macik, *Thromb Haemost* 1987).

The mechanism by which Anti-Inhibitor Coagulant Complex acts in patients with factor VIII antibodies is discussed by Giles (A. R. Giles, *Trans Med Rev* 1987; 1:131–7).

In the same journal the management of patients with factor VIII inhibitors is reviewed (J. M. Lusher, *Trans Med Rev* 1987;1:123–30).

Page 336. Ultraviolet irradiation of human platelets is now undergoing clinical trials.

Chapter 10. Therapeutic Hemapheresis

Page 376. For a good review of our current knowledge of thrombotic thrombocytopenic purpura, see J. J. Byrnes and J. L. Moake. Thrombotic thrombocytopenic purpura and the hemolytic-uremic syndrome: Evolving concepts of pathogenesis and therapy. *Clin Haematol* 1986;15:413–42.

Page 383. "Adaptive immunotherapy" is currently exciting a great deal of interest in experimental cancer therapy. The procedure involves activating the patient's lymphocytes with recombinant interleukin-2, collecting those lymphokine-activated killer (LAK) cells by leukapheresis, and transfusing them back to the patient. Recent progress is given by Rosenberg, et al. (*N Engl J Med* 1987;316:889–97).

Index

A antigen
  in platelet transfusion, 128
  subgroups of, 81–91
A_1 antiserum, preparation of, 88
ABO blood group system, 86–93
  ABH biochemistry, 87–88
  agglutinating antibodies of, 80
  antigens, 81
  biochemistry of, 86–87
  Bombay phenotype, 91–92
    para-, 92–93
  chimerism and, 175
  compatibility
    in bone marrow transplantation, 233–234
    crossmatching, 198
    in cytapheresis, 44
    erythroblastosis fetalis and, 357
    granulocyte transfusion and, 340
    jaundice and, 363–364
    Rh hemolytic disease and, 348, 361
  discovery of, 86
  erythroblastosis fetalis and, 362–364
    antibody characteristics in, 362–363
    diagnosis of, 363–364
    exchange transfusion in, 364
  immunization, 64
  inheritance, 86
  maternofetal incompatibility. *See* Hemolytic disease of newborn
  para-Bombay phenotype, 92–93
  polyagglutinability, 175
  recent blood transfusion and, 175–176
  red cell reactions, 87
  serum reactions, 87
  subgroups
    of A, 88–91
    testing, 156
  testing and typing, 150–156
    agglutinating alloantibody in test serum in, 154, 155

antibody directed at cell-suspending medium ingredient in, 154, 155
antibody to dye in antiserum in, 154, 155
automated test systems for, 148, 149
cell grouping, 151
cold autoagglutinin in, 153, 154
coloring agent in, 154, 155
common reaction patterns, 151
discrepancy resolution, 152–156
in erythroblastosis fetalis, 356–357, 360
in exchange transfusion, 360
forward grouping, 151
  common errors in, 153
mixed-field agglutination, 175–176
polyagglutinability in, 175
problems in, 151–156
quality control in, 159
recent blood transfusion and, 175–176
recent bone marrow transplantation and, 175–176
recipient, 174
reverse grouping, 151–152
  common errors in, 153
rouleaux in, 153–155
serum grouping, 151–152
subgroups, 156
in transfusion reaction, 266
weak or absent agglutinins, 154, 155–156
transfusion to different ABO group, 219–220
Absorption, 199–200
Acid-citrate-dextrose, in blood collection, 40
Acquired immunodeficiency syndrome (AIDS)
  AIDS-related complex, 276
  autologous transfusion and, 3

395

Acquired immunodeficiency syndrome
    (AIDS)—*Continued*
  directed donations and, 3
  donor testing for, 16–19, 279–280
  high-risk donors, 17–19
  HIV antibody test in, 164–165
  homosexuality and, 17, 277–279
  information sheet for donors, 18
  intravenous drug abuse and, 15
  investigating former transfusion recipients for, 280–281
  "look-back" procedure in, 280–281, 392
  plasma exchange and, 384
  predonation information sheet, 18, 32
  prison inmates and, 16
  transfusion-associated, 276–281, 283, 392
    incidence of, 276–277
    prevention of, 277–280
    recipient testing, 280–281
    testing donor blood for, 279–280
    transmission, 277
Acupuncture, hepatitis and, 16
Acutane, donor exclusion for, 22
Adaptive immunotherapy, 393
Agar gel diffusion, in hepatitis testing, 272
Age, donor, 11
Agglutinates, formation theories, 67–68
Agglutination. *See also* Hemagglutination
  antibiotics and, 195
  anticoagulants and, 195
  in antigen-antibody reaction, 66–67
  automated, 149
  bovine albumin and, 195
  drug use and, 195
  microbial contamination and, 196
  mixed-field, 90
    in recipient sample, 175–176
  pseudo-, 196–197
  reading of, 147–148
  saline and, 195
  scoring, 206, 207
Agglutinin, saline, 60. *See also* Saline agglutinin
AIDS. *See* Acquired immunodeficiency syndrome
AIDS-related complex, 276
Air embolism, 261, 265
Alanine aminotransferase testing, 14, 165, 273

Albumin, 314–315
  autoagglutination phenomenon, 195
  bovine, agglutination and, 136–137, 180, 195
  clinical uses for, 315
  in cryoglobulinemia, 374
  in fluid therapy, 215
  in plasma exchange, 372
  as plasma substitute, 380
Alleles, 81
Allergy
  drug, in donor, 21
  food, in donor, 21
  in hemapheresis, 48
  hydroxyethyl starch, 48
  transfusion reaction, 258–259, 265
    prevention of, 259
    treatment of, 258–259
  transfusion transmission of, 21
Alloantibody, versus autoantibody, 182–183
Alloimmunization, 63–65
  by blood group antigens, 63–65
  in bone marrow transplantation, 231
  defined, 63
  in hypertransfusion, 228
  maternal, 348–351
    fetal effects of, 351–352
  multiple transfusion and, 121
  in platelet transfusion, 128
  in renal transplantation, 230
Alpha-methyldopa, agglutination and, 195
2-Aminoethylisothiouronium bromide, 204
Ammonia spirits, 36
Ammonium, plasma, 264
Amniocentesis
  delta OD readings in, 355–356
  for erythroblastosis fetalis, 354–356
Amniotic fluid
  bilirubinoid pigments in, 354–355
  optical-density difference, 355–356
Amorph, defined, 82
Amphotericin B, granulocyte transfusion and, 341
An^a antigen, 113
Anaphylatoxin, biologic activity of, 72
Anaphylaxis
  colloid solutions and, 215
  IgA and, 258
Anemia
  donor, 13–14, 21
  in premature infants, 224
  RBC transfusion in, 213

Anesthesia, hemolytic reaction and, 257
Angina, donor, 22
Ankylosing spondylitis, HLA B27 in, 130
Anthropology, 85
Anti-A_1 antibodies, 88
Anti-A_1 lectin, in polyagglutinability, 175
Antibiotics
  agglutination and, 195
  contaminated blood components and, 262
  donor use of, 27
Antibodies, 57–61
  ABO hemolytic disease and, 362–363
  anamnestic response, 63
  -antigen reaction. *See* Antigen-antibody reaction
  avidity, 76
    hemolytic transfusion reaction and, 76–77
    high-titer low-, 190–191
  bivalent, 60
  blocking, 60
  blood group, 75–77
    avidity, 76–77
    detection of, 159–160
    reactions, 77
    serologic classification of, 60–61
    testing methods, 135–139
    titer, 77
  circulating, 62
  classification of, 60–61
  cold, 60
  complete, 60
  -containing serums, storage of, 77
  cytomegalovirus, testing for, 165
  defined, 55
  detection of, 354
  formation of, 62–63
  frozen, 77
  hemolytic transfusion reactions and, 249, 251–258
    donor plasma, 249, 255–256
    interdonor incompatibility and, 249
    major incompatibility and, 249, 251–255
    minor incompatibility, 249
    recipient plasma, 249, 251–255
  hepatitis, 271–272
  high-titer, low-avidity, 190–191
  HIV, test for, 164–165
  identification of, 354
    in pregnancy, 353
    titration in, 205
  in immune response, 62–63
  immunoglobulins. *See* Immunoglobulins (Ig); *see also specific*
  immunologic memory, 62
  incomplete, 60, 136
  individual formation capacity, 284
  induction period, 62
  labeling, 68
  -mediated reactions, in vitro, 65–69
  platelet, 284–285
  -producing cells. *See* B lymphocytes
  radio-labeled, 74
  RBC hydration shell and, 67–68
  reactivity, inhibition of, 202
  recipient
    hemolytic reaction and, 249, 251-155
    identification of, 183–197
    unexpected, 178–183
  screening
    donor, 159–160
    recipient, 178–179, 183–197
  secondary response, 63
  thawed, 77
  titration, 204–206
    in pregnancy, 354
  unexpected
    detection methods, 179–181
    in donor blood, 160
    identification of, 183–187
    reagent RBC for screening, 181–182
    in recipient blood, 178–183
    special investigation techniques, 199–207
  univalent, 60
  uptake of, pH and, 144
  warm, 60
  white cell, 284–285
Antibody screening test, 159–160
  absorption, 199–200
  antibiotics and, 195
  antibody-coated donor cells, 194–195
  anticoagulants and, 195
  antigen-antibody ratio in, 142–143
  autoantibody in, 192–195
  autologous control in, 183
  Bg antigen in, 190
  bovine albumin and, 195
  centrifugation in, 142
  Chido antigen in, 191
  cold autoagglutinins, 193
  colloidal silica and, 197
  drugs and, 195

Antibody screening test—*Continued*
  elution, 200, 201
  enzyme techniques for, 146–147, 181
  factors influencing sensitivity of, 140–145
  high-titer low-avidity, 190–191
  hydrogen ion concentration in, 143
  incubation temperature in, 141–142
  incubation time in, 140–141
  ionic strength of test mixture in, 144–145
  macromolecular substances in, 144–145
  microbial contamination and, 196
  mixed-field antiglobulin reaction, 194–197
  multiple specificity, 188, 189
  polybrene methods, 181
  polycations in, 145–146
  in pregnancy, 352–353
  protamine methods, 181
  pseudoagglutination, 196–197
  reagent RBC for, 181–182
  recipient, 179–183
  Rodgers antigen in, 191
  at room temperature and below, 180
  rouleaux, 196–197
  saline and, 195
  Sd^a (Sid) antigen in, 192
  single antibody in serum, 186
  terminology for, 199–203
  test mixture ionic strength in, 144
  titration, 204–206
  using bovine albumin, 180
  variable reactivity and dosage, 184–188
  warm autoantibodies, 193
Anticoagulant. *See also specific*
  acid-citrate-dextrose, 40
  agglutination and, 195
  citrate dextrose, 297
  exchange transfusion and, 361
  in leukapheresis, 45–46
  red cell preservation and, 297
  red cell recovery and, 297
Antiemetics, 36
Antigen-antibody complex, 66
Antigen-antibody reaction, 65
  agglutinate formation in, 67–68
    surface hydration theory of, 67–68
    zeta potential theory of, 67
  antibody labeling in, 68
  cell age and, 75
  dosage and, 74
  firm but reversible, 65
  historic background, 55
  immune hemolysis in, 68–69
  in vitro, 65–69
  in vivo, 65
  neutralization of, 68
  precipitation, 66
  quantitative aspects of, 75
  RBC antigens and, 74
  RBC genotype and, 74–75
  serologic manifestations of, 66
  stages of, 65–66
  storage and, 75
  surface hydration theory of, 67–68
  zeta potential theory of, 67
Antigenic determinant, 56. *See also* Antigens; Epitope
Antigens, 56–57
  -antibody reaction. *See* Antigen-antibody reaction
  blood group
    immunization by, 63–65
    testing methods, 135–149
  carrier, 57
  of different blood groups, 81
  dosage effect, 83
  epitope, 56
  equivalence zone, 66
  expression in RBC, 205–206
  hepatitis, 271–272
  hepatitis B surface, tests for, 162–163
  high frequency, 84–85, 113, 114
    antibodies to, 188
    typing and testing, 158
  histocompatibility, 116–130. *See also* HLA system
  immune response, 56–57
  immunogenicity of, 80
  low frequency, 84–85, 112–114
    antibodies to, 188–190
  in maternal alloimmunization, 348
  platelet-specific, 129
  polymorphism, 85
  private, 84
  public, 84
  reactive site, 56
  reciprocally related, 84–85
  red cell surface, 80
  sex-linked, 110–112
  soluble, 66
Antiglobulin test, 80, 137–140
  in antibody detection, 182

direct. *See* Direct antiglobulin test
indirect, 138–139. *See also* Antibody screening test; Crossmatching
mixed-field reaction, 194–195
sources of error in, 139–140
Antihemophilic factor, 322–323
concentrates, HIV infection and, 393
hepatitis and, 274
storage of, 292
Antihistamine, 21, 36
in transfusion reaction, 258–259
Antihypertensive agents, 27–28
Anti-Inhibitor Coagulant Complex, 323
Antimalarial therapy, 19
Antipyretic, in transfusion reaction, 260
Antiserum, centrifugation of, 142
Antithrombin III, 319, 326
Anuria, hemolytic transfusion reaction and, 253
AnWj antigen, 113
Apheresis. *See also* Hemapheresis
complications of, 48
defined, 38
platelet. *See* Platelets, apheresis
Arrhythmia, cardiac, in massive transfusion, 218
Arteriosclerosis, donor, 11
Arthritis
hyperuricemic, 25
rheumatoid, 377–378, 380
Aspirin
donor use of, 27
platelet transfusion and, 336–337
Asthma, in transfusion reaction, 258
At^a antigen, 113
Autoabsorption, 200
Autoagglutination phenonemon, albumin, 195
Autoagglutinin, hydrogen ion concentration and, 143. *See also* Cold agglutinins
Autoantibody
versus alloantibody, 182–183
cold agglutinins, 193
in Goodpasture's syndrome, 375
in myasthenia gravis, 375
testing of, 192–195
warm, 194
Autoimmune disease, 55–56
antigens in, 56
crossmatching and, 199

hemolytic anemia, alpha-methyldopa and, 195
plasma exchange in, 378–379
Autologous transfusion
and children, 391
donation for, 3
preoperative collection, 226–227
Automated blood grouping instruments, 148–149
Automated cell separation. *See* Hemapheresis
Automated test systems, 148–149
Autosome, defined, 80

B antigen and antibody
in erythroblastosis, 361, 364
inheritance, 86
specificity of, 87
subgroups of, 91
B lymphocytes, 56, 61, 65
Babesiosis, transfusional, 20–21, 282, 283
Bacteremia, dental surgery and, 21–22
Bacterial enzyme, in polyagglutinability, 175
Bacterial infection, in polyagglutinability, 196
Bacteriolysis, 68
Bed, donor, 35
Beta-2-microglobulin, testing of donor blood, 279
Bg antigens, 115–116
antibodies to, 115–116, 190
Bi antigen, 113
Bilirubin
in erythroblastosis fetalis, 351
gestational age and, 357
hemoglobin breakdown and, 250
Bilirubinoid pigment, in amniotic fluid, 354–355
Bisexuality, AIDS and, 17, 277–278, 279
Bleeding tendency, 263–264, 265
donor, 27
Blood
components. *See* Blood components
fractions and derivatives, 291, 292
in antithrombin III deficiency, 326
for clotting factor deficiencies, 318–325
in DIC, 325
in factor IX deficiency, 326
official names for, 292

Blood, fractions and derivatives—*Continued*
  in protein C deficiency, 326
  in von Willebrand's disease, 326
  warming, 261–262, 361–362
    microwave for, 218
Blood banks
  bloodmobile, 7–8
  community, 1, 8–9
  computerized records, 8
  hospital, 1
  inventory control in, 8, 241–242
  legislation for, 3
  national organizations, 1
  records, 237
    computerized, 8–9
  satellite drawing station, 8
  as service industry, 1
  types of, 1
Blood cell separators
  in automated hemapheresis, 39–42
  centrifugation systems for, 39–40
  devices for, 39–42
  membrane systems for, 40–42
  in therapeutic hemapheresis, 367
Blood center. *See* Blood banks
Blood collection. *See* Collection of blood
Blood components, 291–341
  contaminated, 262
  fractions and derivatives, 291, 292
  irradiation of, 235
  official names for, 292
  preparation, 291
  recipient as donor, 16
Blood disease, in donor, 26
Blood donation. *See* Donor(s) and donation of blood
Blood groups, 80–130
  alloimmunization, 63–65
  antibodies. *See* Antibodies
  antigen-antibody reactions, 65
    factors affecting, 74–75
  antigens. *See* Antigens; *see also specific*
  automated testing of, 148–149
  discovery, 80
  genetic considerations of, 80–85
  immune response, 61–63
  immunization, 282–285
  immunology of, 55–77
  purpose of, 85
  significance of, 85
  testing methods, 150–159

Blood loss, and laboratory tests, 391
Blood pressure, donor, 23
Blood recipient, and HIV-zero positivity, 392
Blood volume
  loss of, 214–221
    in plasma exchange, 385
    signs and symptoms of, 215
  normal values for, 212
  plasma, 211, 212
  red cell, 211–212
Bloodmobile, 7–8
Body surface area, 330, 331, 333
  of children, 330, 332, 333
Body temperature, donor, 11
Bombay blood type, 91–92
  para-, 92–93
Bone marrow
  aplasia, 234
  B lymphocytes in, 61
Bone marrow transplantation
  donor, 126
  donor program operation principles, 127
  graft-versus-host disease in, 231, 234
  granulocyte transfusion in, 234
  HLA system in, 126–127
  HLA typing for, 231–232
  irradiation of blood components, 234, 235
  MLC-compatible, 126
  plasma exchange in, 379, 380
  posttransplant support in, 234
  pretransplant management in, 231–232
  pretransplant conditioning in, 232–233
  RBC transfusion in, 231–234
  recipient, 175–176
Bovine albumin, agglutination and, 136–137, 180, 195
Bp^a antigen, 113
Bradycardia, donor, 22, 34–35
Brain, bilirubin toxicity in, 351–352
Breast cancer, transfusion in, 234
Bronchodilators, 36
Brucellosis, transmission of, 282, 283
Buffy coat, in centrifugation, 39–40
Bw4 typing, 121, 122
Bw6 typing, 121, 122
Bx^a antigen, 113
By antigen, 113

C. *See* Complement (C) system
C antigen (Rh), 121
  dosage effect, 74
  immunization, 64
  testing for, 157
Cadaver
  blood, 5
  renal transplantation, 125
Calcium-binding agents, complement and, 71–72
Cancer, in donor, 25–26
Cardiac arrest, in massive transfusion, 218, 385
Cardiolipin antigen, 148
Cardiovascular disease, donor, 22
Cardiovascular surgery, bleeding tendency and, 263
Carrier, antigen, 57
Cartwright blood group system
  antigens, 81
  phenotypes, 111
Cascade filtration, in plasma exchange, 369
Ce antiserum, 97–98
Cell-mediated immunity, 55
  T lymphocytes in, 61
Celltrifuge II, 40
Cellular immunity, 56
Centrifugation, 39–40
  in antibody detection tests, 142
  buffy coat formation in, 39–40
  Cobe-IBM 2997, 40
  continuous flow, 39
  counterflow elutriation in, 40
  discontinuous flow, 39
  enzyme techniques and, 146–147
  extracorporeal circuit, 39, 40
  Fenwal CS-3000, 40, 41
  IFC Haemonetics system, 40
  intermittent flow, 39
  speed of, 142
  of whole blood, 291
Centrifuge, speed of, 142
Cerebral palsy, bilirubin encephalopathy and, 352
Cerebrovascular accident, as complication of blood donation, 22, 23
Chagas' disease, transmission of, 282, 283
Chelation therapy, in iron overload, 228
Chemotherapeutic agent, extracorporeal photo-activation of, 381

Chemotherapy
  plasma exchange and, 374
  transfusion in, 234–235
Chickenpox, in donor, 20
Chido blood group system
  antibodies, 191
  antigens, 81
Chido antigen, antibodies to, 191
Chimerism, 175
Chloroquine, for antibody elution, 203–204
Cholera vaccine, 28
Cholesterol, plasma exchange and, 379
Chr^a antigen, 113
Chromosome. *See also* Gene; Genetics
  crossing over, 83
  locus, 81
  sex, 80
  synteny, 84
13-cis-retinoic acid, donor use, 22
Citrate phosphate dextrose, 297–298
  posttransfusion survival and, 301
Citrate phosphate dextrose adenine-1, 298–299
  posttransfusion survival and, 301
Citrate toxicity, 263, 265
  hemapheresis and, 263
  in hemapheresis donor, 47–48
  in massive transfusion, 217
  in plasma exchange, 384–385
Clotting factor deficiency, derivatives and components for, 318–325
Co antibodies, identification of, 185
Coagulation, in extracorporeal circuit, 40
Coagulation factor
  deficiency of, derivatives and components for, 318–325
  half-life of, 319
  in plasma exchange, 372
Coagulation function test, in massive transfusion, 216
Cobe-IBM 2997, 40
Cold agglutinins, 60, 193
  autoagglutinins, crossmatching and, 199
  erythroblastosis fetalis and, 353
  hydrogen ion concentration and, 143
  infectious mononucleosis and, 115
  LW antigen, 115
Cold blood
  in exchange transfusion, 261
  reaction to, 218, 361–362

Cold insoluble globulin, 321
Collection of blood, 30–34
　blood-drawing area, 30
　centrifugation systems in, 39–40
　containers for, 30–31
　donor identification, 32
　donor information, 32
　donor reaction to. *See* Donor reactions
　from infant, 170
　from recipient, 169–174
　hemapheresis in, 37–47
　lesion of, 296
　membrane systems in, 40–42
　nonvenous, from recipient, 170
　phlebotomy, 33–34
　refreshments following, 34
　samples for testing and crossmatching, 31
　venipuncture site for, 32–33
Colloid solutions, 215
　in burn management, 221
Colloidal silica, in pseudoagglutination, 197
Colton blood group system
　antigens, 81
　phenotypes, 111
Community blood bank, 1, 8–9
Complement (C) system, 69–73
　activation
　　alternative pathway, 69
　　classical pathway, 69, 70–71
　　Ig G and, 57
　　immunoglobulin in, 60
　　in vivo, 69
　　polypeptides, 72
　biologic activities of, 72
　in blood group serology, 73
　components of, 69–73
　in immune hemolysis, 69
　serum inactivation, 72
Consent, donor, 11, 32
Container, 30–31
　additive solutions, 301
　position of, 33
　in pseudoagglutination, 197
　in transfusion reaction, 266
Contamination
　of equipment, 166
　in pseudoagglutination, 197
Convulsion, donor, 36
Coombs' test. *See* Antiglobulin test

Copper sulfate test, of donor blood, 13–14
Coronary heart disease
　donor, 22
　hypertension and, 23
Corticosteroids, in leukapheresis, 46
Council of Community Blood Centers, 1
Counterflow elutriation, in centrifugation system, 40
Cr antigen, 113
Creutzfeldt-Jakob disease, 393
Crossing over phenomenon, 83
Crossmatching
　antiglobulin phase of, 198
　autoantibodies and, 199
　defined, 169
　of donor blood, 31
　elution, 201–202
　HLA compatibility and, 124–125
　interdonor incompatibility and, 178
　for platelets, 124–125
　recipient, 197–198
　in renal transplantation, 126
　immunized recipient, 198–199
　urgent transfusion, 199
　titration, 204–206
Cross-reacting HLA antigens (CREGs), 129
Cryoglobulinemia, plasma exchange in, 374, 377
Cryoprecipitate, 319–322
Cryoprecipitation chamber, in plasma exchange, 369
Crystalloid solution
　in fluid volume replacement, 215
Cs^a antigen, 113
Cutaneous T-cell lymphoma, 381
C^w antigen (Rh), 197
　in antibody screening, 181
Cyclosporine
　in bone marrow transplantation, 232
　in renal transplantation, 125
Cytapheresis
　donor selection for, 42–44
　procedures, 42–45
　screening program for, 44
　therapeutic, 382–383
Cytomegalovirus infection
　antibody testing, 165
　in bone marrow transplantation, 231, 234

in donor, 20
neonatal transfusion and, 225
occupational infection, 391
in renal transplantation, 230
transfusional, 275–276, 283

D antigen, 93. *See also* Rh antigens; Rh system
 automated testing system for, 149
 immunization, 63
 testing, 156–157
  in recipients, 176–177
  variable and variant expression of, 94–96
Dane particle, 271
Dental surgery, donor, 21–22
Deoxyribonucleic acid, in genes, 81
Dexamethasone, in granulocyte stimulation, 46
Dextran solution, 215
 in leukapheresis, 45
D-galactosyltransferase, B antigen specificity and, 87
Dh^a antigen, 113
Diabetes mellitus, in donor, 24–25
Dialysis membrane, reactions associated with, 49
Diastolic blood pressure, donor, 23
DIC. *See* Disseminated intravascular coagulation (DIC)
Diego blood group system
 antibodies, identification of, 185
 antigens, 81, 85
 phenotypes, 111
2,3-Diphosphoglycerate
 oxygen release and, 295–296
Diphtheria vaccine, 28
Dipyrone, direct antiglobulin test and, 195
Direct antiglobulin test, 138
 in ABO hemolytic disease, 363
 drug-induced, 195
 of D^u antigen, 157
 error sources in, 138–139
 in erythroblastosis fetalis, 356, 363
 of recipient, 178
Disseminated intravascular coagulation (DIC), 325
 clinical conditions associated with, 325
 components and derivatives in, 320

exchange transfusion in, 229
factor IX complex and, 324
DNA, in genes, 81
Do antibodies, identification of, 185
Dolichos biflorus, 88, 89, 175
Dombrock blood group system
 antigens, 81
 phenotypes, 111
Donor(s) and donation of blood
 advertisements encouraging, 6
 antibody screening, 159–160
 autologous, 3, 391
  AIDS and, 279
 automated testing of, 148–149
 cadaver, 5
 call-up system, 6
 cash-paid, 2
 collection of. *See* Collection of blood
 reactions. *See* Donor reactions
 directed donations, 3–5
  opinions for and against, 4
 disease transmission via, tests for, 160–165
 donor-specific transfusions for renal transplantation, 3, 230
 drawing of, 30
 education about, 5–7
 finding, 5
 identification of, 32
 informed consent, 32
 labeling of donor blood, 167
 laboratory tests of donor blood, 31
  recording results of, 165–166
 leukapheresis, 45–47
 motivation of, 2
 for neonates, 224–225
 postdonation questionnaire, 278
 rare, 236
 recipient-specific, 3–5
 recruitment programs, 5–8
 selection principles. *See* Donor selection
 testing and typing, 135–166
  for AIDS, 279–280
  antibody screening, 159–160
  automated, 148–149
  blood group, 150–159
  disease transmission, 160–166
  hepatitis, 162, 163, 165
  quality control of, 158–159
  sterility, 166

Donor(s) and donation of blood—*Continued*
  unexpected antibodies in, 160
  unit records, 208
  "walking donor" program, 224
Donor reactions, 34–37
  fainting, 34–35
  in hemapheresis, 47–50
  hematoma, 36
  medication for, 36
  to phlebotomy, conditions affecting, 22–29
  prevention of, 37
  record of, 37
  syncope, 34–35
  treatment of, 35–36
  variations in, 35
Donor selection, 10–14
  acupuncture and, 16
  acute respiratory disease and, 25
  age and, 11
  AIDS and, 16–19
  allergies and, 21
  babesiosis and, 20–21
  bleeding tendencies and, 27
  blood diseases and, 26–27
  blood pressure abnormalities and, 23
  cancer and, 25–26
  chickenpox and, 20
  consent, 11
  for cytapheresis, 42–45
  cytomegalovirus and, 20
  dental surgery and, 21–22
  diabetes mellitus and, 24–25
  drug use and, 27–28
    intravenous, 15
  ear piercing and, 16
  epilepsy or fits and, 26
  gastrointestinal disease and, 25
  German measles and, 20
  gout and, 25
  health interview form, 12
  heart disease and, 22–23
  hemoglobin level and, 13–14
  hepatitis history and, 14–15
  hereditary red cell defects and, 21
  immunizations and, 28
  infectious mononucleosis and, 20
  injections and inoculations, 28
  intravenous drug abuse and, 15
  malaria and, 19
  measles and, 20
  medication and, 27–28
  mumps and, 20
  occupation and, 28
  peptic ulcer and, 25
  phlebotomy response, conditions affecting, 22–29
  polycythemia and, 26–27
    secondary, 27
  pregnancy and, 28–29
  previous blood or plasma recipients, 16
  prison inmates and, 16
  protozoal infection and, 20–21
  pulse abnormalities and, 23
  registration form, 12
  responsibility for, 29–30
  rheumatic heart disease and, 22–23
  skin disease and, 22
  surgery and, 23–24
  syphilis and, 20
  tattooing and, 16
  temperature and, 11
  tuberculosis and, 21
  viral infection and, 20
  weight and, 13
  women, 28–29
DP lymphocyte antigens, 121
DQ lymphocyte antigens, 121
DR lymphocyte antibody, detection techniques, 124
DR lymphocyte antigens, 113
  in immune response, 61
  serologic testing of, 122–124
D(Rh) antiserum. *See also* Rh antibody; Rh system
  classification of, 96
  D^u. *See also* D^u type
    automated testing system for, 149
    testing for, 157
  recipient, 176–177
  Rh immune globulin and, 350–351
  Rh33 antigen and, 95
  in Rh-negative mothers, 352
  testing for, 156–157, 352
  titration of, 354
Drug(s)
  abuse. *See* Drug abuse
  in agglutination, 195
  allergy to, donor, 21
  for donor reaction, 36
  donor use, 27–28
    intravenous abuse, 15
    prescribed, 27–28

intravenous abuse
  AIDS and, 277
  removal of, exchange transfusion in, 229
Drug abuse
  AIDs and, 17, 27, 277
  donor, 15
  hepatitis and, 271
D^u type, 94
  high-grade, 95
  low-grade, 95
  qualitative variability of, 95
  quantitative variability of, 95
  testing, 157
    automated, 149
Duffy blood group system, 107–108
  antibody, 108
    polycation detection of, 145
  antigens, 81
  erythroblastosis fetalis and, 353
  IgG antibodies of, 60–61
  immunization, 63
  phenotypes, 108
  typing and testing of, 178
Dyspnea, donor, 22

E antigen (Rh)
  dosage effect, 74
  race and, 100
  testing for, 157
e antigen (Rh)
  dosage effect, 74
  race and, 100
Ear piercing, hepatitis and, 16
Education
  AIDS information sheet for donors, 18
  of blood donors, 5–7
Electrolyte abnormality
  in massive transfusion, 217
  in plasma exchange, 372
  red cell breakdown products and, 302
  transfusion and, 264, 265
Elution, 200, 201
  heat method, 201–202
  last-wash control, 201
Elutriation, counterflow, 40
Embolism, 261, 265
Emergency release form, 223
Emm antigen, 113
Encephalopathy, bilirubin, 351–352, 357

Enzyme
  absorption and, 200
  proteolytic, 181
  in serologic testing, 146–147, 181
Enzyme-linked immunoassay (ELISA)
  of cytomegalovirus antibody, 165
  of hepatitis B core antibody, 163
  of hepatitis B surface antigen, 162, 163
Epilepsy, in donor, 26
Epinephrine, in granulocyte stimulation, 46
Epitope, defined, 56
Er^a antigen, 113
Erythroblastosis fetalis. See Hemolytic disease of newborn
Erythrocytapheresis, therapeutic, 383
Erythrocyte, zeta potential of, 67
Es antigen, 113
Ethylenediaminetetraacetate, complement and, 71–72
Exchange transfusion
  in ABO erythroblastosis, 364
  amniocentesis and, 356
  anticoagulants and, 361
  blood storage and, 361
  blood temperature and, 361–362
  blood warming for, 261–262
  cold bood in, 261
  in disseminated intravascular coagulation, 229
  in drug removal, 229
  in erythroblastosis fetalis, 359–362
    ABO blood group in, 360
    amniocentesis and, 356
    blood group in, 360
    blood storage and, 361
    blood temperature and, 361–362
    maternal blood, 359–360
    Rh type in, 360, 361
    two-volume, 359
  in hyperbilirubinemia in neonates, 228
  intrauterine, 359
  maternal blood in, 359–360
  modified, for anemia, 241
  in neonatal sepsis, 229
  partial, in sickle cell disease, 229
  in respiratory distress syndrome, 229
  two-volume, 359
  ultrasound imaging in, 358
Exercise, granulocyte count and, 46

Factor I, 319
Factor II, 319

Factor V, 319
　deficiency, 320
Factor VII, 319
　deficiency, 320
Factor VIII, 319, 321
　deficiency, 320. *See also* Hemophilia
　with factor VIII antibodies, 320
　inhibitor, plasma exchange and, 376, 377
Factor IX deficiency, 320, 326. *See also* Hemophilia
Factor X, 319
　deficiency, 320
Factor XI, 319
　deficiency, 320
Factor XIII, 319
　deficiency, 320
Fainting, donor, 34–35
Familial hypercholesterolemia, plasma exchange in, 379, 380
Febrile transfusion reaction, 259–260, 265
　prevention of, 260
　treatment of, 260
Fenwal CS-3000 blood cell separator, 40, 41
Fenwal Plasmacell-C membrane collecting device, 43
Fetomaternal hemorrhage, Kleihauer detection technique in, 350
Fetoscopy, direct intravascular transfusion via, 358
Fetus
　hemolytic disease and. *See* Hemolytic disease of newborn
　hydrops. *See* Hydrops fetalis
　pulmonary maturity of, 356
Fibrinogen, 292
Fibronectin, 321
Ficin, in serologic testing, 146
Filtration
　cascade, 369
　membrane plasma separation devices, 368–369
　in on-line cryogelation, 380–381
　RBC transfusion, 238–239
Filtration leukapheresis, 46–47
　reactions to, 49
Fluid volume replacement
　in hemorrhagic shock, 215
　solutions for, 215
Fr^a antigen, 113
Fritz antigen, 113

Fy antibodies, 107–108. *See also* Duffy blood group system
　identification of, 185
Fy antigens, 107. *See also* Duffy blood group system
　enzyme detection of, 147
　typing, 158

G antigen (Rh), 98–100
Gallstone, jaundice due to, 15
Gamma globulin, in immunodeficiency, 258
Gamma STS-M, 149
Ge antigens, 113, 114
Gelatin, modified fluid, 45
Gene, 81
　alleles, 81
　amorph, 82
　cis, 85
　codominant, 83
　independent segregation of, 84
　linkage, 83–84
　linkage disequilibrium, 84
　locus, 81
　recessive, 83
　synteny, 84
　trans, 85
Genetics
　anthropology and, 85
　antigens of high and low frequency, 84–85
　dominance and recessiveness, 83
　genotype, 82
　linkage and synteny, 83–84
　phenotype, 82
　polymorphism, 85
　related and unrelated antigens, 84
　terminology of, 81–82, 85
　zygosity, 81–82
Germ cell, division of, 83
German measles (rubella), in donor, 20
Gf antigen, 113
Globulin
　cold insoluble, 321
　immune. *See* Immune globulin
Glucose-6-phosphate dehydrogenase deficiency, hemolytic reaction and, 256–257
Glycophorin A, 104
　enzyme detection of, 147
Glycophorin B, 104
Glycosyltransferase, 87
　Le gene and, 106

Goodpasture's syndrome, plasma exchange in, 375, 377
Gout, donor, 25
Graft-versus-host disease, 264, 265, 283
  in bone marrow transplantation, 231, 234
  intrauterine transfusion and, 359
  prevention of, 264
Granulocyte, storage, 340
Granulocyte transfusion, 337–341
  in bone marrow transplantation, 234
  compatibility and, 340
  criteria for, 338–339
  dosage, 339–340
  electromechanical infusion device for, 240
  HLA typing for, 45, 128–130
  macromolecular agents and, 46
  reactions and complications of, 340–341
  therapeutic cytapheresis for, 382
Groupamatic G360-C, 149
Guillain-Barré syndrome, plasma exchange in, 376, 377
Gy^a antigen, 113

H antigen, Bombay phenotype and, 91
Hapten, defined, 57
Haptoglobin, 250
Hay fever, in donor, 21
Health interview, donor, 12
Heart attack, donor, 22
Heart failure, neonatal, 357
Heart murmur, in donor, 23
Heart transplantation, HLA typing in, 128
Heibel antigen, 113
Helper T cell, 61
Hemagglutination. *See also* Agglutination
  antigen-antibody reaction and, 74
  low-ionic polycation augmentation test of, 145
  numerical scoring system for, 206, 207
Hemapheresis
  allergic reaction in, 48
  automated, 39–42
  blood donation by, 37–47
  cell depletion in, 49–50
  centrifugation, 39–40
  citrate toxicity in, 47–48, 263
  effect on donor, 47–50
  frequency of, 49–50
  hemolysis in, 48–49
  lymphocyte count following, 50
  manual, 38–39
  membrane systems, 40–42
  platelet count following, 50
  reactions to, 47–49
  steroid reactions in, 48
  therapeutic, 367–368. *See also* Plasma exchange
    complications of, 383–386
      delayed, 385–386
      procedural, 384–385
      vascular, 384
    cytapheresis, 382–383
    diseases treated by, 372–380
    extracorporeal adsorption in, 380–381
    immunoadsorption in, 381, 382
    mortality in, 386
    on-line cryogelation in, 380–381
Hematocrit, transfusion trigger and, 213
Hematoma, at phlebotomy site, 36
Hemizygote, 83
Hemodialysis, membrane systems in, 40–41
Hemodilution
  in myocardial ischemia, 227
  in open-heart surgery, 214
  in plasma exchange, 372
Hemoglobin
  breakdown of, 250
  clearance of, hemolytic transfusion reaction and, 250–251
  free, 250
    red cell storage and, 302–303
  hemolytic transfusion reaction and, 249
  measurement of, 13–14
  oxygen dissociation curve, 294
  saturation, 293
  transfusion and, 249
  in umbilical cord blood, 357
Hemoglobin-dissociation curve, in premature infants, 224
Hemoglobin-haptoglobin complex, 250
Hemoglobinuria, hemolytic transfusion reaction and, 249
Hemolysis, 136
  in antibody testing, 182
  antibody-mediated, 236
  blood pumps and, 240
  contaminated blood components and, 262

Hemolysis—*Continued*
  delayed, 254–255
  immune, 68–69
  Lewis antibodies in, 107
  microwave blood warming and, 218
  posttransplant, 234
  RBC transfusion in, 213
Hemolytic anemia. *See also* Autoimmune disease
  autoimmune, 195
  cold-antibody, plasma exchange in, 379, 380
  microangiopathic, plasma exchange in, 378–379
Hemolytic disease of newborn, 348–364
  ABO, 357, 362–364
    antibody characteristics in, 362–363
    diagnosis of, 363–364
    exchange transfusion in, 364
  ABO typing in, 356–357
  antibody effects on fetus in, 351–352
  bilirubin determination in, 357
  direct antiglobulin test in, 357
  D^u mother in, 350–351
  exchange transfusion in, 359–362, 364
  fetal red cell passage to mother in, 349
  hemoglobin level in, 357
  intrauterine transfusion in, 358–359
  kernicterus and, 351–352, 357
  maternal alloimmunization in, 348–351
  neonatal testing, 356–357
  plasma exchange in, 379, 380
  plasmapheresis in, 357–358
  prenatal diagnosis of, 352–356
    amniocentesis, 354–356
    antibody detection tests, 352–353
    antibody identification, 353
    antibody titration in, 354
    blood typing, 352
    IgG antibody, 353
    ultrasound imaging, 356
  prevention of, 349–350
  Rh antibody in, removal by plasmapheresis, 357–358
  Rh immune globulin in, 349–350
  Rh incompatibility and, 93
  Rh typing in
    neonatal testing for, 357–358
    paternal, 349, 353
  Rh-positive father and, 349, 353
Hemolytic transfusion reaction, 249–258, 265
  anti-A and anti-B, 251
  antibody avidity and, 76–77
  antibody in donor plasma, 249, 255–256
  antibody in recipient plasma, 249, 251–255
  antibody type and, 251–252
  delayed, 76–77, 254–255
  without demonstrable antibody, 255
  diagnosis of, 257
  glucose-6-phosphate dehydrogenase deficiency and, 256–257
  hyperbilirubinemia and, 250
  identification problems in, 253–254
  interdonor incompatibility and, 249
  intravascular, 249
  laboratory test problems in, 254
  major incompatibility, 249, 251–255
    antibody type and, 251–252
    decreased red cell survival, 255
  minor incompatibility, 249
  renal failure and, 253
  signs and symptoms, 252–253
  treatment of, 257–258
Hemolytic-uremic syndrome, plasma exchange in, 376
Hemophilia
  AIDS and, 276
  component therapy for, 322
  with inhibitor, plasma exchange in, 376, 377
Hemorrhagic shock, 214
  fluid volume replacement in, 215
Hemosiderin, deposition in renal tubules, 250
Hemosiderosis, transfusional, 282, 283
Heparin anticoagulant, exchange transfusion and, 361
Hepatitis
  acupuncture and, 16
  alanine aminotransferase testing in, 273
  antibody, 271–272
  antigen, 271–272
  characteristics of, 270
  close contact with, 15
  delta, 269
  donor history of, 14–15
  ear piercing and, 16
  incidence of, 270–271
  infectious, 269
  intravenous drug abuse and, 15
  prevention of, 274–275
  prison inmates and, 16

serum, 269
tattooing and, 16
transfusional, 268–275, 283
  testing for, 165
Hepatitis A, 269
  blood donation and, 14
  posttransfusion, 273
Hepatitis B, 269
  blood donation and, 14
  clinical and serologic changes in, 272
  icteric, 269
  occupational infection, 391
Hepatitis B core antibody, testing, 273–274
Hepatitis B immune globulin, 14
Hepatitis B surface antigen, 14, 272
  testing for, 162–163, 272–273
Hepatitis B vaccine, 28
Hepatitis non-A, non-B, 269
  blood donation and, 14
  immune serum globulin and, 274–275
  surrogate tests for, 163–165
Hetastarch. See Hydroxyethyl starch
Heterozygote, 82
  obligate, 84
Hexadimethrine bromide, in antibody detection, 145
Hey antigen, 113
Hg^a antigen, 113
HI antigen, 193
High-risk donors, 392
Histocompatibility antigens, 116–130
HIV. See Human immunodeficiency virus (HIV)
HLA system, 116–130
  B lymphocyte antigens, 121–124
  Bw4 typing, 121, 122
  Bw6 typing, 121, 122
  C antigens, 121
  cell membrane markers, 56
  class I antigens, 120–121
    in bone marrow transplantation, 232
    in transplantation, 120
  class II antigens, 121–124
    in bone marrow transplantation, 232
    in immune response, 61
    in immunoglobulins, 124
  compatibility test, 124
  crossmatching, 124–125
  cross-reacting groups, 129

DR antigens, 122–124
haplotypes, 118
immunogenetics of, 116–118
mixed lymphocyte culture, 123
MLC antigen, 121–122
older designations of, 117
one-way MLC test, 121
phenotypes, 118
screening, 124–125
specificities, 119
supergene, 116
transfusion and, 128–130
  granulocyte, 128–130
  platelet, 128
transplantation and, 125–130
  bone marrow, 126–127
  heart, 128
  kidney, 125–126
  liver, 128
two-way MLC test, 121–122
typing, 118–121
  in bone marrow transplantation, 231–32
  in granulocyte transfusion, 45, 128–130
  in heart transplantation, 128
  in leukemia, 234
  in liver transplantation, 128
  lymphocyte microcytotoxicity method, 118–120
  in platelet transfusion, 128, 129
  in renal transplantation, 125–126
Homozygote, 82
hr antigens. See Rh antigens
Human immunodeficiency virus (HIV)
  antibody test, 164–165
  antihemophilic factor concentrates and, 393
  donor detection, 19
  occupational infection, 391
  transmission of, 276
Human leukocyte antigen. See HLA system
Human pituitary-derived growth hormone, 393
Human T-cell lymphotropic virus, 276, 392. See also Acquired immunodeficiency syndrome (AIDS)
Humoral immunity, 55, 56
Hy antigen, 113
Hydrocortisone, in granulocyte stimulation, 46

Hydrogen ion concentration
  in antibody detection tests, 143
  red cell breakdown products and, 302
Hydrops fetalis, 351
  ultrasound evaluation of, 356
Hydrostatic force, in plasma exchange, 369
Hydroxyethyl starch
  allergic reaction to, 48
  in fluid volume replacement, 215
  in leukapheresis, 45
Hyperbilirubinemia
  acute hemolysis and, 250
  hemolytic transfusion reaction and, 250
  in neonates, exchange transfusion in, 228
Hypercholesterolemia, familial
  plasma exchange in, 379, 380
Hyperkalemia, 264
Hypertension, donor, 23
Hypertransfusion
  for sickle cell disease, 228
  for thalassemia, 228
Hyperuricemic arthritis, in donor, 25
Hyperventilation, donor, 35
Hyperviscosity syndrome, plasma exchange in, 374, 377
Hypervolemia, in plasma exchange, 384
Hypocalcemia, in massive transfusion, 217
Hypofibrinogenemia, 320
Hypoglycemic agents, 24–25
Hypokalemia, in massive transfusion, 217–218
Hypoproteinemia
  in plasma exchange, 372, 384
  plasma loss and, 38
Hypotension
  donor, 22, 23, 34–35
  in plasma exchange, 384
Hypothermia, calcium in, 217
Hypovolemia, in plasma exchange, 372, 384

I antibody, 114–115
I antigen, 113, 114–115
IBM 2997 centrifuge, 40
Identification
  of donor, 32
  labels. See Labels and labeling
  problems of, 253–254
  of recipient
    at bedside, 171–172
    at laboratory, 173–174
    on administration of transfusion, 174
    wrist label for, 172
Idiopathic thrombocytopenic purpura, plasma exchange in, 380
IFC Haemonetics system, 40
Ig. See Immunoglobulin (Ig)
IH antigen, cold agglutinins and, 193
Immune complex
  extracorporeal adsorption of, 380
  in fulminant crescentic nephritis, 377
  on-line cryogelation of, 380–381
  in rheumatoid arthritis, 378
  in systemic lupus erythematosus, 377
Immune complex disease, extravascular, 377–378
Immune globulin, 316–318
  containing specific antibodies, 317–318
  intramuscular, 316
  intravenous, 316–317
  Rh
    in erythroblastosis fetalis, 349–351
    immunoprophylaxis, 379
    in transfusion, 220
Immune hemolysis, 68–69
Immune response, 61–63
  antibody formation in, 62–63
  B lymphocytes in, 61–62
  macrophage in, 61
  T lymphocyte in, 61
Immunity
  auto-, 55
  cell-mediated, 55
  humoral, 55
Immunization. See also Alloimmunization
  blood group, 282–285
  by blood group antigens, 63–65
  during pregnancy, 350
  frequency, 283–284
  immunogenicity, 282–283
  individual antibody formation capacity, 284
  passive, 349
  platelet antibodies, 284–285
  prevention in, 349–350
  Rh
    in D^u type mother, 350–351
    in erythroblastosis fetalis, 349

with Rh immune globulin, 349
  white cell antibodies, 284–285
Immunoadsorption, 381, 382
  in bone marrow transplantation, 379
Immunocompetence, 264
Immunogenicity, 116–118
  antibody-stimulating activity, 57
  of antigens, 80
Immunoglobulin A
  chemical and physical properties of, 59
  deficiency of, 259
  J chain, 58
  structure of, 58
Immunoglobulin D, chemical and physical properties of, 59
Immunoglobulin E, chemical and physical properties of, 59
Immunoglobulin G
  antibody formation, 62
  bovine albumin agglutination and, 180
  chemical and physical properties of, 59
  complement activation and, 57
  in erythroblastosis fetalis, 353, 363
  placental transfer of, 348
  in plasma exchange, 371
  polycation detection of, 145
  reduction of, 59
  Rh antibodies and, 57–58
  schematic representation of, 58
  subclasses, 57–58
Immunoglobulin M
  antibody formation, 62
  autoantibodies and, 193
  in bone marrow transplantation, 233
  chemical and physical properties of, 59
  J chain, 58
  in plasma exchange, 370–371
  in recipient, 176
  Rh antibodies and, 94
  structure of, 57, 58
Immunoglobulins (Ig), 57–60
  activated complement, 60
  blood group antibodies and, 60
  chemical and physical properties of, 59
  classification of, 59
  constant fragment, 59
  defined, 57
  domains, 57
  Fab fragments, 59
  heavy chain, 57, 59
  hinge region, 58
  kappa, 57
  lambda, 57
  light chain, 57, 59
  placental transfer of, 60
  in plasma exchange, 385
  primary response, 60
  removal from RBC, 203
  secondary response, 60
  structure of, 57
  variable region, 57
Immunologic memory, 62
Immunosuppression
  in myasthenia gravis, 375
  in plasma exchange, 385
  plasma exchange and, 371–372, 373
  in renal transplantation, 229
In^b antigen, 113
Incubation temperature, in antibody detection tests, 141–142
Incubation time, in antibody detection tests, 140–141
Indirect antiglobulin test, 138–139
  bovine albumin potentiation of, 136–137
  enzyme techniques in, 146–147
  error sources in, 139–140
  of MNSs system antibodies, 105
  of Rh antibodies, 181
  in saline medium, 135–136
Infant. *See also* Neonate; Premature infant
  AIDS in, 276–277
  blood collection from, 170
  body surface area of, 332
Infection, in plasma exchange, 385
Infectious mononucleosis
  cold-agglutinin in, 115
  versus hepatitis, 20
  transfusional, 20
Influenza vaccine, 28
Informed consent, donor, 11, 32
Inoculation, donor, 28
Interdonor incompatibility
  hemolytic transfusion reaction and, 256
  minor crossmatching and, 178
International Society of Blood Transfusion Working Party on Terminology of Red Cell Surface Antigens, 80
Interview, donor, 12

Intraoperative blood salvage
  in autologous transfusion, 226
  in RBC transfusion, 227
Intrauterine transfusion
  amniocentesis and, 356
  blood selection for, 358–359
  direct antiglobulin test in, 357
  direct intravascular, 358
  in erythroblastosis fetalis, 358
  exchange, 358
  fetoscopy in, 358
  intravascular, direct, 358
  overtransfusion in, 358
  peritoneal, 356
  ultrasound imaging in, 356, 359
Intravenous drug abuse, 15
  AIDS and, 17, 27, 277
  hepatitis transmission and, 271
In vitro antibody-mediated reactions, 65–69
Irradiation of blood products, 235
Iron overload, in hypertransfusion, 228
Iron supplementation, in autologous transfusion, 227
Isotretinoin, donor use, 22

J chain, immunoglobulin, 58
Jaundice
  in ABO incompatibility, 363–364
  donor, 15
  erythroblastosis fetalis and, 15
  gallstones and, 15
  neonatal, 351–352
Je^a antigen, 113
Jk antibodies, identification of, 185. *See also* Kidd blood group system
Jk antigens, 108. *See also* Kidd blood group system
  dosage effect, 74
  typing, 158
JMH antigen, 113
Jn^a antigen, 113
Jo^a antigen, 113
Jr^a antigen, 113
Js antibodies, identification of, 185
Js antigens, in antibody screening, 181

K antibodies, polycation detection of, 145
K antigens, 101–102
  immunization, 64–65
  removal from RBC, 204
  typing, 158

K antiserum, 102–103
Kell blood group system, 101–103
  antibodies, 102–103
  antigens, 81, 84, 102
    frequency, 102
  discovery, 101
  erythroblastosis fetalis and, 353
  genotype, 82
  IgG antibodies of, 60–61
  immunization, 63
  McLeod phenotype, 109
  phenotype, 82
  typing and testing of, 158
    in recipient, 178
Kernicterus, erythroblastosis and, 357
Kidd blood group system, 108–110
  antibodies, 109–110
    record keeping, 208
  antigens, 81
  complement and, 73
  phenotypes, 109
  typing and testing
    enzyme techniques in, 147
    in recipient, 178
Kidney, transplantation of. *See* Renal transplantation
Kleihauer technique, in fetomaternal hemorrhage, 350
Kn^a antigen, 113
Kp antibodies, identification of, 185
Kp antigens, 197
  in antibody screening, 181
Kx antigen, ZZAPP treatment, 203

Labels and labeling
  antibody, 68
  at bedside, 171–172
  of donor blood, 167
  at laboratory, 173–174
  on administration of transfusion, 174
  prelabeling, 171
  wrist band, 172
Laboratory tests. *See also specific*
  and blood loss, 391
  of donor blood, 31
  in hemolytic transfusion reaction, 254
  interpretations, 165–166
  observations, 165
  pretransfusion, 169, 174–178
  problems of, 254
  of recipient's blood sample, 174–178
  results recording, 165–166

symbols, 166
  in transfusion reaction, 266–268
Lactated Ringer's solution, 215
Lan antigen, 113
Landsteiner-Weiner blood group system, antigens, 81
Landsteiner's law, 86, 87
Langerhans cell, class II antigens in, 124
Le antibodies, identification of, 185. *See also* Lewis blood group system
Lectin, 88, 89
  in polyagglutinability, 175
Legislation, plasmapheresis, 38
Leukapheresis
  ABO groups and, 44
  donor blood modification by, 45–46
  donor steroid stimulation in, 46
  filtration, 46–47
    reactions to, 49
  granulocyte collection by, steroid stimulation of, 46
  HLA type and, 45
  macromolecular agents in, 45–46
  Rh type and, 44–45
Leukemia, therapeutic cytapheresis in, 382
Leukoadhesion, 46–47
  reactions to, 49
Leukocytosis, therapeutic cytapheresis in, 382
Lewis antigens, renal transplant and, 125
Lewis blood group system, 106–107
  antibodies, 107
  antigens, 81
  complement and, 73
  phenotypes, 107
  in renal transplant, 125
Li^a antigen, 113
Liver disease
  with bleeding, 320
  calcium in, 217
  transplantation in. *See* Liver transplantation
Liver function test, in infectious mononucleosis, 20
Liver transplantation
  HLA typing in, 128
  massive transfusion in, 231
  RBC transfusion in, 231
Lke antigen, 113

Look-back procedure for AIDS, 280, 281, 392
Low-birth-weight infant, transfusion for, 225
Low-density-lipoprotein, plasma exchange and, 379
Low-ionic polycation test, 145, 181
Ls^a antigen, 113
Lu antibodies, identification of, 185
Lu antigens, in antibody screening, 181
Lupus erythematosus, plasma exchange, 377, 380
Lutheran blood group system, 110–112
  antigens, 81
  phenotypes, 111
  sex-linked antigen in, 110–112
LW antigen, 105–106
LW blood group system, 105–106
  antibodies, 106, 115
Lymphocytapheresis
  in renal transplant rejection, 379
  in rheumatoid arthritis, 378
Lymphocyte
  B cell. *See* B lymphocytes
  microcytotoxicity of, 118–120
  T cell. *See* T lymphocyte
Lymphocyte count, platelet apheresis and, 50
Lymphocytotoxicity test, 120
Lymphokine-activated killer cells, 393
Lymphoplasmapheresis, in rheumatoid arthritis, 378

M antibody, identification of, 185
M antigen
  dosage effect, 74
  enzyme detection of, 147
  linkage disequilibrium in, 84
M antiserum, 103
Macromolecular agent
  in antibody testing, 181
  in leukapheresis, 45–46
Macrophage, 56, 61
  in immune response, 61
Malaria, transfusion-associated, 15, 19, 281, 283
Massive transfusion, 214–221
  acid-base abnormalities in, 217–218
  blood warming for, 218
  in burn injury, 221
  of changing ABO groups, 219–220
  citrate toxicity in, 217

Massive transfusion—*Continued*
  coagulation function test in, 216
  fluid volume replacement solutions in, 215
  fresh frozen plasma in, 216–217
  in liver transplantation, 221–222
  microaggregate filters for, 221
  platelets in, 216
  of Rh-positive into Rh-negative recipients, 220
  in sickle cell disease, 228
  in thalassemia, 228
  whole blood versus RBC in, 218–219
McC[a] antigen, 113
Measles, in donor, 20
Measles vaccine, 28
Medications. *See* Drug(s); *see also* specific
Meiosis, 83
Membrane system
  for blood cell separation
    hollow-fiber type, 40
    mathematical formulas for, 41
    sandwich, 41
  Fenwal Plasmacell-C, 43
  in hemapheresis, 40–42
Metabolic acidosis, in massive transfusion, 217
Metabolic alkalosis, in massive transfusion, 217, 218
Microaggregate filter, in massive transfusion, 221
Microangiopathic hemolytic anemia, plasma exchange in, 378–379
Microbial contamination, 191, 262. *See also* Viral infection
MicroGroupamatic, 149
Microwave, for blood warming, 218
Milne antigen, 113
Miltenberger subsystem, 103
Mixed lymphocyte culture technique, 121
  in renal transplantation, 126
Mixed venous oxygen content, RBC transfusion and, 213
Mixed-field antiglobulin reaction, 194–195
MLC test, irradiated blood components and, 235
MNSs blood group system, 103–105
  antibodies, 104–105, 180
  antigens, 81, 103

glycophorin A and glycophorin B in, 104
Mo[a] antigen, 113
Modified fluid gelatins (MFG), in leukapheresis, 45
Mononucleosis, infectious. *See* Infectious mononucleosis
Motivation, of blood donors, 2
Multiple sclerosis, plasma exchange in, 378–379, 380
Mumps vaccine, 28
Myasthenia gravis, plasma exchange in, 375, 377
Myocardial infarction, donor, 22
Myocardial ischemia, hemodilution in, 227
Myoglobinemia, 257
Myoglobinuria, 257

N antibody, identification of, 185
N antigen. *See also* MNSs blood group system
  dosage effect, 74
  enzyme detection of, 147
  linkage disequilibrium in, 84
N antiserum, 103
N-acetylgalactosamine, A antigen specificity and, 87
Narcotic use, donor, 15
Ne[a] antigen, 106
Neocyte, defined, 228
Neonate. *See also* Infant; Premature infant
  anemia in, 357
  bilirubin accumulation in, 351–352
  body surface area of, 332
  heart failure, 357
  hemolytic disease of. *See* Hemolytic disease of newborn
  hyperbilirubinemia in, 228
  jaundice in, 351–352
  neutropenia in, 285
  sepsis in, 229
  thrombocytopenia in, 285
Nephritis, fulminant crescentic
  plasma exchange in, 377, 380
Neuromuscular hyperexcitability
  citrate toxicity and, 384
  donor, 35
Neutralization, of antigen-antibody reaction, 68

Neutropenia, in neonate, 285
Neutrophil
  buffy coat, 45
  C5a and, 69–71
  transfusion. *See* Granulocyte transfusion
Nfld antigen, 113

O blood group
  erythroblastosis fetalis and, 361, 364
  exchange transfusion
    in erythroblastosis, 364
  testing and typing, 158
    in exchange transfusion, 360
  transfusion
    exchange, 364
    uncrossmatched, 219–220
Occupation, donor, 28
Ok^a antigen, 113
Oliguria, hemolytic transfusion reaction and, 253
Olympus PK7100, 149
Open-heart surgery
  hemodilution in, 214
  platelet transfusion in, 228
  RBC transfusion in, 227–228
Or antigen, 113
Oral hypoglycemic agents, 24–25
Os^a antigen, 113
Oxygen
  in red cell, 295–296
  tissue, RBC transfusion and, 213–214
Oxygen dissociation curve
  of hemoglobin, 294
  P$_{50}$ value of, 295
Oxygen partial pressure, hemoglobin saturation and, 293
Oxygen tension
  in stored red cells, 293
  tissue, 293
Oxygen transport, red cell storage and, 293
Oxyhemoglobin, formation of, 293

P antibody, identification of, 185
P antigen, 113
P blood group system, 105
  antibodies, 105
  antigens, 81
  complement and, 73
P$_1$ antiserum, 353

P$_{50}$ value, of oxygen dissociation curve, 295
Packed cells. *See* Red blood cell transfusion
Panel, red cell, 183
Papain, in serologic testing, 146
Para-Bombay blood type, 92–93
Parasite infection, transmission of, 19
Partial thromboplastin time, massive transfusion and, 216
Pasteurization, of antihemophilic factor concentrates, 393
Penicillin, 27
  agglutination and, 195
Peptic ulcer, in donor, 25
Peripheral granulocyte count, steroid stimulation of, 46
Pertussis vaccine, 28
pH, in antibody detection tests, 143
Phenacetin, direct antiglobulin test and, 195
Phenotype, defined, 82
Phlebotomy, 33–34
  in autologous transfusion, 226
  donor response to, conditions affecting, 22–29
  instructions following, 32
  skin disease and, 22
  sterility testing for, 166
  vein selection for, 32
Photopheresis, 381
Physical examination, donor, 11
Phytanic acid increase (Refsum's disease), plasma exchange and, 376
Pigment, hemolytic transfusion reaction and, 251
Placental transfer
  antibody, 348
  of immunoglobulins, 60
Plague vaccine, 28
Plasma, 309–312
  collection of. *See also* Collection of blood
    membrane systems for, 42
  diffusion of, 371
  exchange. *See* Plasma exchange
  fresh frozen, 310–312
    in burn management, 221
    in fluid volume replacement, 215
    in liver transplantation, 231
    in thrombotic thrombocytopenic purpura, 376

Plasma—*Continued*
  liquid, 309–310
  products, FDA defined, 309
  plasma protein fraction, 313
    in fluid volume replacement, 215
    in plasma exchange, 372
  recipient as donor, 16
  source, 312
Plasma cell, 61
Plasma exchange, 367–372
  in autoimmune disease, 378–379
  in bone marrow transplantation, 379, 380
  cascade filtration in, 369
  chemotherapy and, 374
  in cold-antibody hemolytic anemia, 379, 380
  complications of, 383–386
    delayed, 385–386
    procedural, 384–385
    vascular, 384
  concurrent immunosuppression in, 371–372
  continuous-flow systems for, 368
  in cryoglobulinemia, 374, 377
  cryoprecipitation chamber for, 369
  diseases treated by, 372–380
  in erythroblastosis fetalis, 379, 380
  extracorporeal adsorption in, 380–381
  in familial hypercholesterolemia, 379, 380
  in fulminant crescentic nephritis, 377, 380
  in Goodpasture's syndrome, 375, 377
  in Guillain-Barré syndrome, 376, 377
  in hemolytic anemia, 379, 380
    microangiopathic, 376
  in hemophilia with inhibitor, 376, 377
  in hyperviscosity syndrome, 374, 377
  in idiopathic thrombocytopenic purpura, 380
  IgG in, 371
  IgM protein in, 370–371
  immune complexes in, 369, 370
  immunosuppression and, 373
  intermittent-flow systems for, 367–368
  membrane plasma separation devices for, 368–369
  method of, 367–372
  in microangiopathic hemolytic anemia, 376
  mortality in, 386
  in myasthenia gravis, 375, 377
  on-line cryogelation in, 380–381
  patient, 372–373
  posttransfusion purpura and, 376, 377
  quantitative considerations in, 369–371
  rational basis for, 373–374
  in Refsum's disease, 376, 377
  in renal transplant rejection, 379, 380
  replacement media, 372
  in Rh hemolytic disease of newborn, 379, 380
  in rheumatoid arthritis, 377–378, 380
  in systemic lupus erythematosus, 377, 380
  in thrombotic thrombocytopenic purpura, 373, 375–376, 377
  in Waldenström's macroglobulinemia, 374
Plasma protein fraction. *See* Plasma
Plasma volume, measurement of, 211
Plasmapheresis. *See also* Plasma exchange
  defined, 38
  manual, 38
  Rh antibody removal by, 357–358
Plasmodium malariae, 19
Plastic blood containers, 30–31
Plasticizers, 31
Platelet count, apheresis and, 49
Platelet transfusion, 330–333
  aspirin and, 336–337
  in bleeding tendency, 263–264
  body surface area and, 331
    in children, 332
  corrected count increment, 330
  crossmatching for, 336, 337
  electromechanical infusion device for, 240
  HLA typing for, 128, 234
  in leukemia, 234
  in open-heart surgery, 228
  percent recovery formula for, 333
  refractoriness and, 333–336
  Rh-positive into Rh-negative recipient, 45
Platelets, 328–337
  antibodies, 284–285
  apheresis, 38
    ABO group and, 44
    blood count changes in, 49
    cytapheresis procedure for, 42–45
    donor lymphocytes and, 50

donor reactions to, 47
Fenwal CS-3000 for, 40, 41
HLA type and, 45
manual, 39
Rh type and, 44–45
aspirin and, 27
collection of, 328–329
crossmatching, 336, 337
deficiency of, 263
maternal antibodies to, 348
preservation of, 292
refractoriness, 333–336
storage, 329
transfusion of. *See* Platelet transfusion
ultraviolet irradiation of, 393
Poliomyelitis vaccine, 28
Pollio antigen, 113
Polyagglutinability, 175
acquired B, 175
microbial contamination and, 196
Polybrene, in antibody testing, 145, 181
Polybrene antiglobulin test, 146
Polycations, in antibody detection, 145–146
Polycythemia
in donor, 26
primary, 211
secondary, 211
in donor, 27
Polycythemia rubra vera, in donor, 26
Polymorphism, defined, 85
Polyvinyl chloride, blood bags, 31
Postperfusion syndrome, 275
Postphlebotomy instructions, 32
Posttransfusion purpura, 285
plasma exchange and, 376, 377
Potassium
red cell breakdown products and, 302
serum, 264
Povidone-iodine, 32
PP_1P^k antibody, identification of, 185
Precipitation, in antigen-antibody reaction, 66
Prednisone, in granulocyte stimulation, 46
Pregnancy
alloimmunization of, 348–351
amniocentesis in, 354–356
antibody detection tests in, 352–353
antibody titration in, 354
blood typing in, 352
cytomegalovirus infection in, 275

donors and, 28–29
erythroblastosis fetalis diagnosis in, 352–356
IgG antibody in, 353
immunization during, 350
immunization prevention in, 349–350
ultrasound in, 356
Premature infant. *See also* Infant; Neonate
cytomegalovirus infection in, 275–276
RBC transfusion for, 222–225
Pretransfusion testing. *See specific topic, e.g.,* Antibody screening test
Priapism, 229
Prison inmates, as donors, 16
Proband, defined, 85
ProGroup System, 149
Propositus, defined, 85
Prostitution, AIDS and, 17, 278
Protamine, in antibody testing, 181
Protein C deficiency, 326
Proteolytic enzyme, in antibody detection, 181
Prothrombin deficiency, 320
Prothrombin time, massive transfusion and, 216
Protozoal infection, transfusional, 20–21
Prozone phenomenon, 67, 142
defined, 66
Pseudoagglutination, 196–197
colloidal silica in, 197
rouleaux in, 196–197
Psychological factors, donor, 34–35
Pt^a antigen, 113
Pulmonary disease
acute, donor, 25
chronic, polycythemia vera and, 27
Pulmonary edema, in transfusion reaction, 258
Pulse abnormality, donor, 23
Pump, RBC transfusion, 240

Quality control, of blood typing procedures, 158–159
Questionnaire, postdonation, 278

Rabies vaccine, 28
Radioimmunoassay, of hepatitis B surface antigen, 162–163
Rapid plasma reagin test, in syphilis, 161–162
Rasm antigen, 113

418 Index

Rb^a antigen, 113
RBC. *See* Red blood cells (RBC)
Rd antigen, 113
Re^a antigen, 113
Recipient, transfusion
  AIDS testing in, 280–281
  blood sample from, 169–174
    antibody testing, 183–197
    collection of, 170–171
    identification of, 171–174
    testing, 174–178
    unexpected antibodies in, 178–183
  bone marrow transplant, 175–176
  crossmatching, 197–199
  as donor, 16
  record keeping for, 208
  unexpected antibodies in, 178–183
    special investigation techniques in, 199–208
Records
  computerized, 8–9
  donor health interview, 12
  donor reaction, 35–36, 37
  Kidd antibody, 208
  laboratory test, 165–166
  serologic testing, 165–166
  of transfusion reaction, 266, 267–268
  of transmissible disease tests, 165–166
Recruitment program, blood donor, 5–8
Red blood cell transfusion, 211–243. *See also* Autologous transfusion
  addition of medication in, 240–241
  in anemia, 213
  in autoimmune hemolytic anemia, 236
  autologous, 226–227
  blood volume and, 211–212
  in burn management, 221
  in children, 237
  cold agglutinins in, 236
  donor-specific, 230
  exchange
    in erythroblastosis, 364
    in hyperbilirubinemia in newborns, 228
    modified, 241
  filters for, 238–239
  frozen-thawed, 303–306
    in bone marrow transplantation, 232, 234
    for neonates, 225
  in hemolytic anemia, 236
  in hydrops fetalis, 351
  in infants, 237
  infusion rate in, 240
  intraoperative salvage, 227
  inventory control in, 241–242
  irradiation of blood components and, 235
  in malignant disease, 234–235
  massive, 214–221
    acid-base abnormalities in, 217–218
    blood warming for, 218
    in burn injury, 221
    citrate toxicity in, 217
    of different ABO groups, 219–220
    fluid volume replacement solutions in, 215
    fresh frozen plasma in, 216–217
    in liver transplantation, 221–222
    microaggregate filters for, 221
    platelets in, 216
    of Rh-positive into Rh-negative recipients, 220
    in sickle cell disease, 228
    in thalassemia, 228
    whole blood versus RBC in, 218–219
  microaggregate formation and, 238–239
  modified exchange, 241
  for patients with multiple antibodies, 236
  needles for, 238
  for neonates, 222–224
  in open-heart surgery, 227–228
  ordering for surgery, 242–243
  plasma volume, 211
  posttransfusion survival, 301
  pump for, 240
  rate of, 241
  red cell volume, 211–221
  in renal transplantation, 230
  replacement rationale, 213–214
  Ringer's lactate in, 238
  special problems in, 214–237
  techniques of, 237–243
  thrombophlebitis in, 237
  in transplant recipients, 229–234
    bone marrow, 231
    liver, 231
    posttransplant support, 234
    pretreatment conditioning, 232–234
    pretreatment management, 231–232
    renal, 229–231
  trigger, 213
  of uncrossmatched blood, 222
    release form for, 223

vein selection for, 237
volume overload and, 236
walking donor program for, 224
washed
   in bone marrow transplantation, 232, 234
   multiple antibodies and, 236
   versus whole blood, 218–219
Red blood cells (RBC). *See also* Autologous transfusion
   agglutination of, 74
   antibody-coated, donor, 194–195
   antigens, 74
   clumping, 67
   collection of, 296
   CPDA-1, 242
   2,3-diphosphoglycerate in, 295–296
   elution, 201–202
   frozen, 303–306
      advantages and disadvantages of, 305–306
      deglycerolization of, 304–305
      high-glycerol method, 304
      leukocyte-poor, 306–308
      low-glycerol method, 304
      thawing, 304–305
   genotype, 74–75
   hereditary defects of, donor, 21
   immunoglobulin removal from, 203
      chloroquine in, 203
      "ZZAPP treatment," 203–204
   inhibition of clotting, 300
   inventory control, 241–242
   Kell system antigen removal from, 204
   last-wash control, 201
   leukocyte-poor, 306–308
      frozen-thawed, 308
      preparation of, 307
      washed cells, 308
   lysis. *See* Hemolysis
   membrane
      complement attack of, 70–71
      sialoglycoproteins of, 104
   oxygen release from, 295–296
   passage of fetal to mother, 349
   posttransfusion survival, 301
   preservation
      additive solutions, 226
      breakdown products, 301, 302
      citrate phosphate dextrose adenine-1 in, 298–299
      citrate phosphate dextrose in, 297–298
      collection for, 296
      2,3-diphosphoglycerate in, 295–296
      functional characteristics and, 293–295
      hydrogen ion concentration and, 302
      storage lesion and, 297
      temperature and, 296–297
   pseudoagglutination, 196–197
   radiolabeled, 211–212
   reagents for antibody screening, 181–182
   rouleaux, 196–197
   sedimentation characteristics of, 45
   storage, 292–295
      breakdown products, 301, 302
      free hemoglobin in, 302–303
      frozen, 303–306
      functional characteristics of, 293–295
      inhibition of clotting, 300
      lesion, 297
      microaggregates and, 238–239
      viability of, 296
   surface antigens, 80
   technetium-labeled, 212
   thawed, 304–305
      leukocyte-poor, 308
   transfusion. *See* Red blood cell transfusion
   volume measurement, 212–213
   washed
      with saline, 201
      unexpected antibodies and, 160
   zeta potential of, 67
Refreshments, postdonation, 34
Refrigeration, of red cells, 296–297
Refsum's disease, plasma exchange in, 376, 377
Regional enteritis, in donor, 25
Release form, uncrossmatched blood, 223
Renal failure
   hemolytic transfusion reaction and, 253
   posttransfusion hemolysis and, 234
Renal transplantation
   cadaver, 125
   crossmatching for, 126
   cytomegalovirus infection and, 230
   donor, 125
   donor-specific transfusion for, 3
   HLA system and, 125–126
   HLA typing in, 126, 229

420 Index

Renal transplantation—*Continued*
  immunosuppressive therapy in, 125
  Lewis antigens in, 125
  MLC test for, 126
  organ procurement agencies, 126
  RBC transfusion in, 229–231
    pretransplant, 229
  rejection of, plasma exchange in, 379, 380
  transfusion in, 229–231
    donor-specific, 230
    immunosuppression and, 229, 285
    pretransplant, 229
    Rh-positive to Rh-negative recipient, 230
Renal tubule, hemosiderin deposition in, 250
Respiratory alkalosis, donor, 35
Respiratory disease
  acute, in donor, 25
  chronic, polycythemia and, 27
Respiratory distress syndrome, exchange transfusion in, 229
Rg antigen, antibodies to, 191
Rh antibody
  blocking, 356
  delayed hemolytic reaction and, 254–255
  enzyme detection techniques, 147
  fetal detection of, 348
  IgG and, 57–58
  maternal, effect on fetus, 351–352
  reactivity of, 94
    recipient, 117
    testing, 157
  in recipient, 177
  removal by plasmapheresis, 357–358
  testing, 157
    in exchange transfusion, 360
  titration of, 354
  typing, 356–357
Rh antigens, 81
  in blacks, 100
  compound, 97–98
  equivalent notation systems of, 99
  fetal, passage to mother, 349
  testing for, 156–157
Rh hemolytic disease. *See* Hemolytic disease of newborn
Rh immune globulin
  in erythroblastosis fetalis, 349–351
  immunoprophylaxis, 379
  in transfusion, 220
Rh immunization, in D^u type mother, 350–351
Rh immunosuppressive therapy, 349
Rh system, 93–101. *See also* Rh antigens
  antibody. *See* Rh antibody
  antigen. *See* Rh antigens
  compound antigens in, 97–98
  D antigen expression, 94–96
  depressions, suppressions, and deletions in, 100–101
  G antigen in, 98–100
  genetics and terminology of, 93–94
  genotype determination, 96–100
  granulocyte transfusion and, 340
  IgG antibodies of, 60–61
  immunization, 63, 348–364
  phenotype, testing, 158
  principal gene alleles in, 98
  Rh_{mod} phenotype, 101
  Rh_{null} phenotype, 100–101
    warm autoantibodies and, 194
  transfusion
    Rh-positive to Rh-negative recipient, 220, 230
    uncrossmatched, 219, 220
  typing and testing
    automated systems for, 148, 149
    controlling test for D, 176–177
    enzyme techniques in, 146, 147
    low-protein test, 146
    recipient, 176–177
    in transfusion reaction, 266
  warm autoantibodies and, 194
Rheumatic fever, in donor, 22–23
Rheumatic heart disease, in donor, 22–23
Rheumatoid arthritis, plasma exchange in, 377–378, 380
Rh-Hr blood group system, 93–94. *See also* Rh system
  equivalent notation system for, 99
Ringer's solution, 215
  in RBC transfusion, 238
Rl^a antigen, 113
Rocky Mountain spotted fever vaccine, 28
Rodgers blood group system
  antibodies, 191
  antigens, 81

S antibody, identification of, 185
S antigen, linkage disequilibrium in, 84
S antiserum, 104–105
  low-frequency antigens and, 112
Sabin vaccine, 28
Saline agglutinin, 60, 135–136, 195
Saline replacement, in pseudoagglutination, 196
Salk poliomyelitis vaccine, 28
Sc antibodies, identification of, 185
Scianna blood group system
  antigens, 81
  phenotypes, 111
Sd^a antigen, 192
Se gene
  nonsecretors, 88
  secretors, 87–88
Seasonal allergy, donor, 21
Secretion and secretors, 87–88
  ABH blood group, 106–107
Sedimentation, of whole blood, 291
Sepsis, neonatal
  exchange transfusion in, 229
Shunt, artificial, in plasma exchange, 384
Sialoglycoprotein
  enzyme detection of, 147
  of RBC membrane, 104
Sickle cell disease
  exchange transfusion in, 229
  hypertransfusion in, 228
  iron overload in, 228
  typing for antigens in, 228
Sickle trait, donor, 21
Sid antigen, 192
Skin cancer, donor, 26
Skin disease, donor, 22
Sl^a antigen, 113
Smallpox vaccine, 28
  history of, 55
Sodium capyrylate, agglutination and, 195
Spirochete infection, transfusional, 20
Steroid, stimulation of donors, 46
Stibophen, direct antiglobulin test and, 195
Stillbirth
  amniocentesis and, 356
  erythroblastosis fetalis and, 352
Storage and preservation of blood, 291–341
  antibody-containing serum, 77
  antigen-antibody reaction and, 75

blood fractions and derivatives, 313–329
blood group antibodies and, 75
for clotting factor deficiencies, 318–325
clotting inhibition for, 300
faulty, 256
granulocyte, 337–341
immune globulin, 316–318
lesion, 297
neutrophils, 337–341
plasma and liquid plasma, 309–312
platelets, 328–337
red blood cell, 291–308
Surface hydration theory of agglutination, 67–68
Surface markers, of human T lymphocytes, 62
Surface phenomenon, in antigen-antibody reactions, 65
Surgery
  blood ordering for, 242–243
  bleeding tendency and, 263
  dental, donor, 21–22
  donor qualification and, 23–24
  major versus minor, 23, 24
Sw^a antigen, 113
Sw (Class I) antigen, 113
Syncope
  delayed, 35
  donation and, 34–35
  donor, 34–35
Synteny, defined, 84
Syphilis
  rapid plasma reagin (RPR) test for, 161–162
  skin lesions in, 22
  testing for, 148, 160
  transfusional, 20, 281–283
  Venereal Disease Reference Laboratory (VDRL) test for, 161–162
Systemic lupus erythematosus, plasma exchange in, 377, 380
Systolic blood pressure, donor, 23

T lymphocyte, 56, 61
  antigen-antibody reactions, 65
  helper, 61
  interleukin-1 and, 61
  suppressor, 61
  surface markers, 62
Tattooing, donor, 16

Tc antigens, 113
Technetium-labeled red blood cell, 212
Technicon AutoAnalyzer, 149
Temperature
  blood. *See* Transfusion reaction
  body. *See* Body temperature
  exchange transfusion and, 361–362
  of red cell storage, 296–297
Tetanus vaccine, 28
Thalassemia
  hypertransfusion in, 228
  iron overload in, 228
  minor, 21
Therapeutic hemapheresis. *See* Hemapheresis, therapeutic
Thrombocytapheresis, defined, 38. *See also* Platelets, apheresis
Thrombocytopenia
  bleeding tendency and, 263
  in neonate, 285
Thrombocytopenic purpura
  idiopathic, 380
  thrombotic, 373, 375–376, 377, 393
Thrombocytosis, therapeutic cytapheresis in, 382
Thrombophlebitis, RBC transfusion and, 237
Thrombotic thrombocytopenic purpura, plasma exchange in, 373, 375–376, 377
Thymus-derived lymphocyte. *See* T lymphocyte
Tissue oxygen, RBC transfusion and, 213–214
Titration, 204–206
  applications of, 205–206
  methods of, 206
Tn polyagglutinability, 175
To^a antigen, 113
Tr^a antigen, 113
Transabdominal puncture, in intrauterine transfusion, 358
Transaminitis, 269
Transfusion
  -associated AIDS, 392
  autologous, 3
  complications of. *See* Transfusion reaction
  exchange. *See* Exchange transfusion
  intrauterine. *See* Intrauterine transfusion

  peritoneal, intrauterine, 356
  reactions to. *See* Transfusion reaction
  recipients as donors, 16
  red blood cell. *See* Red blood cell transfusion
  uncrossmatched
    in hydrops fetalis, 351
    release form, 223
Transfusion equipment, sterility test, 166
Transfusion reaction, 249–285
  acquired immunodeficiency syndrome, 276–281
    incidence of, 276–277
    prevention of, 277–280
    recipient testing, 280–281
    testing donor blood for, 279–280
    transmission, 277, 283
  air embolism, 261, 265
  allergic, 258–259, 265
    prevention of, 259
    treatment of, 258–259
  babesiosis transmission, 20–21, 281–282, 283
  bleeding tendency and, 263–264, 265
  blood group immunization, 282–285. *See also* Immunization
    frequency, 283–284
    immunogenicity, 282–283
    individual antibody formation capacity, 284
    platelet antibodies, 284–285
    white cell antibodies, 284–285
  blood samples, 266
  blood storage and, 361
  brucellosis transmission, 282, 283
  Chagas' disease transmission, 282, 283
  circulatory overload, 260–261, 265
    prevention of, 261
    treatment of, 260–261
  citrate toxicity, 263, 265
    in plasma exchange, 384–385
  cold blood, 218, 261–262, 361–362
  containers, 266
  contaminated blood and, 262
  cytomegalovirus transmission, 275–276, 283
  defined, 249
  definitive, 266–267
  disease transmission, 10–11, 268–282
  electrolyte toxicity and, 264, 265
  embolism, 261, 265

faulty procedure, 256
febrile, 259–260, 265
　babesiosis in, 20–21
　Bg antibodies and, 115–116
　prevention of, 260
　treatment of, 260
graft-versus-host disease and, 264, 265, 283
　prevention of, 264
hemolytic, 249–258, 265
　antibody in donor plasma, 249, 255–256
　antibody in recipient plasma, 249, 251–255
　diagnosis of, 257
　hemoglobin clearance and, 250
　management of, 257–258
　treatment of, 257–258
　unrelated to blood group incompatibility, 256–257
hemosiderosis, 282, 283
hepatitis transmission, 268–275, 283
　testing for, 165
immediate, 265
immunosuppressive, 285
interdonor incompatibility
　hemolytic, 256
　minor crossmatching and, 178
investigation of, 265–268
　blood samples, 266
　containers, 266
　definitive, 266–267
　immediate, 265
　laboratory procedures, 266–268
　records, 266, 267–268
laboratory procedures in, 266–268
major incompatibility, 249, 251–255
　in bone marrow transplantation, 233
malaria transmission, 15, 19, 281, 283
minor incompatibility, 249
　in bone marrow transplantation, 234
　cytapheresis and, 44
overtransfusion, 358
records, 266, 267–268
suspected. *See* Transfusion reaction, investigation of
syphilis transmission, 20, 281, 283
tuberculosis transmission, 21
viral hepatitis transmission, 268–275, 283

Transfusion recipient. *See* Recipient, transfusion
Transfusion service. *See* Blood banks
Transmissible disease tests, 160–165
　alanine aminotransferase, 165
　cytomegalovirus, 165
　hepatitis B core antibody, 163
　hepatitis B surface antigen, 162–163
　human immunodeficiency virus, 164–165
　result recording, 165–166
　syphilis, 161–162
　transfusion-associated hepatitis, 165
Transplantation. *See specific organ*
Trauma
　fluid therapy in, 215
　uncrossmatched blood in, 222
Treponema pallidum, 161
Trisodium citrate, in leukapheresis, 45
Tuberculosis, transfusional, 21
Tumor, solid
　irradiation of blood components in, 235
　transfusion and, 234
Typhoid vaccine, 28
Typhus vaccine, 28

U antibody, identification of, 185
U antigen, 103, 105
Ultrasound, in pregnancy, 356
Umbilical cord blood
　hemoglobin level in, 357
　I antiserum in, 115
Unexpected antibodies
　in donor blood, 160
　identification of, 183–197
　in recipient blood, 178–183
　special investigation techniques, 199–207
Urticaria, 258

V antigen (Rh), in antibody screening, 181
Vaccination, donor, 28
Vascular damage, in plasma exchange, 384
Vascular permeability, complement in, 69–71
Vasodilators, 36
Vasopressor agents, 36
Vasovagal reaction
　antihypertensive agents and, 28

Vasovagal reaction—*Continued*
  in blood donation, 28
  in plasma exchange, 384
Vel antigens, 113, 114
Venereal Disease Reference Laboratory (VDRL) test, in syphilis, 161–162
Venipuncture
  site, 32–33
    for recipient's blood sample, 170
  skin disease and, 22
Vg^a antigen, 113
Viral hepatitis. *See* Hepatitis
Viral infection
  in donor, 20
  in polyagglutinability, 196
  screening tests for, 161
Volume replacement, solutions for, 215
von Willebrand's disease, 326, 327

Waldenström's macroglobulinemia, plasma exchange in, 374
Warfarin, overdose, 320
Warm antibody, 60
Warm autoantibodies, 194
Wb antigen, 113
Wd^a antigen, 113
Weight, donor, 13
Wes antigen, 113
Western Blot technique, 165

White blood cell
  antibodies, 284–285
    maternal, 348
  antigens, maternal antibodies to, 348
  transfusion, Rh-positive into Rh-negative recipient, 45
Whole blood
  plasma separation from, 291–292
  transfusion, citrate toxicity and, 263
Women, donors, 28–29
Wound healing, RBC transfusion and, 213
Wr^a antigen, 113
Wu antigen, 113

X chromosome, Xg^a antigen and, 110–112
Xg^a antibody, identification of, 185
Xg blood group system, 81
  antigens, 80–81
  enzyme testing techniques in, 147
  phenotypes, frequency, 111

Yellow fever vaccine, 28
Yk^a antigen, 113
Yt antibodies, identification of, 185

"ZZAPP treatment," in RBC immunoglobulin removal, 203–204
Zero-risk blood supply, 392
Zygosity, 81–82